Mood and Anxiety Disorders in Wom

Mood and anxiety disorders in women represent an increasingly important area of research
and treatment development. The authors take a broad biopsychosocial and developmental
approach to the issues, beginning with anxiety disorders in adolescence and progressing
through the life phases of women to menopause and old age. All the disorders are covered,
from anxiety and borderline personality disorder to stress and late-life depression. Particular
attention is paid to questions of vulnerability; epidemiological and clinical evidence showing
gender differences in such disorders; aetiological explanations in terms of biological
(including hormonal) as well as psychosocial parameters; and treatment implications.

David Castle is Professorial Fellow at the Mental Health Research Institute of Victoria;
Professorial Fellow in the Department of Psychiatry, University of Melbourne; Consultant
Psychiatrist at the Royal Melbourne Hospital; and Clinical Professor at the School of Psychiatry
and Neurosciences, University of Western Australia.

Jayashri Kulkarni is Professor of Psychiatry, The Alfred, Melbourne, Australia; Professor,
Monash University, Department of Psychological Medicine, Faculty of Medicine, Melbourne,
Australia

Kathryn M. Abel is Senior Lecturer Head for Center for Women's Mental Health Research and
Consultant Psychiatrist at the University of Manchester; and Honorary Senior Lecturer at the
Institute of Psychiatry, London.

Mood and Anxiety Disorders in Women

Edited by

David Castle

Professorial Fellow, Mental Health Research Institute of Victoria
Professorial Fellow, Department of Psychiatry, University of Melbourne
Consultant Psychiatrist, Royal Melbourne Hospital
Clinical Professor, School of Psychiatry and Neurosciences, University of Western Australia

Jayashri Kulkarni

Professor of Psychiatry, The Alfred, Melbourne, Australia
Professor, Monash University, Department of Psychological Medicine, Faculty of Medicine, Melbourne, Australia

Kathryn M. Abel

Senior Lecturer and Honourary Consultant, Centre for Women's Mental Health Research, Division of Psychiatry, University of Manchester, Manchester, UK

Foreword by
Jill Goldstein

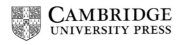

CAMBRIDGE
UNIVERSITY PRESS

CAMBRIDGE UNIVERSITY PRESS
Publishing Division
Science, Technology and Medicine

CAMBRIDGE UNIVERSITY PRESS
Cambridge, New York, Melbourne, Madrid, Cape Town, Singapore, São Paulo

Cambridge University Press
The Edinburgh Building, Cambridge CB2 2RU, UK
Published in the United States of America by Cambridge University Press, New York

www.cambridge.org
Information on this title: www.cambridge.org/9780521

Printed in the United Kingdom at the University Press, Cambridge

A record for this book is available from the British Library

Library of Congress in Publication data

ISBN-13 978-0-521-54753-6 paperback
ISBN-10 0-521-547539 paperback

Every effort has been made in preparing this book to provide accurate and up-to-date information which is in accord with accepted standards and practice at the time of publication. Although case histories are drawn from actual cases, every effort has been made to disguise the identities of the individuals involved. Nevertheless, the authors, editors and publishers can make no warranties that the information contained herein is totally free from error, not least because clinical standards are constantly changing through research and regulation. The authors, editors and publishers therefore disclaim all liability for direct or consequential damages resulting from the use of material contained in this book. Readers are strongly advised to pay careful attention to information provided by the manufacturer of any drugs or equipment that they plan to use.

Contents

Contributors

Dr. Kathryn M. Abel
Senior Lecturer
Centre for Women's Mental Health
Research
Division of Psychiatry,
University of Manchester
Williamson Building
Manchester, M13 9PL,
UK
Honorary Consultant Psychiatrist
Manchester Mental Health & Social Care
Trust, London, UK
Honorary Senior Lecturer
Institute of Psychiatry
London,
UK
kathryn.m.abel@man.ac.uk

Assoc Prof. Nicholas B. Allen
ORYGEN Research Centre and Department
of Psychology
University of Melbourne
35 Poplar Road
Parkville, Vic. 3052
Australia
nba@unimelb.edu.au

Dr. Amanda Baker
Centre for Mental Health Studies
University of Newcastle
Newcastle, NSW 2308
Australia
Amanda.Baker@newcastle.edu.au

Prof. Robert Baldwin
Manchester Mental Health and Social Care
Partnership
York House
Manchester Royal Infirmary
Manchester, M13 9WL, UK
rbaldwin11@aol.com

Anna Barrett
ORYGEN Research Centre and Department
of Psychology
University of Melbourne
35 Poplar Road
Parkville, Vic .3052
Australia
annabarrett101@yahoo.com.au

Prof. Michael Berk
Department of Clinical and Biomedical
Sciences
The University of Melbourne
Kitchener House, The Gelong Hospital,
Ryrie Street
Gelong, Vic. 3220
Australia
mberk@unimelb.edu.au

Assoc Prof. Anne E. Buist
Department of Psychiatry
Austin Health – Heidelberg Repatriation
Hospital
300 Waterdale Road
West Heidelberg, Vic. 3081
Australia
a.buist@unimelb.edu.au

Assoc Prof. Diana Carter
Department of Psychiatry
University of British Columbia, Vancouver,
Canada
Psychiatrist, Reproductive Mental Health
Program BC Women's Hospital
4500 Oak Street, Vancouver, BC V6H 3N1, UK
dcarter@cw.bc.ca

Ms. Jessica Carty
Australian Centre for Posttraumatic
Mental Health
University of Melbourne
Repat Campus, Waterdale Road
Heidelberg, Vic. 3081
Australia
markcc@unimelb.edu.au

Prof. David J. Castle
Collaborative Therapy Unit
Mental Health Research Institute &
The University of Melbourne
155 Oak Street
Parkville, Vic. 3052
Australia
dcastle@mhri.edu.au

Dr. Andrew Chanen
ORYGEN Research Centre
35 Poplar Road
Parkville, Vic. 3052
Australia
achanen@unimelb.edu.au

Prof. Mark Creamer
Australian Centre for Posttraumatic Mental
Health
University of Melbourne
Repat Campus, Waterdale Road
Heidelberg, Vic. 3081
Australia
markcc@unimelb.edu.au

Dr. Betsy Davis
Oregon Research Institute
1715 Franklin Bvd.
Eugene, OR 97403-1983
USA
betsy@ori.org

Prof. Lorraine Dennerstein
Department of Psychiatry
The University of Melbourne
Parkville, Vic. 3010
Australia
ldenn@unimelb.edu.au

Dr. Seetal Dodd
Department of Clinical and Biomedical
Sciences: Barwon Health
The University of Melbourne
P.O. Box 281
Geelong, Vic. 3220
Australia
seetald@barwonhealth.org.au

Dr. Jane Garner
Department of Psychiatry, Chase Farm
Hospital
The Ridgeway
Enfield, Middlesex EN2 8JL
UK
jane.garner@beh-mht.nhs.uk

Dr. Clare Gerada
Royal College of General Practitioners,
Substance Misuse Unit
Hurley Clinic
Kennington Lane SE114BY
England
c.gerada@btinternet.com

Heather B. Howell
Department of Psychiatry
Yale School of Medicine
142 Temple Street, Suite 301
New Haven, CT 06450

Ms. Kristy J. Johns
Clinical Psychology Masters Candidate
Alcohol and Other Drugs Service
Central Coast Health
New South Wales
Australia
kjohns@doh.health.nsw.gov.au

Prof. Jayashri Kulkarni
Director
Alfred Psychiatry Research Centre
The Alfred
Commercial Road
Melbourne, Vic. 3004
Australia
j.kulkarni@alfred.org.au

Dr. Jeanne Leventhal Alexander
Stanford University Department of
Psychiatry, Kaiser Permanente Medical
Group of Northern California
Alexander Foundation for Women's
Health
1700 Shattuck Avenue, # 329
Berkeley, CA 94709,
USA
Jeanne@afwh.org

Dr. Ruth Little
Reproductive Mental Health Program BC
Women's Hospital
4500 Oak Street, Vancouver, BC V6H 3N1
ruthylittle@yahoo.com

Prof. Shaila Misri
Department of Psychiatry & Obs/Gyn
University of British Columbia. Vancouver,
Canada
Director, Reproductive Mental Health
Program BC Women's Hospital
4500 Oak Street, Vancouver, BC V6H 3N1
smisri@cw.bc.ca

Dr. Jane E. Opie
Department of Clinical and Biomedical
Sciences: Barwon Health
The University of Melbourne
P.O. Box 281, Geelong, Vic. 3220
Australia
janeop@barwonhealth.org.au

Dr. Lori E. Ross
Women's Mental Health & Addiction
Research Section
Centre for Addiction & Mental Health
250 College Street, Toronto, Ont. M5T 1R8
Canada
l.ross@utoronto.ca

Dr. Lisa B. Sheeber
Oregon Research Institute
1715 Franklin Bvd., Eugene, OR 97403-1983
USA
lsheeber@ori.org

Prof. Meir Steiner
Department of Psychiatry Behavioural
Neurosciences & Obstetrics & Gynaecology
McMasters University
St Joseph's Healthcare
Hamilton, Ont.
Canada
mst@mcmasters.ca

Dr. Kimberly A. Yonkers
142 Temple Street, New Haven, CT 06510
USA
Kimberly.Yonkers@yale.edu

Dr. Alison L. Warburton
Senior Research Fellow
Centre for Women's Mental Health Research
Division of Psychiatry
University of Manchester
Williamson Building
Manchester M13 9PL
UK
alison.1.warburton@man.ac.uk

Preface

The particular mental health experiences of women have received great attention in recent years. This reflects growing concern about the burden of mental health problems on the lives of women and their families. The most common mental health disorders are anxiety and depression, and women are particularly prone to such disorders. "Mood and Anxiety Disorders in Women" uses a biopsychosocial framework to provide a broad contemporary perspective on mood and anxiety in the context of women's lives. A developmental approach affords an overarching structure for the book, with each chapter examining a particular phase of women's lives. Extensive cross-referencing allows a shared perspective across other developmental stages where appropriate.

Chapter 1 provides an overview of the emotional hurdles facing adolescent girls, with particular reference to how these can contribute to the manifestation of psychological and psychiatric problems at this stage of development. Earlier developmental factors are also discussed.

Picking up on some of these themes, Chapter 2 is concerned with personality disorders and women, with a particular emphasis on why women tend to be more vulnerable to certain personality disorders (notably borderline), and less vulnerable than men to others (notably antisocial personality disorder). Aetiopathogenic parameters, including the role of childhood sexual abuse, as well as diagnostic issues, are addressed.

Chapter 3 turns to substance use disorders in women, covering epidemiological, clinical and therapeutic aspects. It asks why females are less likely than males to abuse alcohol and illicit substances, but places this against the profound impact of substance misuse in women compared to men and the potential impact on their children. The chapter also outlines the particular treatment needs of women who misuse substances, and details what substance use treatment services require, to become "female friendly".

Chapter 4 is an overview of gender differences amongst the anxiety disorders, with special reference to why women seem differentially more prone to certain of these disorders. Women-centred assessment, diagnostic and treatment needs are addressed.

Chapter 5 tackles post-traumatic stress disorder. Gender differences in the exposure to, and the experience of stress are outlined, with an emphasis on those stressors that are more common in women (e.g., rape, childhood sexual abuse, domestic violence). The chapter also considers women's responses to stress, both acutely and in the longer term. Treatment recommendations that are gender-sensitive are presented.

Chapter 6 considers the role of domestic violence in women's lives and the potentially profound impact on women's mental health. The factors associated with risk and disclosure of domestic violence are discussed. The role of mental health professionals in safely engaging women victims of violence are outlined, and potential therapeutic strategies are suggested.

Turning to more biological factors, Chapter 7 provides an overview of the evidence for a role of female gonadal hormones in mood disorders, encompassing basic science and clinical aspects. The aetiology and treatment of the premenstrual syndrome is specifically covered.

The important topic of anxiety and mood disorders during pregnancy and the postpartum period is covered in Chapter 8. There is a special emphasis on postpartum mood disorders. Guidelines for treatment and the role of mother–baby units are specifically covered.

Chapter 9 provides a comprehensive overview of the pharmacological treatment of anxiety and depression during pregnancy and lactation, including practical information and clinical guidelines.

Bipolar affective disorder in women is the topic of Chapter 10. The manifestations of mania in women, and particular risks and vulnerabilities for women during manic episodes, are addressed. Treatment implications, notably use of medications in pregnancy and during breast feeding, are covered, with cross-reference to Chapter 9.

Chapter 11 gives an overview of the biological aspects of the menopause, with reference to those parameters that might affect mental health. The complexity of the menopause and its potential impact on psychosocial functioning are detailed. Adaptive and non-adaptive responses to the menopause are covered, along with guidance for helping women to deal with the changes that occur at this time of life.

Finally, Chapter 12 addresses mood and anxiety disorders in women in late life, encompassing epidemiological and aetiopathological parameters. It considers the potential role of hormones, brain changes and the role of psychosocial parameters in the pathogenesis of depression and anxiety in this life stage. The particular treatment needs of older women are also outlined.

This volume provides a comprehensive and up-to-date overview of mood and anxiety in women taking particular account of the complexity of women's lives and the changes associated with different stages of development. We trust it will be of interest to women in general, as well as being a resource to clinicians, biologists, pharmacologists and all professionals striving to provide high quality, gender sensitive mental health care to women.

Prof. David Castle
University of Melbourne, Melbourne, Australia

Prof. Jayashri Kulkarni
Monash University, Melbourne, Australia

Dr Kathryn M. Abel
*University of Manchester, Centre for Women's Mental
Health Research, Manchester, UK
Manchester Mental Health & Social Care Trust, London, UK
Institute of Psychiatry, London, UK*

Foreword

Depressive and anxiety disorders pose a major public health problem with substantial economic and social burden. As this volume discusses, women have an almost 2-fold risk of these disorders compared to men, a difference that starts in childhood or early adolescence and persists into adulthood. Further, depressive and anxiety disorders have been associated with the development and progression of various forms of physical disease, suggesting the associations of these psychiatric disorders with physical health in general. Thus, understanding the epidemiology and pathophysiology of these disorders, and particularly for women, has important implications for attenuation of suffering worldwide.

In this volume, Drs. Castle, Kulkarni and Abel have gathered multidisciplinary experts, along with themselves, to summarize the current literature on a broad spectrum of topics related to depressive and anxiety disorders in women. This ambitious work not only covers sex differences in mood and anxiety disorders per se, but also in disorders or conditions to which they are related, such as borderline personality disorder (Chanen), incidence and consequences of domestic violence (Warburton and Abel), and substance use disorders (Gerada and colleagues). It is very helpful for investigators in the field to have one volume into which all these data are gathered. Further, there is useful clinical information regarding treatments for these disorders and their interactions with hormonal status in women.

Several neuroendocrine systems have been implicated in the development, prognosis, natural history and treatment of mood and anxiety disorders, including the hypothalamic-pituitary-adrenal (HPA), - gonadal (HPG), and -thyroid (HPT) systems. This volume nicely integrates neuroendocrine factors and their associations with these disorders. This is important for the treatment of these disorders given the higher prevalence of endocrine disorders in mood and anxiety disorders than in the general population, particularly in women. Thus, an understanding of these relationships may promote further inquiry into the development of neuroendocrine modalities of treatment. This is discussed in several chapters in this volume, for example on depression and hormonal fluctuations (Abel and Kulkarni) and during pregnancy and lactation (Buist and colleagues) and the postpartum period (Dodd and colleagues), mood and menopause (Dennerstein and Alexander) and anxiety and depression in older age women (Baldwin and Garner).

The strong international group of authors are well-qualified to present an integrated perspective on mood and anxiety disorders in women. From the epidemiology of sex differences to the psychopharmacology and hormonal clinical trials related to sex differences, their expertise is felt throughout the volume. Historically, this is an important time in which there is a recognized value of investigating sex effects in clinical medicine. The editors have capitalized on this moment and presented a volume that focuses on disorders that have a high prevalence in women and thus are a major public health problem for families and our society. Further, the book offers hope that the development of new treatment modalities will take into consideration sex-specific needs.

Jill M. Goldstein, Ph.D.
Professor of Psychiatry
Department of Psychiatry
Harvard Medical School
Director of Research,
Connors Center for Women's
Health & Gender Biology
Division of Women's Health
Brigham & Women's Hospital

Pubertal development and the emergence of the gender gap in mood disorders: A developmental and evolutionary synthesis

Nicholas B. Allen[1], Anna Barrett[1], Lisa Sheeber[2], Betsy Davis[2]

[1]ORYGEN Research Centre and Department of Psychology, University of Melbourne, Australia
[2]Oregon Research Institute, Eugene, OR, USA

This book addresses mood and anxiety disorders in women. It takes a broad developmental approach, aimed at understanding and offering appropriate treatment for women with such disorders. The primary aim of this first chapter is to examine the emergence of the gender gap in depressive disorders at puberty, and to compare alternative theories as to the factors that underpin gender differentiation in depression at this developmental stage. These models are synthesised using an evolutionary perspective on gender differences to integrate the insights provided by socialisation, life stress, and biological models of pubertal development. Anxiety and anxiety disorders are addressed only peripherally, given the relative paucity of research in this area.

The emergence of gender differences in affective disorders during adolescence

Perhaps the most robust finding in psychiatric epidemiology is that the rate of unipolar depression is higher among females than it is among males (Weissman et al., 1996). Females are nearly twice as likely as males to experience case-level depression diagnoses (Kessler et al., 1994; McGrath et al., 1990; Nolen-Hoeksema, 1990; Weissman & Klerman, 1977), and this finding holds true across a variety of cultures and racial/ethnic groups (Gater et al., 1998). Furthermore, studies of non-clinical depressed mood states have shown that females experience more symptoms during episodes of depressed mood than do males (Wilhelm et al., 1998). Although studies have generally found that there are not gender differences in depression in prepubescent children, by 15 years of age females are twice as likely as males to have experienced a major depressive episode (e.g., Hankin et al., 1998). This places the gender disparity in depressive disorders firmly within the domain of developmental psychopathology, and specifically those developmental processes associated with early adolescence. An understanding of the developmental processes that underlie the emergence of this gender difference may have implications for understanding vulnerability to depression throughout the life cycle.

While anxiety disorders have also been shown to be more common in females (Yonkers & Gurguis, 1995; and see Chapter 4), there is comparatively less research on the causes and developmental pattern of gender differences in anxiety. Lewinsohn et al. (1998) found that retrospective reports of anxiety disorders indicated that the gender gap in such disorders emerges much earlier in life than it does in depression; by age six, females are twice as likely as males to have experienced an anxiety disorder. Given that the early emergence of anxiety disorders is thought to be a marker of risk for later depressive disorder (Parker et al., 1999), the gender gap in anxiety may be a developmental precedent for the gender disparity in depressive disorder that emerges in adolescence. In what follows, we concentrate explicitly on depression and depressive disorders.

The gender gap: fact or artefact?

Before examining theories to account for the gender difference in the prevalence of depression, it is important to establish that the female preponderance is not artefactual. Two major reporting artefacts have been cited as potentially contributing to the reported gender gap in depression; a help-seeking artefact, and a recall artefact. The *help-seeking artefact* refers to a perceived reticence in males to seek treatment or advice for depressive symptoms, which could explain the preponderance of females reporting for treatment. However, in a comparison of data from two worldwide multicentre studies conducted by the Cross National Collaborative Group and the World Health Organization, Kuehner (2003) found that the rates of depression identified in community samples were in accord with those reported from primary care settings. The *recall artefact* postulates that women's recall is biased in favour of past negative affective states, and thus women report a higher rate of lifetime depression. Kuehner (1999) conducted a controlled test of this by comparing men and women's reports of depressive symptomatology during a depressive episode, and their recall of these symptoms 6 months later. He found no recall artefact: there was no disparity in the reported severity of symptoms at times one and two, between males and females.

A third suggested artefact is that the higher rate of sexual abuse and rape experienced by girls and young women accounts for subsequent depression rates, although it is worth noting that is this does not constitute an artefact per se, but rather a potential aetiological explanation for the gender difference in mood disorders. Kessler (2000) did find that after rape and sexual trauma were controlled for in a population database, the gender difference in a first episode of depression was halved. However, when traumatic experiences more likely to be experienced by men were also controlled for, the female preponderance was restored. Findings such as these suggest that the increased prevalence of depression in females is not due to artefact.

Theories of the emergence of the gender gap during early adolescence

The gender intensification hypothesis

The *gender intensification hypothesis* (Hill & Lynch, 1983; Wichstrom, 1999) suggests that gender role orientations become more differentiated between the sexes over the adolescent years, as a result of exacerbated gender socialisation pressures during this time. For women, these pressures, both direct and in the form of social learning, are primarily thought to occur through observation of their parents' marital relations, which emphasise lesser public power and greater responsibility for the domestic sphere and care as part of the female gender role (Obeidallah et al., 1996) and through the socialising effects of parenting behaviours (Sheeber et al., 2002). The hypothesised effect of these socialisation experiences is the promotion of assumptions that emphasise collectivity, and a lower sense of self-esteem amongst females. These tendencies, in turn, contribute to the increase in depressive symptoms in women. The consequence of this intensified gender typing, according to these theorists, is that deficits in efficacy and instrumentality, reflected in low levels of traditionally masculine personality characteristics, may place young adolescent girls at higher risk for depression through greater exposure to experiences that promote learned helplessness (Obeidallah et al., 1996).

One important source of socialisation experiences is parenting behaviours throughout childhood and adolescence. Based on reviews of clinical and developmental literature, Hops (Hops et al., 1990; Hops, 1992, 1996) posited two paths by which parents may inadvertently increase their daughters' risk for depressive symptomatology and disorder. First, familial socialisation processes may serve to normalise and encourage girls' expression of depressive-like behaviours (e.g., sadness; self-derogation). Second, differential parental reinforcement of gender-typic behaviours may lead girls to display less instrumental and more relationship-focused behaviours, both of which are related to theoretically derived and empirically supported risk factors for depression. These gender-typic behavioural patterns, learned in early childhood and reinforced across time, are hypothesised to hamper girls' ability to meet the normative challenges of adolescence, thus contributing to the increased prevalence of depressive symptomatology among girls in this developmental stage.

There is some evidence that girls may be differentially socialised to display depressive behaviours during childhood. In a recent review on parental socialisation of emotion, Eisenberg et al. (1998) found that although parents do not typically report reacting differently to girls' and boys' emotional displays, observational data suggest that there are indeed differences, "albeit perhaps less than one might expect". In particular, a series of studies indicated that parents put more pressure on boys to control their emotions and "unnecessary" crying. Block (1983) reported that parents were quicker to respond to crying in girls than in boys. Parents' meta-messages about the acceptability of emotional expressions are apparently clear to children in that boys expect their parents to disapprove of their expression of sadness more so than girls (Fuchs & Thelen, 1988).

Parents' reactions to children's negative emotions may also provide them with gender-differentiated strategies for regulating negative affect. Although the data are limited, some evidence suggests that boys may be encouraged to use distraction and problem-solving more so than are girls (Eisenberg et al., 1998). In fact, one study indicated that school-age children expected fathers to respond to boys' emotional expressions with problem-solving and mothers to respond to girls' by focusing on feelings (Dino et al., 1984). Similarly, in a review of the origins of ruminative coping styles, Nolen-Hoeksema (1998) indicates that failure to teach girls active coping strategies for dealing with negative affect contributes to girls' greater use of ruminative styles of responding to depressed moods. Further, she suggests that to the extent girls are told that they are naturally emotional, they may have lower expectations that their behaviour can influence their affective experiences.

It has also been proposed that parents socialise girls to be more relationship-oriented and less instrumental than boys, and that this may in turn result in the socialisation not of depressive behaviours themselves, but rather risk factors for depression. Huston (1983) reported that girls receive more encouragement for dependency and affectionate behaviour. They are also reported to receive more support for nurturant play (Ruble et al., 1993). Interestingly, Block (1983) reported that in Baby X studies in which infants are "assigned" a gender (i.e., the same baby is labelled a "boy" and a "girl" in interactions with different participants), adults provided more reinforcement for nurturant play when the baby was said to be a girl; such evidence is compelling in that Baby X studies control for gender differences in children's actual behaviour. On a related theme, evidence suggests that mothers encourage girls more than boys to have concern for others, share, and behave prosocially (see Keenan & Shaw, 1997 for a review). Additionally, they may be less attentive to girls' assertive behaviour (Kerig et al., 1993). Parents may also impede the development of girls' sense of mastery by limiting their activities and freedom. In a 1983 review of the literature, it was reported that mothers were more likely to give unnecessary assistance to girls than to boys, and were more likely to reward frustration with physical comfort (Block, 1983).

There is also modest evidence that girls have lower self-evaluations of their own efficacy and that such evaluations are related to depressive symptomatology

(Avison & McAlpine, 1992; Ohannessian et al., 1999). In a recent review, Ruble et al. (1993) reported that preadolescent girls report lower expectations for success, more maladaptive attributions for success and failure, and poorer self-esteem, than age-matched boys. Though gender differences did not emerge in all of the studies reviewed by Ruble et al., the direction of effects was consistent when gender differences were observed. However, it is important to remain cognizant of the likelihood that disturbances in perceived self-competence may be sequelae rather than causes of depressive symptomatology. Two recent longitudinal studies by Cole et al. (1998, 1999) suggest that children's underestimates of their own competence emerge as a function of depressive symptomatology and that controlling for depression eliminates the observed gender differences in estimation of their competencies.

Thus, although these data suggest that parents' early gender-differentiated social-isation of children's emotional and social behaviours may have effect on children's ability and motivation to regulate emotion, large gaps remain in the literature. In particular, the largely cross-sectional studies do not provide evidence that these parental behaviours are predictors and not consequences of children's sex-typed behaviours. For example, if girls display more sadness and boys more anger, it would be reasonable to hypothesise that parents' tendency to discuss sadness with girls and anger with boys emerged consequent to the children's behavioural propensities. Similarly, it is not clear whether parents' tendency to be more emo-tion focused in response to young girls emotions and problem focused in response to young boys, doesn't reflect girls' earlier verbal and emotional development (Keenan & Shaw, 1997). Additionally, as a caveat it is important to keep in mind that the research discussed herein focuses on parents' responses to children's nor-mative emotional expressions. Though we consider it reasonable to construe depres-sive symptomatology as being at one end of a continuum of normative affective expression, the connection between early socialisation of depressive-like behav-iours and subsequent depressive functioning is, at this point, quite speculative.

Moreover, in a meta-analysis of research dating back to the 1950s, Lytton and Romney (1991) concluded that although there is modest evidence of parental encouragement for sex-typed activities, the evidence does not support overall dif-ferences in parental restrictiveness or encouragement of either achievement or dependency as a function of child gender. Hence, it appears that the evidence for the shaping of differential activities for girls and boys is stronger than that for other areas of gender-socialisation.

Limitations of the gender intensification hypothesis

Aside from the limited number of studies that would allow strong causal inferences to be drawn regarding socialisation and the emergence of the gender gap in mood disorders, there is also some literature that is inconsistent with this hypothesis.

Studies documenting the trajectories of children's own gender role concepts have shown that the rigidity of children's gender stereotypes tends to *lessen* as adolescence approaches. These studies have also found that boys are likely to labour under more rigid self-imposed sex-types than girls (Banerjee & Lintern, 2000). Also, gender intensification theorists cite the emergence of the gender gap at adolescence as support for their argument; however, as will be discussed below, the onset of the gender difference in depression is not predicted by age as such, but rather by pubertal status of the individual (Angold et al., 1998). If female depression is a consequence of a broad societal pressure applied to girls when they reach a certain age or stage of schooling, this should not be the case.

Another problematic finding with regards to gender intensification theories of adolescent depression is that the rates of female depression have not lessened over the last 50 years (Weissman et al., 1996). While the feminist movement has yet to yield true gender equality, it is clear that the status and opportunities that adolescent girls may expect at present far outstrip those available 50 years ago. Gender intensification theories would logically predict that a rise in the financial and social power of women would be accompanied by a commensurate fall in depression onset at that developmental stage, where the assumption of adult female roles is hypothesised to be paramount to adolescent girls' sense of self-worth and efficacy. This matter, however, may not be as straightforward as it first appears. If the socialisation of female roles in terms of reduced instrumentality and increased sensitivity to social relationships has not changed fundamentally over time, then the increased opportunity for females may actually increase the gap between their behavioural repertoire and the demands placed on them. Nevertheless, the lack of change in the gender gap in rates of depression over a period of dramatic historical change in the type and range of roles socialised in young women does seem puzzling if gender socialisation is the key process driving this phenomenon.

Another contradiction within these theories is their heavy emphasis on the timing of gender intensification as a corollary to the timing of the emergence of the gender gap in affective disorders. As noted above, social learning and gender typing have been shown to begin in the first few years of life. If identification with a feminine stereotype is as strongly linked to depression as some of these theorists suggest, the finding that the rates of depression in prepubertal children are equal between genders is counter-intuitive (Gelman et al., 2004). A more sophisticated version of the gender intensification hypothesis posits that what is socialised in females during childhood are reductions in instrumentality and increased experiences of helplessness and dependency (see above; Sheeber et al., 2002). These socialisation experiences then constitute a diathesis that interacts with the developmental demands of early adolescence to create greater risk for depression in females. However, even this very plausible view of the role of socialisation pressures during adolescence needs to explain what it is about the developmental demands of early adolescence that is specifically associated with the emergence of depressive disorders in vulnerable females (as opposed to, say, anxiety where gender differences are seen much earlier in life (Lewinsohn et al., 1998)).

Finally, although the degree of gender gap in depressive disorders is unevenly distributed, such that women in disadvantaged sectors of society (e.g., women of colour, women living in poverty, single mothers, and those with less than a high school education) are disproportionately affected (Everson et al., 2002), the fact that the gender gap is also reliably observed in more privileged social groups also casts doubt on the validity of a theory which posits membership of a devalued social group as the primary causative influence on depression.

Gender roles and individual differences in personality

Investigations into developmental changes in gender identity often use self-report measures of traits traditionally thought to be more characteristic of males than females, or vice versa. In the Personal Attributes Questionnaire, for example, the "masculine" item endorsements include: *independent, active, competitive, making decisions easily, self-confident, not giving up easily*, and *standing up well under pressure* (Spence et al., 1974). The finding that high scores on these traits are protective against depression certainly seem to be robust (e.g., Hoffman et al., 2004), but the assumption that these are indeed inherently masculine traits may need re-evaluation. When these traits are considered in their own right, decoupled from their description as "masculine", the feminist argument becomes circular, in claiming that, for example, low self-confidence leads to depression, which is in part indexed by low self-confidence (Barrett & White, 2002).

One way to reframe the relationship between gender roles and depressive phenomena is by taking into account the correlation between sex role inventory scores, and broader personality traits. For example, Francis and Wilcox (1998) found that high scores on the Bem sex role inventory (Bem, 1974) masculinity scale were associated with low neuroticism and high extraversion, whereas high scores on femininity were associated with high neuroticism. Neuroticism has previously been identified as a candidate temperament trait that may place some individuals at higher risk for depression and anxiety, and is also reliably found to be higher in females (Fanous et al., 2002). O'Shea (2002, cited in Parker & Brotchie, 2004) found that, though female adolescents did record higher neuroticism scores than males, high neuroticism was a strong predictor of first onset depression, regardless of gender. In fact, adjustment for neuroticism scores greatly attenuated the gender differential in first onset depression in this sample. This suggests that it may be neuroticism, rather than gender role per se, that confers risk for depression, although this still begs the questions as to why female gender and typical female gender role descriptions are associated with greater levels of neuroticism.

Pubertal development and the diathesis for affective disorder

The relevance of pubertal changes to the developmental examination of the gender gap lies primarily in the potential role of hormonal changes at puberty as catalytic agents for the development of depression in those females placed at risk by temperamental predisposition. Angold et al. (1998) found that the transition to Tanner stage III (an index of body shape change) of puberty predicted the increase in rates of diagnostic and statistical manual of mental disorders (DSM-IV) unipolar depression in girls, exhibiting a much larger effect on rates of depression than chronological age. This supports the view that changes in rates of depression at adolescence are specifically related to the physical changes of puberty, rather than to broad psychosocial factors common to girls at a particular stage of adolescence. However, it does not rule out the possibility that societal pressures are the primary precipitators of depression, but are prompted not by age but by the visible manifestations of puberty. This problem was later clarified by the addition of hormonal variables into the model (Angold et al., 1999), which eliminated the effect of morphological status, strongly implicating the effects of oestrogen in the development of depression in adolescent girls.

At puberty, females' hormonal levels begin to fluctuate cyclically over a broader spectrum than males'. Oestrogen in particular is recognised as playing an important role in mediating females' sensitivity to stress. Oestrogen apparently acts as an anxiolytic, and thus the cyclical withdrawal of oestrogen that occurs shortly prior to menstruation may be analogous to the physiological effects of anxiolytic withdrawal, creating a greater sensitivity in menarcheal and adult females to the anxiogenic and depressogenic effects of negative life events. At the onset of puberty for males, on the other hand, the increase of testosterone has been found to have a protective effect against depression and anxiety, although it tends to increase aggressive and risk-taking behaviours (Seeman, 1997).

It is important to note that the cyclical release and withdrawal of oestrogen alone is not suggested to be the causative factor for the sudden increase in the incidence of depressive episodes in adolescent girls. Rather, this cycle is thought to form a biological kindling which increases the stress reactivity of at-risk individuals to negative life events. In this respect, negative perceptions of gender role expectations or a socialised limitation in the behavioural repertoire of females may indeed come into play as proximal risk factors, but are regarded as precipitants of the development of mood disorder in girls who are, by nature of temperament and biology, already at risk. In other words, the interaction of temperament and hormonal change may create a vulnerability diathesis upon which social factors may act as a catalyst to generate gender difference in rates of depression.

In support of the putative interaction between pubertal oestrogen changes and negative life events, Brooks-Gunn and Warren (1989) found that while pubertal oestrogen level rise accounted for 4% of variance in increased negative affect reported by adolescent girls, the joint contributions of oestrogen rise and negative life events accounted for 17% of the variance. It would appear that the onset of puberty sensitises young women to the stress of negative life events, and possibly desensitises young men, via the protective influence of testosterone. Prepubertal boys and girls tend to show similar correlations between number of life stressors and depressive affect. However, after the onset of puberty, the relationship between stress and negative affect strengthens for young women, and declines almost to elimination in young men (Angold et al., 1999).

Pubertal change and interpersonal stressors

Given the hypothesis that the relation between pubertal hormone changes and depression in females is mediated by negative life events, it is notable that the majority of stressors preceding the onset of adolescent depression are of an interpersonal quality (Cyranowski et al., 2000). Consistent with this observation, it has been proposed that the relationship between the quality of family relationships and depressive symptoms may be stronger for females than males (Kavanagh & Hops, 1994). During adolescence females tend to gain independence more slowly from their families (Huston & Alvarez, 1990) and have relationships that are both more disclosing and more conflictual with their parents than do males (Montemayor, 1983; Noller, 1994). Many studies using self-report measures have in fact found a stronger negative correlation between cohesive and supportive family relationships and depressive symptoms amongst girls than boys (Avison & McAlpine, 1992; Rubin et al., 1992; Slavin & Rainer, 1990; Windle, 1992), although a study by Sheeber et al. (1997), which included observational as well as self-report measures of family functioning, found that the relationship between family functioning and depression was equivalent for males and females. This suggests that the stronger link between family processes and depression amongst females may be primarily determined by the way depressed states affect female *perceptions* of the family environment rather than objectively observable features.

The correspondence between the findings of a specific association between interpersonal stress and risk for depression on the one hand, and the evidence of increased affiliative proclivities amongst females, (both as compared to males, and after menarche) on the other, led Cyranowski et al. (2000) to examine potential biological substrates for female affiliative behaviour. Non-human mammal research has strongly implicated the hypothalamic neuropeptide oxytocin in affiliative and care-giving behaviours (Depue & Lenzenweger, 2001). Oxytocin transmission is thought to be regulated by oestrogen and progesterone levels, giving rise to the idea of a hormonally driven pubertal increase in affiliative proclivity for females (Cyranowski et al., 2000). This potential connection between pubertal development and an increase in biologically controlled sensitivity to social stressors allows for a synthesis of psychosocial, biological, and stress-response precipitants to adolescent onset depression, with the important caveat that the role of oxytocin in human female affiliative behaviour is yet to be fully understood. Although the formation of affiliative networks is in itself a protective factor against depression, the increased desire and need for these relationships, as well as the burden of increased care-taking within relationships, may mean that affiliative failures form potent stressors for girls who are temperamentally at risk, as has been emphasised by recent evolutionary models of depression.

An evolutionary synthesis of pubertal influences on vulnerability to depressive disorders

Many theorists have argued that depressed states are most essentially related to reductions of positive affect (anhedonia being a key defining feature), and that the regulators of positive affect are embedded in *social* cognition and behaviour (e.g., Allen & Badcock, 2003; Joiner & Coyne, 1999; Gilbert, 1989, 1992; Gotlib & Hammen, 1992; Watson, 2000). Critical to a functional or evolutionary view of depression is the proposition that there are various biological processes that guide individuals to enact certain social or interpersonal roles, including gender roles. There are many clues in the research literature to suggest that social processes (both in terms of social cognition and interpersonal behaviour) play a critical role in the aetiology and maintenance of depressed states in both genders. Critical empirical observations here include findings demonstrating that depression is often precipitated by interpersonal events (as noted above), and that interpersonal processes often mediate the exacerbation or resolution of depressive episodes (Joiner et al., 1999). Stressful interpersonal contexts are amongst the most reliable antecedents of depressed states (e.g., Kendler et al., 2003; Monroe et al., 1999) and certain interpersonal behaviours, such a excessive reassurance seeking, are strong and specific predictors of risk for depression (Joiner & Metalsky, 2001).

A recently proposed model of the function of depressed states seeks to explain why there is such a close link between social cognition, social behaviour, and depressive phenomena. The *social-risk* hypothesis of depression (Allen & Badcock, 2003) suggests that depressed mood (i.e., down regulation of positive affect and confident engagement in the world) evolved to facilitate a risk-averse approach to social interaction in situations where individuals perceive their social resources (e.g., status, affection, friendship, power) to be at critically low levels. Thus, whereas positive affect encourages engagement in a range of activities, most especially social ones, reduced positive affect discourages such engagement. In this sense depressed mood was (in the evolutionary past) a defensive–protective strategy designed to reduce such activities, especially those with uncertain pay offs.

There are in fact a whole range of social activities and social roles wherein people have to make decisions about how costly or risky it is to develop or maintain the relationships, taking into consideration the risks that result from the possibility that others might not want to develop or maintain such a relationship in return. Clearly roles are co-constructed between self and other(s) and attempts to develop or maintain a role relationship is not without risks and potential costs. For example, co-operating in a group of exploiters might mean they benefit at one's expense, and competing for status and access to resources with others who are more powerful might elicit attacks or rejections. Thus it is important that individuals evaluate risks against benefits in whatever goal or role they are pursuing.

The social-risk hypothesis suggests that depressed mood evolved as a salient mediator between estimates of social risk and social behaviour. In other words, positive moods will fall when people evaluate that they have suffered a defeat or rejection that forces a reappraisal of their role pursuits. This risk-assessing/mood regulating mechanism affects social-perceptual processes such that the individual becomes hypersensitive to indications of social risk. In the area of social behaviour, the mechanism affects both communicative behaviour (signalling in order to reduce threats and to elicit safe forms of support), and resource acquisition behaviours (a general reduction in behavioural propensities towards high-risk social investments that may result in interpersonal conflict or competition). It is interesting to note that recent work on self-esteem has conceptualised a similar process called a "sociometer," which monitors others' reactions and alerts individuals to the possibility of social exclusion (Leary et al., 1995).

Sexual selection and vulnerability to depression

Buss (1995) has proposed that sexual selection defines the domains in which the sexes have faced different adaptive challenges, and therefore should explain those psychological sex differences that appear to exist at a species-wide level. The primary theory of the differential selective pressures facing males and females is referred to as "parental investment theory," and was originally proposed by Trivers (1972). The central idea of parental investment theory is that in mammals, including humans, the *minimal* requirements for successful reproduction differ dramatically between the sexes. For males, only the sex act and the contribution of easily replenished sperm are required, whereas for females there is a long period of gestation (and its associated limitations and vulnerabilities), along with intensive care of offspring during infancy and childhood. This means that some of the fundamental reproductive-adaptive tasks facing each of the sexes are different: for males these tasks include gaining sexual access to females, identifying reproductively valuable females, and ensuring paternity certainty; for females these tasks include identifying males who are able *and* willing to invest resources in her (especially during her extended pregnancy), and their offspring (Buss, 1994, 1995).

Sexual selection has been used to understand the emergence of sex differences in a variety of areas of human behaviour (e.g., Buss, 1994; Daly & Wilson, 1983; Geary, 1996; Symons, 1979). Particularly relevant to the arguments presented here is the conceptualisation of gender differences in inhibitory control of behaviour presented by Bjorklund and Kipp (1996). These authors point out that parental investment theory not only predicts that females must be able to choose well-resourced and dependable partners, but that the consequences of abandonment in mating (and other) relationships are potentially more damaging to their inclusive fitness as compared to males, given the difference in resources required for each of the sexes to enter into new reproductive relationships.

Eibl-Eibesfeldt (1989) observed that the need for enhanced female social sensitivity may not have applied only to mating relationships, but that the social style of females has also provided the primary basis for the long-term stability of social groups. Indeed, given that the major reproductive task predicted for females by parental investment theory is to gain investment and protection for herself and her offspring, the quality and consistency of this investment has probably been more critical than from whom it is obtained. This would suggest that quality of social relationships in general (i.e., not simply mating relationships) is more critical for females than males. Consistent with this, Essock and Mcguire (1985) have pointed out that females invest more energy in the initiation and maintenance of non-kin social support networks. Bjorklund and Kipp (1996) linked this investment to selective pressures to carefully choose and maintain relationships. Their review of the evidence is consistent with this assertion and indicates that females exhibit greater inhibitory control in social, cognitive and behavioural realms. In short, the evolutionary challenges predicted by parental investment theory and evolutionary views of sex differences would require females to exercise greater caution in negotiating the social ecology than males. The view that gender differences in depression are related to sexual selection mechanisms is also consistent with the data indicating that depression is only more common in females during their reproductive years (Bebbington et al., 1998).

Research on sex differences in social cognition has supported the prediction that females are more sensitive to the negative social implications of information. For instance, Ruble et al. (1993) reviewed the evidence and suggested that females are more susceptible than males to self-evaluative concerns, particularly negative behavioural and evaluative reactions to failure. Roberts and Nolen-Hoeksema (1994) have likewise found that women's self-evaluations were more reliant on the views of others than were men's self-evaluations. At a more general level, there are clear sex differences in being object-oriented versus people-oriented, with females showing a strong tendency to be more people-oriented (Geary, 1996; McGuiness, 1993). Clearly, according to the social-risk hypothesis, greater sensitivity to (and processing of) feedback regarding social performance would be expected to result in more frequent activation of depressed states, given that depressed states are understood to be instigated by a perception of loss of social value.

Another aspect of the greater female dependence on relationships to achieve fitness-enhancing goals is that females may be more constrained than males from exiting relationships (even very unsatisfactory ones) without compromising their pursuit of important goals (McGuire & Troisi, 1998). This may result in situations of chronic social threat, which may provide signals that continually engage and escalate depressive mechanisms.

Conclusions

In sum, our evolutionary synthesis explains a number of key features of the gender gap in depressive disorders. The social-risk hypothesis (Allen & Badcock, 2003), when combined with predictions from evolutionary theory regarding social and cognitive differences between the sexes, does predict a greater likelihood of depressed states amongst females that may be linked to evolved reproductive biology. Evolutionary theory predicts that females will be more likely to perceive social threats and make negative self-evaluations based on interpersonal feedback, and that this gender difference (which is predicted by parental investment theory) is therefore likely to emerge during reproductive phases of the lifespan. It is during these years that depression has been shown to be more common amongst females. This evolutionary synthesis therefore suggests that the emergence of the gender gap in depression at adolescence cannot be attributed solely, or even primarily, to the influence of gender socialisation processes, but these processes will interact with prepotent evolved gender differences to influence the emergence of the gender gap in mood disorders. The basic measures of masculinity and femininity that drive much of the gender socialisation theory on this topic are confounded with known risk factors for depression (such as personality) and even depression itself. An alternative conceptualisation of these characteristics suggests that they reflect variations of temperament, most particularly in measures of neuroticism or even subclinical depression. Neuroticism is then posited as a temperamentally anxiogenic and depressogenic trait, which may place some girls more at risk than others, prior to the onset of puberty. This trait vulnerability may be exacerbated by the cyclical withdrawal of oestrogen after menarche.

Furthermore, it has been suggested that the hormonal changes that occur as part of pubertal development directly contribute to females' heightened sensitivity to social circumstances. This may be linked to evidence that interpersonal events provide the vast majority of precipitating life stressors before a first episode onset of depression in adolescents. Given the specific link between depressed states (as opposed to, e.g., anxious states) and perceptions of social threat predicted by evolutionary views such as the social-risk hypothesis, it is not surprising that these hormonal changes appear to be the strongest predictor of the emergence of gender differences in rates of depression (Angold et al., 1999).

Our arguments here are an attempt to synthesise a range of disparate literatures into a more integrative view of the role of gender in depressive disorders. We hope that this point of view not only helps to provide a new perspective on the developmental and psychopathological processes that underlie these phenomenon, but also may inform attempts at early intervention and prevention. Clearly pubertal females represent one of the most well identified groups for indicated prevention and early intervention efforts in mood disorders. When female gender is associated with other risk factors, such as social disadvantage (Everson et al., 2002), early puberty (Graber et al., 1997), or maternal depression (Sheeber et al., 2002), cohorts at very high risk for the emergence of depressive symptoms and disorders can be identified. The design of these interventions strategies, however, needs to be informed by a sophisticated understanding of the interplay between biological processes, socialisation pressures, life events, and individual differences. Indeed, we would emphasise that the evolutionary view we have proposed does not imply that biological processes have primacy, but rather points the way towards understanding how biology can profoundly interact with socialisation experiences and life stress to create a diathesis for depressive disorder. This has also been emphasised by recent findings that have shown that pubertal timing in girls can be influenced by life stress, especially those associated with paternal investment (Belsky et al., 1991; Ellis, 2004). These perspectives open up new directions for both research and intervention in females suffering from depressive disorders.

REFERENCES

Allen, N.B., & Badcock, P.B.T. (2003). The social risk hypothesis of depressed mood: Evolutionary, psychosocial, and neurobiological perspectives. *Psychological Bulletin, 129*, 887–913.

Angold, A., Costello, E.J., Erkanli, A., & Worthman, C.M. (1999). Pubertal changes in hormone levels and depression in girls. *Psychological Medicine, 29*(5), 1043–1053.

Avison, W.R., & McAlpine, D.D. (1992). Gender differences in symptoms of depression among adolescents. *Journal of Health and Social Behavior, 33*, 77–96.

Banerjee, R., & Lintern, V. (2000). Boys will be boys: The effect of social evaluation concerns on gender-typing. *Social Development, 9*(3), 397–408.

Barrett, A.E., & White, H.R. (2002). Trajectories of gender role orientations in adolescence and early adulthood: A prospective study of the mental health effects of masculinity and femininity. *Journal of Health and Social Behavior, 43*(4), 451–468.

Bebbington, P.E., Dunn, G., Jenkins, R., Lewis, G., Brugha, T., Farrell, M., & Meltzer, H. (1998). The influence of age and sex on the prevalence of depressive conditions: Report from the National Survey of Psychiatric Morbidity. *Psychological Medicine, 28*, 9–19.

Belsky, J., Steinberg, L., & Draper, P. (1991). Childhood experience, interpersonal development, and reproductive strategy: An evolutionary theory of socialization. *Child Development, 62*, 647–670.

Bem, S.L. (1974). The measurement of psychological androgyny. *Journal of Consulting and Clinical Psychology, 42*, 155–162.

Bjorklund, D.F., & Kipp, K. (1996). Parental investment theory and gender differences in the evolution of inhibition mechanisms. *Psychological Bulletin, 120*, 163–188.

Block, J.H. (1983). Differential premises arising from differential socialization of the sexes: Some conjunctures. *Child Development, 54*, 1335–1354.

Brooks-Gunn, J., & Warren, M.P. (1989). Biological and social contributions to negative affect in young adolescent girls. *Child Development, 60*(1), 40–55.

Buss, D.M. (1994). *The evolution of desire: Strategies of human mating.* New York: Basic Books.

Buss, D.M. (1995). Psychological sex differences: Origins through sexual selection. *American Psychologist, 50*, 164–168.

Cole, D.A., Martin, J.M., Peeke, L.G., Seroczynski, A.D., & Hoffman, K. (1998). Are cognitive errors of underestimation predictive or reflective of depressive symptoms in children: A longitudinal study. *Journal of Abnormal Psychology, 107*(3), 481–496.

Cole, D.A., Martin, J.M., Peeke, L.A., Seroczynski, A.D., & Fier, J. (1999). Children's over- and underestimation of academic competence: A longitudinal study of gender differences, depression, and anxiety. *Child Development, 70*(2), 459–473.

Cyranowski, J.M., Frank, E., Young, E., & Shear, K. (2000). Adolescent onset of the gender difference in lifetime rates of major depression. *Archives of General Psychiatry, 57*(1), 21–27.

Daly, M., & Wilson, M. (1983). *Sex, evolution, and behavior,* 2nd edn. Boston: Willard Grant Press.

Depue, R.A., & Lenzenweger, M.F. (2001). A neurobehavioral dimensional model. In: Livesley, & W. John (Eds.), *Handbook of personality disorders: Theory, research, and treatment* (pp. 136–176). New York, NY, USA: Guilford Press.

Dino, G.A., Barnett, M.A., & Howard, J.A. (1984). Children's expectations of sex differences in parents' responses to sons and daughters encountering interpersonal problems. *Sex Roles, 11*(7–8), 709–717.

Eisenberg, N., Cumberland, A., & Spinrad, T.L. (1998). Parental socialization of emotion. *Psychological Inquiry, 9*(4), 241–273.

Ellis, B. (2004). Timing of pubertal maturation in girls: An integrated life history approach. *Psychological Bulletin, 130*, 920–958.

Essock Vitale, S., & Mcguire, M.T. (1985). Women's lives from an evolutionary perspective II: Patterns of helping. *Ethology and Sociobiology, 6*, 155–173.

Everson, S.A., Maty, S.C., Lynch, J.W., & Kaplan, G.A. (2002). Epidemiologic evidence for the relation between socioeconomic status and depression, obesity, and diabetes. *Journal of Psychosomatic Research, 53*, 891–895.

Fanous, A., Gardner, C., Prescott, C., Cancro, R., & Kendler, K. (2002). Neuroticism, major depression and gender: A population-based twin study. *Psychological Medicine, 32*, 719–728.

Francis, L.J., & Wilcox, C. (1998). The relationship between Eysenck's personality dimensions and Bem's masculinity and femininity scales revisited. *Personality and Individual Differences, 25*(4), 683–687.

Fuchs, D., & Thelen, M.H. (1988). Children's expected interpersonal consequences of communicating their affective state and reported likelihood of expression. *Child Development, 59*(5), 1314–1322.

Gater, R., Tansella, M., Korten, A., Tiemens, B., Mavreas, V., & Olatawura, M. (1998). Sex differences in the prevalence and detection of depressive and anxiety disorders in general health care settings. *Archives of General Psychiatry, 55*, 405–413.

Geary, D.C. (1996). Sexual selection and sex differences in mathematical abilities. *Behavioral and Brain Sciences, 19*, 229–284.

Gelman, S.A., Taylor, M.G., & Nguyen, S.P. (2004). Mother-child conversations about gender. *Monographs of the Society for Research in Child Development, 69*(1), vii–127.

Gilbert, P. (1989). *Human nature and suffering.* Hove: Lawrence Earlbaum Associates.

Gilbert, P. (1992). *Depression: The evolution of powerlessness.* New York: Guilford.

Gotlib, I.H., & Hammen, C.L. (1992). *Psychological aspects of depression: Towards a cognitive interpersonal integration.* Chichester: John Wiley and Sons.

Graber, J.A., Lewinsohn, P.M., Seeley, J.R., & Brooks-Gunn, J. (1997). Is psychopathology associated with the timing of pubertal development? *Journal of the American Academy of Adolescent and Child Psychiatry, 36*, 1768–1776.

Hankin, B.L., Abramson, L.Y., Moffitt, T.E., Silva, P.A., McGee, R., & Angell, K.E. (1998). Development of depression from preadolescence to young adulthood: Emerging gender differences in a 10-year longitudinal study. *Journal of Abnormal Psychology, 107*, 128–140.

Hill, J.P., & Lynch, M.E. (1983). The intensification of gender-related role expectations during early adolescence. In: J. Brooks-Gunn, & A.C. Petersen (Eds.), *Girls at puberty: Biological and psychosocial perspectives* (pp. 201–228). New York: Plenum.

Hoffman, M., Powlshta, K., & White, K. (2004). An examination of gender differences in adolescent adjustment: The effect of competence on gender role differences in symptoms of psychopathology. *Sex Roles, 50*, 795–810.

Hops, H. (1992). Parental depression and child behaviour problems: Implications for behavioural family intervention. *Behaviour Change, 9*(3), 126–138.

Hops, H. (1996). Intergenerational transmission of depressive symptoms: Gender and developmental considerations. In: C. Mundt, M.J. Goldstein, K. Hahlweg, & P. Fiedler (Eds.), *Interpersonal factors in the origin and course of affective disorders* (pp. 113–128). London: Gaskell/Royal College of Psychiatrists.

Hops, H., Sherman, L., & Biglan, A. (1990). Maternal depression, marital discord, and children's behavior: A developmental perspective. In: G.R. Patterson (Ed.), *Depression and aggression in family interaction* (pp. 185–208). Hillsdale, NJ: Lawrence Erlbaum.

Huston, A.C. (1983). Sex-typing. In: P.H. Mussen (Ed.), *Handbook of child psychology* (pp. 387–467). New York: Wiley.

Huston, A., & Alvarez, M. (1990). The socialization context of gender role development in early adolescence. Montemayor, & Raymond (Eds.); Adams, & Gerald, R. (Eds.); et al. (1990). *From childhood to adolescence: A transitional period? Advances in adolescent development: An annual book series* (pp. 156–179),Vol. 2. Thousand Oaks, CA, USA: Sage Publications, Inc. 308 pp.

Joiner, T.E., & Coyne, J.C. (1999). *The interactional nature of depression: Advances in interpersonal approaches.* Washington DC: American Psychological Association.

Joiner, T.E., Coyne, J.C., & Blalock, J. (1999). On the interpersonal nature of depression: Overview and synthesis. In T.E. Joiner & J.C. Coyne (Eds.). *The interactional nature of depression: Advances in interpersonal approaches.* Washington DC: American Psychological Association.

Joiner, T.E., Metalsky, G.I., Lew, A., & Klocek, J. (1999). Testing of casual mediation component of Beck's theory of depression: Evidence for specific mediation. *Cognitive Therapy and Research, 23,* 401–412.

Joiner Jr, T.E., & Metalsky, G.I. (2001). Excessive reassurance seeking: delineating a risk factor involved in the development of depressive symptoms. *Psychological Science, 12*(5), 371–378.

Kavanagh, K., & Hops, H. (1994). Good girls? Bad boys? Gender and development as contexts for diagnosis and treatment. In: T.H. Ollendick, & R.J. Prinz (Eds.), *Advances in clinical child psychology* (pp. 45–79). New York: Plenum.

Kendler, K., Hettema, J., Butera, F., Gardner, C., & Prescott, C. (2003). Life event dimensions of loss, humiliation, entrapment, and danger, in the prediction of onsets of major depression and generalised anxiety. *Archives of General Psychiatry, 60,* 789–796.

Keenan, K., & Shaw, D. (1997). Developmental and social influences on young girls' early problem behavior. *Psychological Bulletin, 121*(1), 95–113.

Kerig, P.K., Cowan, P.A., & Cowan, C.P. (1993). Marital quality and gender differences in parent-child interaction. *Developmental Psychology,* (29), 931–939.

Kessler, R.C. (2000). *Gender differences in major depression: Epidemiological findings.* Washington, DC: American Psychiatric Publishing, Inc.

Kessler, R.C., McGonagle, K.A., Zhao, S., Nelson, C.B., Huges, M., Eshman, S., Wittchen, H-U., & Kendler, K.S. (1994). Lifetime and 12-month prevalence of DSM-III-R psychiatric disorders in the United States. *Archives of General Psychiatry, 51,* 8–19.

Kuehner, C. (1999). Gender differences in the short-term course of unipolar depression in a follow-up sample of depressed inpatients. *Journal of Affective Disorders, 56*(2–3), 127–139.

Kuehner, C. (2003). Gender differences in unipolar depression: an update of epidemiological findings and possible explanations. *Acta Psychiatrica Scandinavica, 108*(3), 163.

Lewinsohn, P.M., Gotlib, I.H., Lewinsohn, M., Seeley, J.R., & Allen, N.B. (1998). Gender differences in anxiety disorders and anxiety symptoms in adolescents. *Journal of Abnormal Psychology, 107,* 109–117.

Leary, M.R., Tambor, E.S., Terdal, S.K., & Downs, D.L. (1995). Self-esteem as an interpersonal monitor: The sociometer hypothesis. *Journal of Personality and Social Psychology, 68,* 519–530.

Lytton, H., & Romney, D.M. (1991). Parents' differential socialization of boys and girls: A meta-analysis. *Psychological Bulletin, 109*(2), 267–296.

McGrath, E., Keita, G.P., Strickland, B.R., & Russo, N.F. (1990). *Women and depression: Risk factors and treatment issues.* Washington DC: American Psychological Association.

McGuiness, D. (1993). Gender differences in cognitive style: Implications for mathematics performance and achievement. In: L.A. Penner, G.M. Batsche, H.M. Knoff, & D.L. Nelson (Eds.), *The challenge of mathematics and science education: Psychology's response.* Washington DC: American Psychological Association.

McGuire, M.T., & Troisi, A. (1998). Prevalence differences in depression among males and females: Are there evolutionary explanations? *British Journal of Medical Psychology, 71,* 479–491.

Monroe, S.M., Rohde, P., Seeley, J.R., & Lewinsohn, P.M. (1999). Life events and depression in adolescence: Relationship loss as a prospective risk factor for first-onset of major depressive disorder. *Journal of Abnormal Psychology, 108,* 606–614.

Montemayor, R. (1983). Parents and adolescents in conflict: All of the families some of the time and some families most of the time. *Journal of Early Adolescence, 3,* 83–103.

Nolen-Hoeksema, S. (1990). *Sex differences in depression.* Palo Alto, CA: Stanford University Press.

Nolen-Hoeksema, S. (1998). Ruminative coping with depression. In: J. Heckhausen & C.S. Dweck (Eds.), *Motivation and self-regulation across the life span.* (pp. 237–256). New York: Cambridge University Press.

Noller, P. (1994). Relationships with parents in adolescence: Process and outcome. Montemayor, & Raymond (Eds.); Adams, & Gerald R. (Eds.); et al. (1994). *Personal relationships during adolescence. Advances in adolescent development: An annual book series* (pp. 37–77), Vol. 6. Thousand Oaks, CA, USA: Sage Publications, Inc. vii, 254 pp.

Obeidallah, D.A., McHale, S.M., & Silbereisen, R.K. (1996). Gender role socialization and adolescents' reports of depression: Why some girls and not others? *Journal of Youth and Adolescence, 25*(6), 775–785.

Ohannessian, C.M., Lerner, R.M., Lerner, J.V., & von Eye, A. (1999). Does self-competence predict gender differences in adolescent depression and anxiety?. *Journal of Adolescence, 22,* 397–411.

Parker, G.B., & Brotchie, H.L. (2004). From diathesis to dimorphism: The biology of gender differences in depression. *Journal of Nervous and Mental Disease, 192*(3), 210–216.

Parker, G., Wilhelm, K., Mitchell, P., Austin, M., Roussos, J., & Gladstone, G. (1999). The influence of anxiety as a risk to early onset depression. *Journal of Affective Disorders, 52,* 11–17.

Roberts, T.A., & Nolen-Hoeksema, S. (1994). Gender comparisons in responsiveness to other's evaluations in achievement settings. *Psychology of Women Quarterly, 18,* 221–240.

Rubin, C., Rubenstein, J.L., Stechler, G., Heeren, T., Halton, A., Housman, D., & Kasten, L. (1992). Depressive affect in "normal" adolescents: Relationship to life stress, family, friends. *American Journal of Orthopsychiatry, 62*(3), 430–441.

Ruble, D.N., Greulich, F., Pomerantz, E.M., & Gochberg, B. (1993). The role of gender-related processes in the development of sex differences in self-evaluation and depression. *Journal of Affective Disorders, 29,* 97–128.

Seeman, M.V. (1997). Psychopathology in women and men: Focus on female hormones. *American Journal of Psychiatry, 154*(12), 1641–1647.

Sheeber, L., Hops, H., Alpert, A., Davis, B., & Andrews, J. (1997). Family support and conflict: Prospective relations to adolescent depression. *Journal of Abnormal Child Psychology, 25*(4), 333–344.

Sheeber, L.B., Davis, B., & Hops, H. (2002). Gender specific vulnerability to depression in children of depressed mothers. In: S. H. Goodman, & I. H. Gotlib (Eds.), *Children of depressed parents: Mechanisms of risk and implications for treatment* (pp. 253–274). Washington, DC: American Psychological Association.

Slavin, L.A., & Rainer, K.L. (1990). Gender differences in emotional support and depressive symptoms among adolescents: A prospective analysis. *American Journal of Community Psychology*, *18*(3), 407–421.

Spence, J., Helmreich, R., & Stapp, J. (1974). The Personal Attributes Questionnaire: A measure of sex role stereotypes and masculinity-femininity. *Catalogue of Selected Documents in Psychology*, *4*, 43–44.

Symons, D. (1979). *The evolution of human sexuality*. New York: Oxford University Press.

Trivers, R.L. (1972). Parental investment and sexual selection. In: B. Campbell (Ed.), *Sexual selection and the descent of man: 1871–1971*, Chicago: Aldine.

Watson, D. (2000). *Mood and Temperament*. The Guilford Press: New York.

Weissman, M.M., & Klerman, G.L. (1977). Sex differences and the epidemiology of depression. *Archives of General Psychiatry*, *34*, 98–111.

Weissman, M.M., Bland, R.C., Canino, G.J., Faravelli, C., Greenwald, S., Hwu, H.G., et al. (1996). Cross-national epidemiology of major depression and bipolar disorder. *Journal of the American Medical Association*, *276*(4), 293–299.

Wichstrom, L. (1999). The emergence of gender difference in depressed mood during adolescence: The role of intensified gender socialization. *Developmental Psychology*, *35*, 232–245.

Wilhelm, K., Parker, G., & Asghari, A. (1998). Sex differences in the experience of depressed mood state over fifteen years. *Social Psychiatry and Psychiatric Epidemiology*, *33*, 16–20.

Windle, M. (1992). A longitudinal study of stress buffering for adolescent problem behaviors. *Developmental Psychology*, *28*, 522–530.

Yonkers, K.A., & Gurguis, G. (1995). Gender differences in the prevalence and expression of anxiety disorders. In: M.V. Seeman (Ed.), *Gender and psychopathology* (pp. 113–130), Washington, DC: American Psychiatric Press.

2

Borderline personality disorder: Sex differences

Andrew M. Chanen

ORYGEN Research Centre, Department of Psychiatry, University of Melbourne, Melbourne, Victoria, Australia

Borderline personality disorder (BPD) is a severe mental disorder, characterised in the Diagnostic and Statistical Manual of Mental Disorders (DSM-IV-TR (APA, 2000)) by a pervasive pattern of instability of interpersonal relationships, self-image and affects and marked impulsivity. It is the most common and the most serious of the personality disorders (PDs) in clinical practice (Work Group on Borderline Personality Disorder, 2001). BPD is associated with considerable distress, psychosocial impairment, morbidity and mortality (Work Group on Borderline Personality Disorder, 2001) and is of particular relevance to this volume because, according to DSM-IV-TR, it is one of three PDs (along with histrionic and dependent PDs) diagnosed more frequently in women. This chapter provides an overview of sex differences in BPD, covering clinical presentation, longitudinal course, aetiological factors and neurobiological underpinnings.

Diagnostic features

The DSM-IV describes nine diagnostic criteria for BPD, with a cut-point of five to achieve "caseness". These criteria include
1 frantic efforts to avoid real or imagined abandonment,
2 a pattern of unstable and intense interpersonal relationships,
3 identity disturbance,
4 impulsivity,
5 recurrent deliberate self-harm,
6 affective instability,
7 chronic feelings of emptiness,
8 inappropriate, intense anger and
9 transient, stress-related paranoid ideation or severe dissociative symptoms.

This categorical approach to the diagnosis of PDs has been the subject of trenchant criticism. Diagnoses, including BPD have been described as "convenient fictions that inadequately describe complex psychopathology and have very limited relevance to treatment planning" (Ball, 2001, p. 148) and empirical studies have failed to support such categories (Livesley, 2001). There is emerging consensus that individual differences in PDs are best described using a dimensional model (Widiger & Simonsen, 2005a, b) and that the most robust evidence supports the use of the Five Factor Model (FFM) (Costa & Widiger, 2002) or analogous systems (Widiger, 1998a). However, the exact form of any model to replace the current DSM system is still the subject of considerable debate (Livesley, 2003; Widiger & Simonsen, 2005b).

In an attempt to make more sense of the features underlying BPD, the nine DSM-IV criteria for BPD are sometimes grouped into four domains (Lieb et al., 2004), namely, affective (anger, emptiness and affective instability), cognitive (transient psychotic symptoms and identity disturbance), behavioural (deliberate self-harm and impulsivity) and interpersonal (fear of abandonment and unstable relationships). However, factor analytic studies of the DSM BPD criteria set have yielded a three-factor solution consisting of disturbed relatedness (unstable relationships, identity disturbance, emptiness and stress-related paranoid ideation), emotional dysregulation (affective instability, inappropriate anger and avoidance of abandonment) and behavioural dysregulation (impulsivity and deliberate self-harm) (Sanislow et al., 2002; Skodol et al., 2002a).

Possible sources of sex differences

There has been considerable debate about whether reported sex differences in PDs, including BPD, in clinical samples reflect true biological, psychological or social differences between men and women or whether they are an artifact of sampling or diagnostic biases (Skodol & Bender, 2003; Widiger, 1998b). DSM-IV reports that borderline, histrionic and dependent PDs occur more frequently in females, whereas schizoid, schizotypal, paranoid, antisocial, narcissistic and obsessive–compulsive PDs are more often diagnosed in men. BPD and antisocial personality disorder (ASPD) are most notable for the degree of gender difference, with the female to male ratio for the former being 3:1 and the latter being 1:3. This, along with their shared underlying traits, has prompted researchers to ask whether these disorders might in fact be two sides of the same coin (Paris, 1997).

Widiger has conducted a number of reviews of this literature (Hartung & Widiger, 1998; Widiger, 1998b; Widiger & Spitzer, 1991) and has provided a comprehensive description of the sources of bias potentially contributing to the observed sex differences (Widiger, 1998b). These include

1 biased diagnostic constructs,
2 biased thresholds for diagnosis,
3 biased application of diagnostic criteria,

4 biased sampling of the population,

5 biased assessment instruments,

6 biased diagnostic criteria.

Although most of the literature relating to these issues has focused upon histrionic and dependent PDs, these issues have been comprehensively discussed in relation to BPD by Skodol and Bender (2003).

A *biased diagnostic construct* refers to sexist stereotyping of behaviour. Biased diagnostic criteria are the opposite of stereotyping, that is, the behaviours consistent with one's gender role might be assessed as less pathological. This has been debated for decades but received particular prominence with Kaplan's (1983) critique of the DSM-III. In this, she argued that stereotyped feminine behaviour would attract a DSM-III diagnosis (biased diagnostic construct), such as dependent or histrionic PD, whereas stereotyped masculine behaviour would not. There are limited data investigating this contention. One study (Henry & Cohen, 1983) failed to find a significant difference in the diagnosis of BPD using a male and female version of a case description from the DSM-III casebook. In a second study of 277 normal undergraduate and graduate students, the same authors found that males self-reported more characteristics of BPD than did female students, leading the authors to conclude that certain behaviours might only be labelled as pathological when they occur in women.

Sprock et al. (1990) asked 50 undergraduate students (33 female) who were unfamiliar with the DSM or the criteria for PDs, to sort the 142 DSM-III-R PD criteria along a dimension from features most characteristic of men to those most typical of women. Inappropriate anger was seen as strongly masculine, whereas all other diagnostic criteria were generally seen as feminine. When the anger item was removed, the remaining criteria were weighted toward the feminine end of the male–female dimension. They speculate that men and women might present with different BPD symptom patterns.

Klonsky et al. (2002) examined this issue from a different perspective. They asked whether people who are rated masculine or feminine by themselves and their peers more often meet the criteria for PDs. They found no difference in the prevalence of self-reported BPD in their sample of 665 undergraduate students (60% women). Interestingly, college students who rated themselves as behaving unlike their gender (i.e., feminine men and masculine women) endorsed more features of BPD. Furthermore, feminine-acting men exhibited the highest degrees of personality pathology across all DSM-IV PDs. This appears to contradict Kaplan's (1983) thesis. However, in another study of college students, Morey et al. (2002) found that PD characteristics seen as more problematic for a woman tend to be those that are more prevalent in women and vice versa. This suggests that extremes of sex-type behaviours are more likely to be seen as problematic.

Biased thresholds for diagnosis occur if there is a different point at which a diagnosis would be given to a woman, compared to a man. Sprock (1996) tested this hypothesis by asking undergraduate students to rate the degree of abnormality of the DSM-III-R PD criteria set for men, for women and a third group where the gender was unspecified. For BPD, inappropriate anger was rated as more abnormal for females than males and recurrent suicidal threats were rated less abnormal for males than for females or the gender-unspecified condition. There was no significant effect of instruction or of participant gender for the overall diagnosis of BPD. There was a significant interaction between instruction condition and participant gender. Male participants rated women with the BPD criteria as more abnormal than men with the same criteria.

Funtowicz and Widiger (1995, 1999) asked whether PDs that are more commonly diagnosed in women require less dysfunction to meet diagnostic threshold. They assessed the thresholds for the diagnosis of female and male-typed DSM-III-R PDs in 431 college students (240 female) using two self-report measures of PD and three inventories of personality dysfunction (Funtowicz & Widiger, 1995). They found no difference in the diagnostic thresholds for female and male-typed PDs. The same authors (Funtowicz & Widiger, 1999) also studied clinical psychologists' ratings of the degree of impairment and distress associated with the criteria for six PDs, including BPD, and reached the same conclusion. They found no significant difference in the overall level of dysfunction associated with the diagnostic criteria for female-typed PDs compared to male-typed PDs, suggesting that there was no bias against women.

Biased application of diagnostic criteria refers to the unequal application of criteria to one sex or the other. There is considerable empirical support for this bias in regard to PDs in general (Widiger, 1998b). Clinicians have been demonstrated to adhere poorly to the diagnostic criteria in both DSM-III (Morey & Ochoa, 1989) and DSM-III-R (Blashfield & Herkov, 1996) when making PD diagnoses. Although the agreement was better for BPD than for many other PDs in these studies, female patients were more likely to receive baseless diagnoses of BPD from female clinicians in both studies. A more recent study (Morey et al., 2002) did not find any gender differences in self-rated BPD criteria in college students. Furthermore, BPD criteria were rated to be as problematic for males as females.

Biased sampling of the population might also be called the "clinician's illusion" (Cohen & Cohen, 1984). This leads to attribution of the characteristics of patients who are currently ill to the entire population ever contracting the illness. In relation to BPD, this might reflect women's higher rates of help seeking (Skodol & Bender, 2003).

Most of the studies of sex differences reported above are derived from clinical samples (Widiger & Weissman, 1991). Two studies, one using a diagnostic algorithm derived from the Diagnostic Interview Schedule in the Epidemiologic Catchment Area Study (Swartz et al., 1990) and the other using a screening questionnaire (Ekselius et al., 1996) in a convenience sample of 531 people (including 176 healthy volunteers) have found a significantly higher proportion of women with DSM-III and DSM-III-R BPD respectively. This latter study also examined sex differences at the level of the individual DSM-III-R BPD criteria. Two criteria (suicidal behaviour and emptiness) were endorsed more often by males. Unstable relationships, affective instability, inappropriate anger and fear of abandonment were endorsed significantly more often by females.

More recently, there have been some advances made in population level research, with the use of representative samples and standard, interview-based diagnostic instruments (Samuels et al., 2002; Torgersen et al., 2001). There has also been one national study (Jackson & Burgess, 2000). Torgersen et al. (2001) estimated the pooled prevalence of BPD in 10 previous community samples to be 1.24%. Their own study is the most methodologically sound of the epidemiological studies in adults. It was conducted in a representative community sample in Oslo, Norway and found a weighted prevalence of BPD of 0.7%, with no statistically significant difference between men and women. In the only national survey in the literature, Jackson and Burgess (2000) found no significant gender differences for ICD-10 BPD but a greater proportion of men with ICD-10 impulsive PD. This finding should be interpreted with caution because, as with the study by Ekelsius (1996), diagnoses were made using a screening instrument with limited psychometric data.

The prevalence of BPD in adolescence has received little attention. Studies have generally been methodologically flawed. However the two main studies suggest a prevalence somewhere between a weighted population estimate of 0.9% (Lewinsohn et al., 1997) and a sample estimate of 7.8% (Bernstein et al., 1993). While one review has suggested that the prevalence of BPD in the latter study is higher in adolescent females (Lieb et al., 2004), this difference was not statistically significant. Grilo et al. (1996) found that female adolescent psychiatric inpatients were more likely than males to meet criteria for BPD.

Biased assessment instruments refers to the items used in instruments themselves applying to one sex more than the other. There does not appear to be any literature on this form of bias in relation to instruments for measuring BPD. The more general PD literature supports that there are biases more often on scales that involve disorders more often diagnosed in men (Widiger, 1998b), such as narcissistic and ASPDs.

In summary, although a number of biases may be operating to explain some of the gender variance in vulnerability to and expression of BPD, it seems that females are at heightened risk of this disorder. We now consider the clinical presentation of BPD and explore gender differences in that domain.

Clinical presentation

Paris, Zweig-Frank and colleagues published a series of papers comparing men with the BPD diagnosis (Paris et al., 1994b, 1996; Zweig-Frank et al., 1994a, b) to men with other PDs, which mirror findings in females with BPD. Compared to non-BPD participants, men with BPD experienced more frequent and more severe childhood sexual abuse (CSA), a longer duration of physical abuse, increased rates of early separation or loss and a higher paternal control score (Paris et al., 1994b), as measured on the parental bonding instrument (Parker et al., 1979). They also found men with BPD to be higher in levels of hostility and to make more frequent use of maladaptive and image distorting defences (Paris et al., 1996), compared to men without BPD. Furthermore, they also found dissociative features to be more common in men with BPD than in men with other PDs (Zweig-Frank et al., 1994a), a finding supported more recently by Timmerman and Emmelkamp (2001). Finally, a range of psychological risk factors, including adverse childhood experiences, did not differentiate between men with BPD who self-mutilated and those who did not (Zweig-Frank et al., 1994b).

There are few studies directly comparing men and women with BPD. Zanarini and colleagues' study (Zanarini et al., 1998a, b) of 379 inpatients (296 females and 83 males) with BPD found lifetime substance use disorder and ASPD to be more common among men and lifetime eating disorders to be more common among women. They suggest that men and women with BPD "specialised" in different disorders of impulse. These findings are supported by data from the Collaborative Longitudinal Study of Personality Disorders (CLPS, see below) (D.M. Johnson et al., 2003) and by a study of private practice outpatients in the USA (Zlotnick et al., 2002), which compared 105 women and 44 men with BPD, diagnosed by structured interview. The main point of difference between these studies is that two studies found post traumatic stress disorder (PTSD) to be more common among females with BPD (D.M. Johnson et al., 2003; Zanarini et al., 1998a) and one (Zlotnick et al., 2002) found no sex differences. The finding of significant co-occurrence for ASPD is also supported by two studies by Grilo et al. (2002a, b).

Cross-sectional baseline data from the CLPS (D.M. Johnson et al., 2003) comparing 175 women with 65 men with BPD (all inpatients at recruitment) found men with BPD to be more likely to present with substance use disorders, along with schizotypal, narcissistic and ASPDs. Women with BPD were more likely to present with PTSD, eating disorders and the BPD criterion of identity disturbance. The authors emphasise that men and women with BPD display more similarities than differences. They also comment that the sex differences found in BPD are consistent with sex differences found in epidemiological studies of psychopathology (e.g., higher rates of substance use in males and higher rates of eating disorders and PTSD in women), suggesting that they are not unique to BPD. More likely, they relate to males' tendency to display *externalising* forms of pathology and women's tendency to display *internalising* pathology. Interestingly, many sex differences normally found in epidemiological samples (e.g., higher rates of affective and (non-PTSD) anxiety disorders in women), were not found in this sample, prompting the intriguing suggestion that BPD pathology might attenuate the expression of usual sex differences in psychopathology.

Golomb et al. (1995) comment that one possible source of sex differences in rates of BPD in clinical samples might be from the clinical heterogeneity of the disorder. The studies above would suggest that in samples of patients with eating disorders one would expect to find a higher rate of BPD in females whereas in samples of substance users one would expect the reverse to be true. While Golomb et al. failed to find any sex differences in rates of BPD in depressed outpatients, Carter et al. (1999) studied 225 depressed outpatients and found males to be significantly more likely to meet criteria for BPD.

In summary, while some sex differences in the clinical presentation of BPD are well supported by data, these do not appear to be specific to BPD and appear to reflect sex differences in psychopathology found in the general population. Most striking is that women and men with BPD display more similarities than differences, a fact which often seems to be overlooked in clinical practice and which appears to contribute to the misdiagnosis of BPD in men (D.M. Johnson et al., 2003). With this in mind, we now turn to examine the temporal stability and longitudinal course of BPD.

Temporal stability and longitudinal course

There are several reviews of the stability of PDs in adult clinical populations (Grilo & McGlashan, 1999; Grilo et al., 2000; McDavid & Pilkonis, 1996; Perry, 1993; Sanislow & McGlashan, 1998; Zimmerman, 1994) and some studies in community samples (J.G. Johnson et al., 1997; Lenzenweger, 1999; Trull et al., 1998). Apart from ASPD, BPD is the best studied of the DSM PDs in this regard. McDavid and Pilkonis (1996) reviewed 10 studies of BPD with follow-up durations ranging from a few weeks to 15 years. Despite concerns about methodological flaws in many of these studies (McDavid & Pilkonis, 1996; Zimmerman, 1994), the data suggest that interview-based assessments of BPD have only moderate stability (a mean of 56% retaining their BPD diagnosis at follow-up) in adults, even when measured dimensionally (Ferro et al., 1998; J.G. Johnson et al., 1997). In a more recent brief review of 17 small-scale studies of the short-term course of BPD, Zanarini et al. (2003) found five studies reporting diagnostic stability. At 1–7 years after initial assessment, 4–53% (median 33%) of participants no longer reached the diagnostic threshold for BPD. These authors' own data (Zanarini et al., 2003) reported on 290 inpatients with BPD followed over 6 years. They found a progressive decline in DSM-III-R BPD symptom counts. At 2-year follow-up, 34.5% fell below diagnostic threshold. This increased to 49.4% at

4 years and 68.6% at 6 years. Over the entire 6-year follow-up period, 73.5% fell below diagnostic threshold at some stage. Impulsivity symptoms declined most quickly, followed by cognitive and interpersonal symptoms, followed by affective symptoms. They did not examine sex differences in this study. Data from the CLPS has also been published and suggests high levels of 1-year rank order stability for BPD (Shea et al., 2002). However, only 41% of participants remained above diagnostic threshold for BPD over the 12-month period. Again, sex differences were not examined.

Stability of DSM-III-R PD in the transition from teenage to adulthood has been reported from the Children in the Community Study (Bernstein et al., 1993; Crawford et al., 2001; J.G. Johnson et al., 2000), where moderate to high levels of stability have been found across the DSM clusters and high levels of stability were found in particular in cluster B (Crawford et al., 2001). In clinical samples, the Yale Adolescent Follow-Up Study found low stability of categorical PD over 2 years in adolescent inpatients (Mattanah et al., 1995) and low to moderate stability for dimensional PD ratings (Grilo et al., 2001). Chanen et al. (2004) examined the 2-year stability of categorical and dimensional PD in 101, 15–18-year-old psychiatric outpatients. Of those with any categorical PD diagnosis at baseline, 74% still met criteria for a PD at follow-up, with marked gender differences (83% of females and 56% of males). The sample size prevented any analysis of gender differences in specific PDs. Kappa for BPD was low, while rank order and mean-level dimensional stability for BPD was moderate.

Thus, the published studies of longitudinal course of BPD mostly do not specifically address the issue of gender difference. This is probably because most studies are in clinical samples, meaning that most participants with this PD are female. It is striking, however, that so many people with PDs tend to "lose" their diagnosis over time by falling below definitions of "caseness" for the disorder. The data of Chanen et al. (2004) suggest this might be more likely for males than females in older adolescents. However, it is noteworthy that large-scale community-based studies of the traits underlying PD have not found any significant sex differences in mean level or rank order stability over lengthy follow-up periods (Caspi et al., 2005). Further research is required, notably to explore what particular features of particular PDs might change differentially with time in males and females. In the absence of such comprehensive data, we turn to a consideration of aetiological parameters in BPD, with a view to whether there are clues there to the gender divergence in the disorder.

Aetiology

Data from Torgersen et al. (2000) support the substantial heritability of BPD. They studied all DSM-III-R PDs in 92 monozygotic and 129 dizygotic adult twin pairs, using a structured clinical interview and found a heritability estimate of 0.69 for BPD. The issue remains, though, how this translates into differential rates for males and females. As Widiger (1998b) comments, "Resolution of the sex bias controversy has been hindered in part by the absence of a theoretical model of personality disorder that proposes differential sex prevalence rates." (p. 98). Widiger suggests that trait-based models of PD, in particular the FFM (Wiggins, 1996), might provide some assistance in this respect. If PDs were extreme, maladaptive variants of normal personality traits, then the prevalence of PDs would be expected to mirror any differential sex prevalence of the factors and facets of the FFM. In fact, in the literature on normal personality, consistent sex differences have been obtained for most of the domains and facets of the FFM (Widiger, 1998b) and for some other trait measures (Jang et al., 1998). Furthermore, there are also significant sex differences in the magnitude of heritability of those traits and some evidence of sex-specific genetic effects (Jang et al., 1998).

These workers (Jang et al., 1998) have pursued this further. Using their model of personality dysfunction, which yields 18 basic and four higher-order dimensions (analogous to four of the FFM dimensions, excluding "openness" (Livesley et al., 1998)), they asked 681 volunteer twin pairs from the general population to complete the Dimensional Assessment of Personality Pathology (DAPP-BQ). Their data showed that most PD traits measured by the DAPP-BQ are heritable in both sexes and suggested sex-specific genetic influences underlying 14 of the 18 DAPP-BQ dimensions. Conversely, no sex-specific environmental influences were found across any of the dimensions. For the four higher-order dimensions, all genetic influences were sex-specific, with no sex-specific environmental influences demonstrated.

Livesley et al. (1998) note that the higher-order dimension of Emotional Dysregulation (comprising submissiveness, cognitive dysregulation, identity problems, affective lability, oppositionality, anxiousness, suspiciousness, social avoidance and insecure attachment) is analogous to DSM-IV BPD but broader in scope than the DSM construct, more akin to Kernberg's borderline personality organisation (Kernberg, 1967) and Linehan's (1993) description of BPD. It is noteworthy that both rejection (interpersonal hostility and judgemental attitudes) and stimulus seeking (sensation seeking, impulsivity and recklessness) do not load on to Emotional Dysregulation but rather on to Dissocial Behaviour.

With specific regard to the DAPP traits hypothesised to underlie BPD, Bagge and Trull (2003) assessed the relationships between the 18 lower-order DAPP-BQ traits and DSM-IV PD symptoms (measured on the Personality Diagnostic Questionnaire-4 (PDQ-4)) in a sample of 315 undergraduate psychology students. They found strong support for DSM-IV BPD being comprised of cognitive dysregulation, identity problems, affective lability, anxiousness, suspiciousness, insecure attachment, self-harm, stimulus seeking, rejection and conduct problems.

Relating these data to Jang and colleagues' study (Jang et al., 1998), above, submissiveness was the only trait that did not have a significant heritable component in males and likewise for cognitive dysregulation, suspiciousness and self-harm in females. Sex-specific genetic effects were detected for all traits, except insecure attachment. There was no evidence to support sex-specific, non-shared environmental influences for any traits underlying BPD. It is also noteworthy that callousness and conduct problems, along with their higher-order factor, dissocial, were not significantly heritable in females.

Despite compelling evidence supporting the relationship between CSA and adult psychopathology (Fergusson et al., 1996a; Mullen et al., 1993) and that this relationship appears to be causal (Kendler et al., 2000), the role of CSA and other forms of childhood adversity (Edwards et al., 2003) in the aetiology of specific disorders, including BPD, remains controversial, as CSA is neither necessary nor sufficient for the development of the disorder (J.G. Johnson et al., 1999; Paris, 1998; Zanarini et al., 2000). Childhood adversity, especially severe childhood abuse is common in BPD (Zanarini et al., 1997, 2000, 2002). In epidemiological studies of community samples, CSA is more common in females (Fergusson et al., 1996b). This appears also to be the case in BPD (Paris et al., 1994a, b) and this fact might contribute to the differential sex prevalence of BPD. However, CSA and other forms of childhood adversity are not uncommon in males (D.M. Johnson et al., 2003).

Epidemiological evidence is accumulating that genotypes can moderate children's sensitivity to environmental insults (Caspi et al., 2002, 2003). There is also evidence emerging in studies of adults that an individual's personality plays an important role in influencing exposure to some forms of environmental adversity (Jang et al., 2003; Kendler et al., 2003). Moreover, this relationship appears to be largely mediated by common familial factors that predispose both to temperamental difficulties and to environmental adversity.

Using similar logic to Widiger (1998b) (see above), Skodol and Bender (2003) highlight biological developmental differences and differential socialisation between boys and girls as possible contributors to the differential sex prevalence of PDs. To date, there are no specific data in this domain relating to BPD.

Overall, the aetiological underpinnings of sex differences in PDs in general and BPD in particular are complex, with multi-level interactions of genetic and environmental (familial and social) parameters acting at certain vulnerable stages of neural, emotional and social development. Furthermore, the very way the person temperamentally predisposed to BPD interacts with other people and the world in general elicits certain responses that serve to reinforce the pathology. For example, impulsivity might lead to exposure to sexual trauma or violence, which in turn might lead to insecure relationships. Such "interactionist" models must be the basis of future aetiological research.

Neurobiology

Finally, we review briefly the literature on the neurobiology of BPD, again with particular emphasis on sex differences. It should be emphasised that most studies in the area have been predominantly of females and that very few studies have been designed to address gender differences comprehensively.

Converging lines of evidence suggest involvement of frontal and limbic structures and circuits in adults with BPD (Lieb et al., 2004; Skodol et al., 2002b). Structural and functional imaging studies have allowed regional localisation of this dysfunction to cortical inhibitory areas, including the orbitofrontal cortex (OFC), ventro-medial frontal cortex and anterior cingulate cortex (Skodol et al., 2002b). Imaging studies have also demonstrated reduced metabolic activity in orbital and medial prefrontal regions associated with impulsive aggression in BPD and ASPD (Skodol et al., 2002b). Moreover, the orbitofrontal and cingulate cortices show a blunted response to serotonergic probes (New et al., 2002). Structural magnetic resonance imaging (MRI) studies in female adults with BPD demonstrate bilateral amygdala and hippocampal volume reduction (Driessen et al., 2000; Schmahl et al., 2003b; Tebartz van Elst et al., 2003). An early, methodologically compromised study (Lyoo et al., 1998) showed reduced frontal lobe volumes in a mixed gender sample, compared to controls. More recently, a study in females found reduction of the left orbitofrontal and right anterior cingulate cortices (Tebartz van Elst et al., 2003). However, a voxel-based morphometric study by one of these groups (Rusch et al., 2003) found only grey matter volume loss in the left amygdala with no prefrontal changes.

These structural studies have been supported by functional and metabolic imaging studies. One functional MRI (fMRI) study (Herpertz et al., 2001) found greater amygdala activation bilaterally in six female BPD patients, without co-occurring Axis I disorder, compared with healthy controls, while viewing aversive pictures compared to neutral pictures. Another found BPD patients to have significantly greater left amygdala activation to the facial expressions of emotion (versus a fixation point), compared with healthy controls (Donegan et al., 2003). A magnetic resonance spectroscopy (MRS) study (Tebartz van Elst et al., 2001) found evidence of subtle prefrontal neuropathology in terms of reduced N-acetylaspartate (NAA) concentrations in the dorsolateral prefrontal cortex of patients with BPD. NAA is mainly produced in neurons and is regarded as a putative marker of number and volume of neurons (Rudkin & Arnold, 1999).

Three positron emission tomography (PET) studies have found prefrontal cortical hypometabolism in BPD compared to healthy controls (De la Fuente et al., 1997; Soloff et al., 2000, 2003b). Another found increased activation of dorsolateral prefrontal cortex and anterior prefrontal cortex when BPD patients were presented with scripts designed to evoke memories of abandonment (Schmahl et al., 2003a).

Neuropsychological investigation suggests a dysfunctional prefrontal circuit in impulsive aggression (Best et al., 2002). There is evidence of a range of neuropsychological impairments in people with BPD in attention, memory, visuospatial function and emotional processing (Rogers, 2003) but these have been inconsistently replicated and have not been demonstrated to be specific to BPD. One study found that female patients with BPD had difficulties tolerating delayed rewards, compared to healthy controls (Dougherty et al., 1999). Another found that, compared to healthy controls, non-depressed patients with BPD were impaired on a planning task and showed impaired decision-making involving choices between uncertain rewards and punishments (Bazanis et al., 2002). These tasks have been shown to be sensitive to orbitofrontal dysfunction.

These data demonstrate a potential neurobiological circuit of relevance for BPD traits involving the OFC and medial temporal cortex. It is hypothesised that concurrent pathology affecting the prefrontal cortex (PFC) and limbic structures might be a neural correlate of affective and impulsive aggressive behaviour, irrespective of the underlying psychiatric disorder (Tebartz van Elst et al., 2003). The impact of gender on either vulnerability to or expression of these pathologies remains unclear.

Another approach in neurobiological studies is to focus upon subgroups of BPD, such as those with impulsive aggression, in an attempt to delineate relevant endophenotypes (Siever et al., 2002; Skodol et al., 2002b). Most of the above studies have been conducted in groups homogeneous for sex and have limited power to detect sex differences. Despite this, sex differences have been reported in serotonergic functioning in BPD (Leyton et al., 2001; Soloff et al., 2003a). Leyton et al. (2001) studied 13 medication-free patients with BPD (eight female) using a PET scanning technique that indexes serotonin synthesis capacity, and compared them to 11 healthy controls (five female). Males with BPD had significantly lower serotonin synthesis in corticostriatal sites, including the medial frontal gyrus, anterior cingulate gyrus, superior temporal gyrus and corpus striatum; however, in females with BPD these changes were seen in fewer regions.

Soloff et al. (2003a) conducted a study specifically looking for sex differences in central serotonergic function in BPD. They used a fenfluramine challenge test in 64 BPD subjects (44 female) and 57 controls (21 female). Male BPD participants had significantly diminished prolactin responses compared to healthy controls but female BPD participants did not. Measures of impulsivity and aggression were inversely related to prolactin responses among male but not female subjects. This led them to conclude that sex differences in central serotonergic function may contribute to variations in impulsivity in BPD.

Thus, the neurobiology of BPD is beginning to inform our understanding of sex differences in the disorder, most notably with respect to serotonergic mechanisms. However, studies are mostly not designed to address specific sex-related issues and further work is required in this area.

Conclusions

We have reviewed sex differences in BPD, and conclude that, a number of potential biases aside, the disorder is more common in females. How this relates to inherent differences in the aetiological and neurobiological parameters and/or the way females and males interact with the environment, remains unclear. This is a fruitful area for future research. Such work can be usefully informed by reference to other aspects of gender differences in development and in vulnerability to anxiety and depressive disorders, as outlined in other chapters of this volume.

REFERENCES

APA. (2000). *Diagnostic and statistical manual of mental disorders* (Vol. IV-Text Revision). Washington: American Psychiatric Association.

Bagge, C.L., & Trull, T.J. (2003). DAPP-BQ: Factor structure and relations to personality disorder symptoms in a non-clinical sample. *Journal of Personality Disorders, 17*(1), 19–32.

Ball, S.A. (2001). Reconceptualizing personality disorder categories using personality trait dimensions: Introduction to special section. *Journal of Personality, 69*(2), 147–153.

Bazanis, E., Rogers, R.D., Dowson, J.H., Taylor, P., Meux, C., Staley, C., et al. (2002). Neurocognitive deficits in decision-making and planning of patients with DSM-III-R borderline personality disorder. *Psychology of Medicine, 32*(8), 1395–1405.

Bernstein, D.P., Cohen, P., Velez, C.N., Schwab-Stone, M., Siever, L.J., & Shinsato, L. (1993). Prevalence and stability of the DSM-III-R personality disorders in a community-based survey of adolescents. *American Journal of Psychiatry, 150*(8), 1237–1243.

Best, M., Williams, J.M., & Coccaro, E.F. (2002). Evidence for a dysfunctional prefrontal circuit in patients with an impulsive aggressive disorder. *Proceedings of the National Academy of Sciences of the United States of America, 99*(12), 8448–8453.

Blashfield, R.K., & Herkov, M.J. (1996). Investigating clinician adherence to diagnosis by criteria: A replication of Morey and Ochoa (1989). *Journal of Personality Disorders, 10*(3), 219–228.

Carter, J.D., Joyce, P.R., Mulder, R.T., Sullivan, P.F., & Luty, S.E. (1999). Gender differences in the frequency of personality disorders in depressed outpatients. *Journal of Personality Disorders, 13*(1), 67–74.

Caspi, A., McClay, J., Moffitt, T.E., Mill, J., Martin, J., Craig, I.W., et al. (2002). Role of genotype in the cycle of violence in maltreated children. *Science, 297*(5582), 851–854.

Caspi, A., Roberts, B.W., & Shiner, R.L. (2005). Personality development: Stability and change. *Annual Review of Psychology, 56,* US: Annual Reviews, 453–484.

Caspi, A., Sugden, K., Moffitt, T.E., Taylor, A., Craig, I.W., Harrington, H., et al. (2003). Influence of life stress on depression: Moderation by a polymorphism in the 5-HTT gene. *Science, 301*(5631), 386–389.

Chanen, A., Jackson, H.J., McGorry, P.D., Allot, K.A., Clarkson, V., & Yuen, H.P. (2004). Two-year stability of personality disorder in older adolescent outpatients. *Journal of Personality Disorders, 18*(6), 526–541.

Cohen, P., & Cohen, J. (1984). The clinician's illusion. *Archives of General Psychiatry, 41*(12), 1178–1182.

Costa, P.T., & Widiger, T. (Eds.). (2002). *Personality disorders and the five-factor model of personality*, 2nd edn. Washington, DC: American Psychological Association.

Crawford, T.N., Cohen, P., & Brook, J.S. (2001). Dramatic-erratic personality disorder symptoms: I. Continuity from early adolescence into adulthood. *Journal of Personality Disorders, 15*(4), 319–335.

De la Fuente, J.M., Goldman, S., Stanus, E., Vizuete, C., Morlan, I., Bobes, J., et al. (1997). Brain glucose metabolism in borderline personality disorder. *Journal of Psychiatric Research, 31*(5), 531–541.

Donegan, N.H., Sanislow, C.A., Blumberg, H.P., Fulbright, R.K., Lacadie, C., Skudlarski, P., et al. (2003). Amygdala hyperreactivity in borderline personality disorder: Implications for emotional dysregulation. *Biological Psychiatry, 54*(11), 1284–1293.

Dougherty, D.M., Bjork, J.M., Huckabee, H.C., Moeller, F.G., & Swann, A.C. (1999). Laboratory measures of aggression and impulsivity in women with borderline personality disorder. *Psychiatry Research, 85*(3), 315–326.

Driessen, M., Herrmann, J., Stahl, K., Zwaan, M., Meier, S., Hill, A., et al. (2000). Magnetic resonance imaging volumes of the hippocampus and the amygdala in women with borderline personality disorder and early traumatization. *Archives of General Psychiatry, 57*(12), 1115–1122.

Edwards, V.J., Holden, G.W., Felitti, V.J., & Anda, R.F. (2003). Relationship between multiple forms of childhood maltreatment and adult mental health in community respondents: Results from the adverse childhood experiences study. *American Journal of Psychiatry, 160*(8), 1453–1460.

Ekselius, L., Bodlund, O., von Knorring, L., Lindstrom, E., & Kullgren, G. (1996). Sex differences in DSM-III-R, axis II-personality disorders. *Personality & Individual Differences, 20*(4), 457–461.

Fergusson, D.M., Horwood, L., & Lynskey, M.T. (1996a). Childhood sexual abuse and psychiatric disorder in young adulthood: II. Psychiatric outcomes of childhood sexual abuse. *Journal of the American Academy of Child & Adolescent Psychiatry, 35*(10), 1365–1374.

Fergusson, D.M., Lynskey, M.T., & Horwood, L. (1996b). Childhood sexual abuse and psychiatric disorder in young adulthood: I. Prevalence of sexual abuse and factors associated with sexual abuse. *Journal of the American Academy of Child & Adolescent Psychiatry, 35*(10), 1355–1364.

Ferro, T., Klein, D.N., Schwartz, J.E., Kasch, K.L., & Leader, J.B. (1998). 30-month stability of personality disorder diagnosis in depressed outpatients. *American Journal of Psychiatry, 155*(5), 653–659.

Funtowicz, M.N., & Widiger, T.A. (1995). Sex bias in the diagnosis of personality disorders: A different approach. *Journal of Psychopathology & Behavioral Assessment, 17*(2), 145–165.

Funtowicz, M.N., & Widiger, T.A. (1999). Sex bias in the diagnosis of personality disorders: An evaluation of DSM-IV criteria. *Journal of Abnormal Psychology, 108*(2), 195–201.

Golomb, M., Fava, M., Abraham, M., & Rosenbaum, J.F. (1995). Gender differences in personality disorders. *American Journal of Psychiatry, 152*(4), 579–582.

Grilo, C.M., Anez, L.M., & McGlashan, T.H. (2002a). DSM-IV axis II comorbidity with borderline personality disorder in monolingual hispanic psychiatric outpatients. *Journal of Nervous & Mental Disease, 190*(5), 324–330.

Grilo, C.M., Becker, D.F., Edell, W.S., & McGlashan, T.H. (2001). Stability and change of DSM-III-R personality disorder dimensions in adolescents followed up 2 years after psychiatric hospitalization. *Comprehensive Psychiatry, 42*(5), 364–368.

Grilo, C.M., Becker, D.F., Fehon, D.C., Walker, M.L., et al. (1996). Gender differences in personality disorders in psychiatrically hospitalized adolescents. *American Journal of Psychiatry, 153*(8), 1089–1091.

Grilo, C.M., & McGlashan, T. (1999). Stability and course of personality disorders. *Current Opinion in Psychiatry, 12*(2), 157–162.

Grilo, C.M., McGlashan, T.H., & Skodol, A.E. (2000). Stability and course of personality disorders: The need to consider comorbidities and continuities between axis I psychiatric disorders and axis II personality disorders. *Psychiatric Quarterly, 71*(4), 291–307.

Grilo, C.M., Sanislow, C.A., & McGlashan, T.H. (2002b). Co-occurrence of DSM-IV personality disorders with borderline personality disorder. *Journal of Nervous & Mental Disease, 190*(8), 552–554.

Hartung, C.M., & Widiger, T.A. (1998). Gender differences in the diagnosis of mental disorders: Conclusions and controversies of the DSM-IV. *Psychological Bulletin, 123*(3), 260–278.

Henry, K.A., & Cohen, C.I. (1983). The role of labeling processes in diagnosing borderline personality disorder. *American Journal of Psychiatry, 140*(11), 1527–1529.

Herpertz, S.C., Dietrich, T.M., Wenning, B., Krings, T., Erberich, S.G., Willmes, K., et al. (2001). Evidence of abnormal amygdala functioning in borderline personality disorder: A functional MRI study. *Biological Psychiatry, 50*(4), 292–298.

Jackson, H.J., & Burgess, P.M. (2000). Personality disorders in the community: A report from the Australian national survey of mental health and wellbeing. *Social Psychiatry & Psychiatric Epidemiology, 35*(12), 531–538.

Jang, K.L., Livesley, W., & Vernon, P.A. (1998). A twin study of genetic and environmental contributions to gender differences in traits delineating personality disorder. *European Journal of Personality, 12*(5), 331–344.

Jang, K.L., Stein, M.B., Taylor, S., Asmundson, G.J.G., & Livesley, W.J. (2003). Exposure to traumatic events and experiences: Aetiological relationships with personality function. *Psychiatry Research, 120*(1), 61–69.

Johnson, D.M., Shea, M., Yen, S., Battle, C.L., Zlotnick, C., Sanislow, C.A., et al. (2003). Gender differences in borderline personality disorder: Findings from the collaborative longitudinal personality disorders study. *Comprehensive Psychiatry, 44*(4), 284–292.

Johnson, J.G., Cohen, P., Brown, J., Smailes, E., & Bernstein, D.P. (1999). Childhood maltreatment increases risk for personality disorders during early adulthood. *Archives of General Psychiatry, 56*(7), 600–606.

Johnson, J.G., Cohen, P., Kasen, S., Skodol, A.E., Hamagami, F., & Brook, J.S. (2000). Age-related change in personality disorder trait levels between early adolescence and adulthood: A community-based longitudinal investigation. *Acta Psychiatrica Scandinavica, 102*(4), 265–275.

Johnson, J.G., Williams, J.B.W., Goetz, R.R., Rabkin, J.G., et al. (1997). Stability and change in personality disorder symptomatology: Findings from a longitudinal study of HIV+ and HIV− men. *Journal of Abnormal Psychology, 106*(1), 154–158.

Kaplan, M. (1983). A woman's view of DSM-III. *American Psychology, 38*(7), 786–792.

Kendler, K.S., Bulik, C.M., Silberg, J., Hettema, J.M., Myers, J., & Prescott, C.A. (2000). Childhood sexual abuse and adult psychiatric and substance use disorders in women: An epidemiological and cotwin control analysis. *Archives of General Psychiatry, 57*(10), 953–959.

Kendler, K.S., Gardner, C.O., & Prescott, C.A. (2003). Personality and the experience of environmental adversity. *Psychological Medicine*, *33*(7), 1193–1202.

Kernberg, O. (1967). Borderline personality organization. *Journal of the American Psychoanalytic Association*, *15*(3), 641–685.

Klonsky, E.D., Jane, J.S., Turkheimer, E., & Oltmanns, T.F. (2002). Gender role and personality disorders. *Journal of Personality Disorders*, *16*(5), 464–476.

Lenzenweger, M.F. (1999). Stability and change in personality disorder features: The longitudinal study of personality disorders. *Archives of General Psychiatry*, *56*(11), 1009–1015.

Lewinsohn, P.M., Rohde, P., Seeley, J.R., & Klein, D.N. (1997). Axis II psychopathology as a function of axis I disorders in childhood and adolescence. *Journal of the American Academy of Child and Adolescent Psychiatry*, *36*(12), 1752–1759.

Leyton, M., Okazawa, H., Diksic, M., Paris, J., Rosa, P., Mzengeza, S., et al. (2001). Brain regional α-[^{11}C]methyl-L-tryptophan trapping in impulsive subjects with borderline personality disorder. *American Journal of Psychiatry*, *158*(5), 775–782.

Lieb, K., Zanarini, M.C., Schmahl, C., Linehan, P.M.M., & Bohus, P.M. (2004). Borderline personality disorder. *The Lancet*, *364*(9432), 453.

Linehan, M. (1993). *Cognitive-behavioural treatment of borderline personality disorder*. New York, NY: Guilford Press.

Livesley, W.J. (2001). Commentary on reconceptualizing personality disorder categories using trait dimensions. *Journal of Personality*, *69*(2), 277–286.

Livesley, W.J. (2003). Diagnostic dilemmas in classifying personality disorder. [references]. In: Phillips, Katherine First, Michael (Eds.), et al. (2003). *Advancing DSM: Dilemmas in psychiatric diagnosis* (pp. 153–189). Washington, DC: American Psychiatric Association.

Livesley, W.J., Jang, K.L., & Vernon, P.A. (1998). Phenotypic and genetic structure of traits delineating personality disorder. *Archives of General Psychiatry*, *55*(10), 941–948.

Lyoo, I.K., Han, M.H., & Cho, D.Y. (1998). A brain MRI study in subjects with borderline personality disorder. *Journal of Affective Disorders*, *50*(2–3), 235–243.

Mattanah, J.J.F., Becker, D.F., Levy, K.N., Edell, W.S., et al. (1995). Diagnostic stability in adolescents followed up 2 years after hospitalization. *American Journal of Psychiatry*, *152*(6), 889–894.

McDavid, J.D., & Pilkonis, P.A. (1996). The stability of personality disorder diagnoses. *Journal of Personality Disorders*, *10*(1), 1–15.

Morey, L.C., & Ochoa, E.S. (1989). An investigation of adherence to diagnostic criteria: Clinical diagnosis of the DSM-III personality disorders. *Journal of Personality Disorders*, *3*(3), 180–192.

Morey, L.C., Warner, M.B., & Boggs, C.D. (2002). Gender bias in the personality disorders criteria: An investigation of five bias indicators. *Journal of Psychopathology & Behavioral Assessment*, *24*(1), 55–65.

Mullen, P.E., Martin, J.L., Anderson, J.C., Romans, S.E., et al. (1993). Childhood sexual abuse and mental health in adult life. *British Journal of Psychiatry*, *163*(Dec), 721–732.

New, A.S., Hazlett, E.A., Buchsbaum, M.S., Goodman, M., Reynolds, D., Mitropoulou, V., et al. (2002). Blunted prefrontal cortical 18fluorodeoxyglucose positron emission tomography response to meta-chlorophenylpiperazine in impulsive aggression. *Archives of General Psychiatry*, *59*(7), 621–629.

Paris, J. (1997). Antisocial and borderline personality disorders: Two separate diagnoses or two aspects of the same psychopathology? *Comprehensive Psychiatry*, *38*(4), 237–242.

Paris, J. (1998). Does childhood trauma cause personality disorders in adults? *Canadian Journal of Psychiatry*, *43*(2), 148–153.

Paris, J., Zweig-Frank, H., Bond, M., & Guzder, J. (1996). Defense styles, hostility, and psychological risk factors in male patients with personality disorders. *Journal of Nervous & Mental Disease*, *184*(3), 153–158.

Paris, J., Zweig Frank, H., & Guzder, J. (1994a). Psychological risk factors for borderline personality disorder in female patients. *Comprehensive Psychiatry*, *35*(4), 301–305.

Paris, J., Zweig Frank, H., & Guzder, J. (1994b). Risk factors for borderline personality in male outpatients. *Journal of Nervous and Mental Disease*, *182*(7), 375–380.

Parker, G., Tupling, H., & Brown, L.B. (1979). A parental bonding instrument. *British Journal of Medical Psychology*, *52*(1), 1–10.

Perry, J.C. (1993). Longitudinal studies of personality disorders. *Journal of Personality Disorders*, *7*(Supplement), 63–85.

Rogers, R.D. (2003). Neuropsychological investigations of the impulsive personality disorders. *Psychology Medicine*, *33*(8), 1335–1340.

Rudkin, T.M., & Arnold, D.L. (1999). Proton magnetic resonance spectroscopy for the diagnosis and management of cerebral disorders. *Archives of Neurology*, *56*(8), 919–926.

Rusch, N., van Elst, L.T., Ludaescher, P., Wilke, M., Huppertz, H.J., Thiel, T., et al. (2003). A voxel-based morphometric MRI study in female patients with borderline personality disorder. *Neuroimage*, *20*(1), 385–392.

Samuels, J., Eaton, W.W., Bienvenu, O., Brown, C., Costa, P.T., & Nestadt, G. (2002). Prevalence and correlates of personality disorders in a community sample. *British Journal of Psychiatry*, *180*(6), 536–542.

Sanislow, C.A., Grilo, C.M., Morey, L.C., Bender, D.S., Skodol, A.E., Gunderson, J.G., et al. (2002). Confirmatory factor analysis of DSM-IV criteria for borderline personality disorder: Findings from the collaborative longitudinal personality disorders study. *American Journal of Psychiatry*, *159*(2), 284–290.

Sanislow, C.A., & McGlashan, T.H. (1998). Treatment outcome of personality disorders. *Canadian Journal of Psychiatry*, *43*(3), 237–250.

Schmahl, C.G., Elzinga, B.M., Vermetten, E., Sanislow, C., McGlashan, T.H., & Bremner, J.D. (2003a). Neural correlates of memories of abandonment in women with and without borderline personality disorder. *Biological Psychiatry*, *54*(2), 142–151.

Schmahl, C.G., Vermetten, E., Elzinga, B.M., & Bremner, J.D. (2003b). Magnetic resonance imaging of hippocampal and amygdala volume in women with childhood abuse and borderline personality disorder. *Psychiatry Research: Neuroimaging*, *122*(3), 193–198.

Shea, M.T., Stout, R., Gunderson, J., Morey, L.C., Grilo, C.M., McGlashan, T., et al. (2002). Short-term diagnostic stability of schizotypal, borderline, avoidant, and obsessive–compulsive personality disorders. *American Journal of Psychiatry*, *159*(12), 2036–2041.

Siever, L.J., Torgersen, S., Gunderson, J.G., Livesley, W., & Kendler, K.S. (2002). The borderline diagnosis III: Identifying endophenotypes for genetic studies. *Biological Psychiatry*, *51*(12), 964–968.

Skodol, A.E., & Bender, D.S. (2003). Why are women diagnosed borderline more than men? *Psychiatric Quarterly*, *74*(4), 349.

Skodol, A.E., Gunderson, J.G., Pfohl, B., Widiger, T.A., Livesley, W., & Siever, L.J. (2002a). The borderline diagnosis I: Psychopathology, comorbidity, and personality structure. *Biological Psychiatry*, *51*(12), 936–950.

Skodol, A.E., Siever, L.J., Livesley, W., Gunderson, J.G., Pfohl, B., & Widiger, T.A. (2002b). The borderline diagnosis II: Biology, genetics, and clinical course. *Biological Psychiatry*, *51*(12), 951–963.

Soloff, P.H., Kelly, T.M., Strotmeyer, S.J., Malone, K.M., & Mann, J.J. (2003a). Impulsivity, gender, and response to fenfluramine challenge in borderline personality disorder. *Psychiatry Research*, *119*(1–2), 11–24.

Soloff, P.H., Meltzer, C.C., Becker, C., Greer, P.J., Kelly, T.M., & Constantine, D. (2003b). Impulsivity and prefrontal hypometabolism in borderline personality disorder. *Psychiatry Research*, *123*(3), 153–163.

Soloff, P.H., Meltzer, C.C., Greer, P.J., Constantine, D., & Kelly, T.M. (2000). A fenfluramine-activated FDG-PET study of borderline personality disorder. *Biological Psychiatry*, *47*(6), 540–547.

Sprock, J. (1996). Abnormality ratings of the DSM-III-R personality disorder criteria for males vs. Females. *Journal of Nervous & Mental Disease*, *184*(5), 314–316.

Sprock, J., Blashfield, R.K., & Smith, B. (1990). Gender weighting of DSM-III-R personality disorder criteria. *American Journal of Psychiatry*, *147*(5), 586–590.

Swartz, M., Blazer, D., George, L., & Winfield, I. (1990). Estimating the prevalence of borderline personality disorder in the community. *Journal of Personality Disorders*, *4*(3), 257–272.

Tebartz van Elst, L., Hesslinger, B., Thiel, T., Geiger, E., Haegele, K., Lemieux, L., et al. (2003). Frontolimbic brain abnormalities in patients with borderline personality disorder – a volumetric magnetic resonance imaging study. *Biological Psychiatry*, *54*(2), 163–171.

Tebartz van Elst, L., Thiel, T., Hesslinger, B., Lieb, K., Bohus, M., Hennig, J., et al. (2001). Subtle prefrontal neuropathology in a pilot magnetic resonance spectroscopy study in patients with borderline personality disorder. *Journal of Neuropsychiatry & Clinical Neurosciences*, *13*(4), 511–514.

Timmerman, I.G., & Emmelkamp, P.M. (2001). The relationship between traumatic experiences, dissociation, and borderline personality pathology among male forensic patients and prisoners. *Journal of Personality Disorders*, *15*(2), 136–149.

Torgersen, S. (2000). Genetics of patients with borderline personality disorder. *Psychiatric Clinics of North America*, *23*, 1–9.

Torgersen, S., Lygren, S., Oien, P. A., Skre, I., Onstad, S., Edvardsen, J., et al. (2000). A twin study of personality disorders. *Comprehensive Psychiatry*, *41*(6), 416–425.

Torgersen, S., Kringlen, E., & Cramer, V. (2001). The prevalence of personality disorders in a community sample. *Archives of General Psychiatry*, *58*(6), 590–596.

Trull, T.J., Useda, J., Doan, B.-T., Vieth, A.Z., Burr, R.M., Hanks, A.A., et al. (1998). Two-year stability of borderline personality measures. *Journal of Personality Disorders*, *12*(3), 187–197.

Widiger, T.A. (1998a). Four out of five ain't bad. *Archives of General Psychiatry*, *55*(10), 865–866.

Widiger, T.A. (1998b). Sex biases in the diagnosis of personality disorders. *Journal of Personality Disorders*, *12*(2), 95–118.

Widiger, T.A., & Simonsen, E. (2005a). Alternative dimensional models of personality disorder: Finding a common ground. *Journal of Personality Disorders*, *19*(2), 110–130.

Widiger, T.A., & Simonsen, E. (2005b). Introduction to the special section: The American psychiatric association's research agenda for the DSM-V. *Journal of Personality Disorders, 19*(2), 103–109.

Widiger, T.A., & Spitzer, R.L. (1991). Sex bias in the diagnosis of personality disorders: Conceptual and methodological issues. *Clinical Psychology Review, 11*(1), 1–22.

Widiger, T.A., & Weissman, M.M. (1991). Epidemiology of borderline personality disorder. *Hospital & Community Psychiatry, 42*(10), 1015–1021.

Wiggins, J.S. (Ed.). (1996). *The five-factor model of personality: Theoretical perspectives.* New York, NY: Guilford Press.

Work Group on Borderline Personality Disorder (2001). Practice guideline for the treatment of patients with borderline personality disorder. *American Journal of Psychiatry, 158 (suppl)*(10), 1–52.

Zanarini, M.C., Frankenburg, F.R., Dubo, E.D., Sickel, A.E., Trikha, A., Levin, A., et al. (1998a). Axis I comorbidity of borderline personality disorder. *American Journal of Psychiatry, 155*(12), 1733–1739.

Zanarini, M.C., Frankenburg, F.R., Dubo, E.D., Sickel, A.E., Trikha, A., Levin, A., et al. (1998b). Axis II comorbidity of borderline personality disorder. *Comprehensive Psychiatry, 39*(5), 296–302.

Zanarini, M.C., Frankenburg, F.R., Hennen, J., & Silk, K.R. (2003). The longitudinal course of borderline psychopathology: 6-year prospective follow-up of the phenomenology of borderline personality disorder. *American Journal of Psychiatry, 160*(2), 274–283.

Zanarini, M.C., Frankenburg, F.R., Reich, D., Marino, M.F., Lewis, R.E., Williams, A.A., et al. (2000). Biparental failure in the childhood experiences of borderline patients. *Journal of Personality Disorders, 14*(3), 264–273.

Zanarini, M.C., Williams, A.A., Lewis, R.E., Reich, R.B., Vera, S.C., Marino, M.F., et al. (1997). Reported pathological childhood experiences associated with the development of borderline personality disorder. *American Journal of Psychiatry, 154*(8), 1101–1106.

Zanarini, M.C., Yong, L., Frankenburg, F.R., Hennen, J., Reich, D.B., Marino, M.F., et al. (2002). Severity of reported childhood sexual abuse and its relationship to severity of borderline psychopathology and psychosocial impairment among borderline inpatients. *Journal of Nervous & Mental Disease, 190*(6), 381–387.

Zimmerman, M. (1994). Diagnosing personality disorders: A review of issues and research models. *Archives of General Psychiatry, 51*(3), 225–245.

Zlotnick, C., Rothschild, L., & Zimmerman, M. (2002). The role of gender in the clinical presentation of patients with borderline personality disorder. *Journal of Personality Disorders, 16*(3), 277–282.

Zweig-Frank, H., Paris, J., & Guzder, J. (1994a). Dissociation in male patients with borderline and non-borderline personality disorders. *Journal of Personality Disorders, 8*(3), 210–218.

Zweig-Frank, H., Paris, J., & Guzder, J. (1994b). Psychological risk factors and self-mutilation in male patients with BPD. *Canadian Journal of Psychiatry, 39*(5), 266–268.

Substance use and abuse in women

Clare Gerada[1], Kristy Johns[2], Amanda Baker[3] and David Castle[4]

[1]Hurley Clinic, Kennington Lane, London, UK
[2]Alcohol and Other Drugs Service, Central Coast Health, NSW, Australia
[3]Centre for Mental Health Studies, University of Newcastle, NSW, Australia
[4]Mental Health Research Institute and University of Melbourne, Parkville, Victoria, Australia

Over the last century, in most Western countries, women have made many great strides in social equality, including winning the right to vote and to equal wages. This chapter describes how and why women may also be gaining ground on their male counterparts in the consumption of alcohol and illicit substances. While women have "come a long way" (a phrase employed in a cigarette advertising campaign in the 1980s) in their drug use, researchers and treatment providers have been slow to identify women's treatment needs, and to develop newer services sensitive to the needs of women with substance abuse or dependence. Thus, we also describe the characteristics of women-sensitive services and recommend that existing services adopt these features. Mostly we concentrate on alcohol abuse and dependence, as alcohol is the substance that has been most well studied in terms of gender differences; many of the general findings extrapolate to other drugs. We do not explicitly address nicotine dependence here.

Epidemiology and clinical issues

Epidemiology of substance use and abuse: gender differences

Surveys of substance abuse and dependence in the general population fairly consistently show overall rates in females to be lower than those in males. For example, the United States (US) Epidemiological Catchment Area (ECA) Study (Helzer et al., 1991) reported an overall rate for alcohol abuse and dependence of 13.6%, with a male:female ratio of around 5:1 (males 23.8%, females 4.6%). The National Comorbidity Study, also conducted in the USA, found alcohol use disorders to afflict 20.1% of males and 8.2% of females, a rate ratio of 2.5:1 (Anthony et al., 1994). In the National Longitudinal Alcohol Epidemiologic Survey (NLAES; Grant et al., 1994, Grant, 1997), interviews were conducted with 42,862 people over 18 years of age: 13.3% of respondents were found to have had a lifetime alcohol use problem, with gender-specific rates being 18.6% for males and 8.4% for females (rate ratio 2.2:1).

For drugs other than alcohol, gender ratios vary according to age and type of drug. Thus, the cross-sectional household survey conducted by the US National Institute of Drug Abuse (1993) (cited by Lex, 1995) found the highest rates for cannabis and cocaine to be amongst males in the 18–25-year age group: for cannabis, 14.5% of males reported use in the previous month, versus 7.5% of females, whilst the respective rates for cocaine were 2.9% and 0.8%. In the younger age groups, overall rates were lower, but females and males were, roughly, equally likely to have used cannabis or cocaine in the previous month. Rates of heroin use were much lower, with around 1.2% of men and 0.6% of women having ever used.

Studies in countries other than the USA have also reported higher general population rates of alcohol and other drug use in males than females. For example, in the United Kingdom Psychiatric Morbidity Survey (Jenkins et al., 1998; Meltzer et al., 1995), dependence on illicit drugs was reported by 2.9% of men and 1.4% of women. In the Australian National Survey of Mental Health and Wellbeing (Andrews et al., 1999), 12-month prevalence rates for any substance use disorder were 11.1% for males and 4.5% for females. More males than females were dependent on alcohol (5.1% of males, 1.9% of females) and cannabis (2.5% of males and 0.7% of females), but there were no significant gender differences in rates of dependence on opiates and sedatives (0.2% of each sex dependent on opiates, and 0.4% on sedatives).

It is important to note, however, that there are significant cross-cultural differences in the relative risk of substance abuse and dependence amongst men and women. This is most striking when looking at societal attitudes to women drinking alcohol. In an overview of studies that used the Diagnostic Interview Schedule (DIS) to assess alcohol use at a population level, male:female ratios were found to range from 5.4:1 in the USA, through 9.8:1 in Puerto Rico, to 29:1 in Taiwan (Helzer et al., 1990). As Hill (2000) notes, very few societies actually preclude women from drinking alcohol altogether, and in some parts of the world (e.g. parts of Africa), women play a major role in the manufacture and sale of alcohol. Indeed, amongst the Sioux Indians, alcohol use appears more common amongst women than men (quoted by Hill (2000), p. 463).

One of the trends that will be noted from the studies reported above from Western countries, is that of a general narrowing of the gap between the sexes in terms of rates of substance use disorders over time. Changes in the social role of women over the past decades is likely to have influenced the gender gap in substance use and abuse. Male:female ratios of prevalence estimates of substance use are narrowing in many countries. There is a trend among boys and girls in their teens toward comparable rates of use and initiation for alcohol, cocaine, heroin, and tobacco.

These studies might reflect methodological differences between studies over the years, but also seems to underscore a true rise in rates of such problems in women, particularly young women. For example, the British General Household Surveys (see Marshall, 2000, p. 200) revealed that in 1986, 10% of females and 25% of males drank more than 14 units of alcohol a week; by 1996, the rate in females had risen to 14%, whilst the rate in males had remained constant.

Another way of looking at this issue is by assessing studies specifically of young people. For example, in the 2000 National Household Survey on Drug Abuse (NHSDA; see Greenfield & O'Leary (2002), p. 467) in the USA, 16.2% of males and 16.5% of females aged 12–17 years reported alcohol use in the month prior. This again suggests that young women are at increasing risk of initiating alcohol use at a young age.

Comorbidity and long-term course: differences between the sexes

There is clinically important co morbidity between psychiatric illness and substance misuse disorders, particularly in women. Women with affective and anxiety disorders are more likely to present with alcohol or drug abuse/dependence than are women without such disorders. In turn, substance-misusing women are more likely to experience significant depression and anxiety (Chander & McCaul, 2003). It is always difficult to tease apart cause and effect in terms of this sort of co-aggregation of disorders, but it appears that depression and substance use have relatively discrete heritabilities (see Hill, 2000).

Certainly alcohol (and other drugs) can be used to deal with symptoms of depression and anxiety, such as insomnia, social anxiety, and so on. Also, the imbibed substance can affect mood; for example, alcohol can lead to dysphoria, and cannabis can cause panic attacks, expressly in women (Thomas, 1996). Thus, the interactions are complex, and probably work both to precipitate and maintain both sets of disorders (Hill, 2000; Kavanagh et al., 2003). There is some evidence to suggest that in women, depression is more likely to antedate substance use, whilst in men it follows on from such use. Also, in a 3-year follow-up study, Schutte et al. (1997) found that increased depressive symptoms predicted increased alcohol intake in women. What is important is that depression and anxiety disorders are over-represented in women (see Chapters 4 and 7) and that women might be more likely to present with depressive and anxiety symptoms rather than substance use per se (see Marshall, 2000). Thus, careful questioning about substance use should be part of the clinical assessment of such women.

Antisocial personality disorder (APD) is another psychiatric condition strongly associated with substance abuse and dependence. Rates of APD are, of course, higher in males than females, but rates of APD of up to 29% have been reported in female drug users; the rate in their male counterparts was 53% (cited in Lex, 1995). Another issue relates to whether the antisocial behaviours antedate or are consequent upon substance use. In a study of the temporal relationship between these two problems,

Table 3.1. Characteristics of substance use and abuse in women

---

- Overall rates of use tend to be lower than in men, although the differential is narrowing in young people;
- Tend to start using later in life, than men;
- Once started using, tend to go on to dependence more quickly than men (so-called "telescoping" effect);
- Tend to use smaller quantities of substances than men (this might reflect differences in amount required for the same physiological effect);
- Are more likely to drink alone;
- Are more likely than men to have a regular pattern of substance use, with fewer binges;
- Appear more likely to experience certain physical health consequences, than men.

Lex et al. (1994) found that the interactions are complex but that in some women the substance use appears to precipitate and maintain the antisocial behaviours.

Drug use, especially illegal use, is largely a phenomenon of youth, late adolescence, and early adulthood. Women tend to start using substances at a later age than males, though as outlined above, it appears that recent trends are towards women increasingly starting to use substances at a young age, such that amongst adolescents the sex difference in alcohol and illicit drug abuse rates is narrowing (Substance Abuse and Mental Health Services Administration, 1994). For all classes of illicit drugs, men are significantly more likely than women to meet lifetime criteria for dependence, once having used drugs. There are, however, striking differences between different drugs, such that among non-medical users of psychotropics women are significantly more likely than men to develop dependence (Kandel et al., 1986).

It also seems to be the case that women progress more rapidly than men to problem drinking, and also tend to suffer the medical consequences of alcohol use after a shorter period of exposure to a smaller amount of alcohol (Blume, 1992). This is in part at least a consequence of increased chronic concentrations of alcohol in women compared to men (Blume, 1997). Medical problems include hepatic cirrhosis, alcoholic cardiomyopathy, and cognitive impairment. Female drinkers also show elevated rates of breast cancer, hypertension and stroke, and reproductive pathology including amenorrhoea, anovulation, and possibly early menopause. Table 3.1 outlines other characteristics of substance use in women.

Why are rates of substance abuse lower in women than men, but the course worse in women?

Biological parameters

In terms of *biological parameters*, genetic factors appear to operate roughly equally for males and females, though Cloninger et al. (1981) have proposed an early-onset male form of alcoholism that tends to run in families. Other researchers (see Hill, 2000) have suggested that some women with severe early-onset alcoholism have a particularly high familial loading for alcohol use and abuse, underlining the heterogeneity of these problems.

Women have different fat distributions and lower effective volumes of distribution than men, resulting in higher blood levels of the imbibed substance (Jones & Jones, 1976). For cannabis, whose psychomimetic moiety, tetrahydrocannabinol (THC), is particularly lipophyllic, females' greater proportional fat results in a relatively slower clearance rate (Beyer & Conahan, 2003).

Also, gut levels of the alcohol dehydrogenase enzyme, involved in the metabolism of alcohol, tends to be lower in women (Frezza et al., 1990). The consequence of this is the "first pass" effect is reduced in females, resulting in the actual blood alcohol levels being higher per unit consumed.

Psychosocial issues

Broad societal factors may be pertinent to differential rates of substance use amongst men and women. As articulated above, this is evidenced by rates of alcohol use, which vary markedly across cultures with differential attitudes to alcohol use amongst women. There is also some evidence that family parameters might impact differentially upon females (see Hill, 2000).

It is well known that depression and anxiety afflict females more than males (see Chapters 4 and 7). As discussed above, there is some contention about how far depression drives substance use, and thus impacts negatively on the long-term course of the substance use disorder. Longitudinal studies suggest that depression and anxiety (notably social anxiety) at school age or during college is associated, in girls, with an elevated risk of alcohol use problems in adulthood (e.g. Fillmore et al., 1979; Jones, 1971). What certainly seems to be the case is that the "telescoping" effect of disease progression in alcohol abuse tends to be more marked in women who are depressed before the onset of alcohol abuse (Smith & Cloninger, 1981). It has also been shown that women with premenstrual dysphoria are at particular risk of an escalation of substance use during the premenstrual period (Tobin et al., 1994).

Adverse life events and family problems are also more likely to act as precipitants of substance use in women than men (Copeland & Hall, 1992). Sexual abuse is increasingly recognised as a causal, or at least a contributory, risk factor for substance abuse (Winfield et al., 1990). Females are clearly more at risk than males to childhood sexual abuse and again such a history might leave victims possibly at heightened risk of engaging in dangerous long-term substance use.

Thus, there are a number of factors that appear pertinent in the mediation of gender difference in substance use and abuse. The precise constellation of factors operating in any given person is, of course, highly individual and should be seen in a broad biopsychosocial framework.

Substance use and abuse in women: a life phase approach

Youth and adolescence

The findings of increasing rates of alcohol use by young women is a cause for particular concern, given their propensity to more rapid progression to problem drinking and to adverse medical consequences of drinking, as outlined above. Peer pressure undoubtedly plays an important part in the initiation of alcohol and other substance use, notably in the teens where there is pressure to "belong" (see Marshall, 2000). Also, the fact that so much teen socialising revolves around substance use makes it difficult for young people to avoid. Added to this is the anxiolytic effect of alcohol (and cannabis in low dose), which enhances socialisation.

It is probable that Western societies sanction alcohol use by women more than they did even a few decades ago. Thus, young women feel arguably less stigmatised regarding the use of alcohol. The fact that alcohol and other drugs tend to result in disinhibition leaves young women at particular risk for sexual exploitation, with the potential consequences of sexually transmitted diseases, including HIV/AIDS, and unplanned pregnancies. Disinhibition in conjunction with impairment of cognition associated with alcohol and other drugs such as cannabis increase risk-taking behaviours, including driving whilst intoxicated.

Excessive use of alcohol and other substances in the teens can also adversely affect educational attainment. In particular, there are concerns that the cognitive impairment associated with cannabis consumption (at least in the short term), and the amotivational effect of use of high doses, can impair the ability and motivation to learn new information (see Castle & Solowij, 2004). This can have long-term effects for the individual, and some evidence points to women being more vulnerable than men to cognitive impairment (notably impaired visuospatial recall) consequent upon heavy cannabis use (see Pope et al., 1997).

Another problem for young women using large quantities of alcohol and other substances is that the cost associated can leave them resorting to prostitution and crime in order to afford their habit. Thus, the US Bureau of Justice Statistics National Update (1991; quoted by Lex, 1995) reported that 34% of female prison inmates were under the influence of drugs at the time of their offence, and that 39% had used drugs regularly in the month prior to the offence. In the UK, Maden et al. (1990) reported a 400% increase in drug-related offences in women over the period 1979 to 1988.

The reproductive years

Relationship issues can have an important negative impact on substance use in women. For example, women are more likely than men to begin using in the context of a male partner who uses (males are more likely to begin in a peer group setting) (Wilsnack & Wilsnack, 1995). It is not uncommon for the male partner with a drug problem to further pressure the partner to increase her use. Thus, Kandel (1984) found that, for women living with a spouse or partner, the male partners' level of substance use had a greater impact on levels of use, than did peers' use. Furthermore, there is an increased risk of arguments and physical altercations whilst intoxicated (see Chapter 6). Wilsnack et al. (1986) reported that women who drink are more likely to experience sexual aggression, and that this is compounded if the male partner also drinks. Kantor and Strauss (1989), in a survey of battered wives, found high rates of cannabis use amongst the male perpetrators.

Work and financial areas can also be impacted by alcohol and other drug use. Work absenteeism and inability to function effectively at work, can result in loss of employment and the associated difficulties of loss of income. In their prospective study of teenagers followed up to their mid-20s, Kandel et al. (1986) found job instability to be associated with cannabis and other illicit drug use in both men and women. There was a positive correlation between amount of cannabis used at baseline, and periods unemployed over the follow-up period.

The impact of substance abuse on reproductive fitness in women is evidenced by higher rates of amenorrhoea and anovulatory cycles (Blume, 1997). There is also some evidence suggesting elevated rates of spontaneous abortion amongst substance-using women, including nicotine smokers (Weissman, 1999). Unwanted pregnancies and poor antenatal care compound these problems. Furthermore, women who have drug habits are at risk of poor nutrition, with subsequent increased risk for certain foetal abnormalities (e.g. folate deficiency leading to increased risk of spina bifida). Increased rates of physical illness and infections, notably HIV, also leave the foetus vulnerable. Heroin use in pregnancy can cause neonatal addiction and withdrawal, which if untreated can prove fatal (see Greenfield & O'Leary, 2002).

The foetal alcohol syndrome is a particular concern, being estimated to afflict anything from 0.03% to 0.3% of live births (Abel & Sokol, 1991). Its features are well established, and encompass (Jones et al., 1973; see Greenfield & O'Leary, 2002):

• delayed prenatal and postnatal growth,
• microcephaly,
• maxillary hypoplasia,
• abnormal palmar creases,
• cardiac abnormalities,
• capillary haemangiomas.

Substance abuse can also impact more broadly on mother–infant interactions, with the potential for neglect and abuse, and overall suboptimal outcomes for the child.

Middle age and later life

As women approach middle age and later life, the physical consequences of long term substance abuse begin to take their toll. Thus, elevated rates of liver disease, cardiomyopathy, brain damage, and breast cancer are evident in women who drink to excess (see Marshall, 2000). There is also an increased risk of premature death, including through physical complications of drug abuse as well as suicide (Lindberg & Agren, 1988).

There is also evidence that role-loss in middle age, associated with children leaving home, can lead women to either begin or increase their substance use, notably alcohol. Other women feel "trapped" in their social role, and turn to alcohol to alleviate their boredom and frustration. Women who suffer relationship breakdowns are also prone to substance use, with rates of abuse being higher amongst separated and divorced women, compared to their married counterparts (Wilsnack et al., 1994). In later life, death of a spouse may be associated with depression and consequent alcohol use.

Women in later life appear more likely than men to internalise shame and guilt associated with alcohol use, and also experience more familial and social pressure not to seek help for substance abuse problems (see Marshall, 2000). Thus, they often do not directly seek help for their problems, and their substance abuse is not picked up by general practitioners and other health professionals, to whom they may present with physical health of other mental health problems, such as depression. This leads us to a consideration of treatment issues for women with substance abuse problems.

Treating drug and alcohol problems in women

Barriers to treatment for women

Women face significant barriers to gaining access to substance abuse treatment (Marsh et al., 2000). These include (see also Table 3.2):
- the rarity of programmes oriented to the needs of women;
- stigmatisation and child protection issues;
- poor social support networks;
- poor child care and transport facilities;
- weaknesses in maternity services to deal with pregnancy and drug use;
- negative attitudes by health professionals;
- ineffective interagency cooperation and communication.

Substance abuse treatment services are often not designed to meet the special needs of women (Marsh et al., 2000). Existing treatment models have largely been developed by and for men, and continue to be refined on the basis of research largely conducted on male subjects (Swift et al., 1996). Over the last decade, greater

Table 3.2. Factors influencing drug service provision for female drug users, from Becker and Duffy (2002)

Lack of childcare and transport facilities	One of women's main area of dissatisfaction with treatment services involves lack of childcare facilities. Childcare and other domestic responsibilities and lack of transport have been identified as key barriers to accessing services.
Stigmatisation and child protection issues	Fears that children will be removed from them prevents women from admitting to their drug-using problem.
Lack of women only services	Some women feel intimidated talking in mixed counselling groups – usually dominated by men.
Lack of provision for ethnic minority women	Accessing services may be more difficult for ethnic minority women than white women.
Poor social support networks	Support from significant others, especially partners, appears to be an important influence on whether women present and remain in treatment. Women, if they inject drugs, are more likely to have a drug-using partner who also injects.
Weakness in maternity services	Pregnant drug users receive conflicting and confusing advice and information from maternity units. Findings from a survey of all the National Health Service maternity units in England and Wales showed that only 29% of units had formal links with local drug agencies and over 50% (57%) routinely admitted babies of drug using women to high dependency units (Morrison C. (1995). Maternity services for drug misusers in England and Wales: a national survey. *Health Trends, 27*(1), 15–17).
Negative attitudes of health professionals	Research has identified that health professionals as having negative views of drug taking women.

emphasis has been placed on conceptualising women as different from men in terms of their drug use histories, parenting responsibilities, victimisation histories, and difficulty accessing treatment (see above). However, little consideration has been given to these differences, nor to a systematic assessment of the barriers to accessing services, in planning and providing substance abuse treatment programmes (Swift et al., 1996).

Treatment needs

In a review of the literature on alcohol treatment programmes, Shand et al. (2003a) noted a lack of gender differences in outcomes among dependent drinkers, but noted that men and women may have different treatment needs. The same is likely to pertain to illicit drug use. The needs of female alcohol and illicit drug users who enter treatment might encompass serious physical and mental health problems, including:

- poor nutrition and low weight;
- low self-esteem;
- depression;
- the sequelae of physical and sexual abuse;
- if pregnant, premature delivery, low birth weight, and neonatal dependence and withdrawal;
- blood borne viruses, including Hepatitis A, B, C and HIV;
- sexually transmitted diseases including chlamydia and gonorrhoea.

To meet these complex needs, treatment services need to make strong links with key partners in other agencies, such as mental health services, benefit services, housing departments, and social services. Organisations can encourage women to access them by addressing child-care issues, assisting in transport and providing safe "women only" spaces. This may require re-distribution of existing funding or the provision of additional funding.

Following their review of gender differences in alcohol treatment outcomes, Shand et al. (2003a) graded clinical recommendations based on the strength of the evidence (Shand et al., 2003b). Strong recommendations were made for:

1 clinician sensitivity to issues particular to women;
2 provision of a safe therapeutic environment;
3 provision of information and opportunities to address physical and mental health issues and sexual and physical assault;
4 referral to other specialist services where necessary.

Moderate recommendations were made for:

1 strategies to improve women's awareness of services and decrease fears about entering treatment, thereby improving recruitment;
2 the availability of a range of services for women;
3 choice regarding therapist gender.

Engagement in treatment

Perhaps the single most important issue is to attract women into treatment, from where work can be done in reducing the harms and risks associated with substance misuse. People vary in their motivation for and stages of behaviour change (Prochaska & DiClemente, 1986), and it is helpful to respond to women's reasons for seeking substance abuse treatment and the barriers to their doing so. Connors et al. (2001) recommend that in order to help women move from contemplation to action, health care professionals should:

- apply screening instruments that have been validated with women;
- minimise barriers to treatment entry and retention;
- provide brief interventions employing motivational strategies such as the decisional balance (e.g. Miller & Rollnick, 2002) as a means of increasing motivation for and commitment to treatment.

Retention in treatment

Retention in substance abuse treatment is the largest and most consistent predictor of positive outcomes (Hubbard et al., 1997; Simpson et al., 1997). Studies have found that the longer a client remains in treatment, the better the chance that reductions in substance abuse and improvements in functioning will be maintained over time (Knight et al., 2001). Those who stay in programmes for long periods have been found to have lower rates of drug use and criminal behaviour and higher rates of employment and school attendance than those who stay for only short periods (Bale et al., 1980; DeLeon & Schwartz, 1984; Simpson, 1979).

The high rate of treatment dropout for women with drug and alcohol problems is of great concern to clinicians and researchers (Copeland & Hall, 1992) as there is a powerful association between dropping out and negative outcome (Stark, 1992). Dropouts from substance abuse treatment fare poorly, are a source of frustration for the clinician and constitute a major expense for treatment organisations (Stark, 1992). The apparent inability of treatment providers to engage and retain the majority of clients with substance dependence problems makes it highly desirable to identify those people who might be expected to benefit most from a particular treatment (Copeland & Hall, 1992). Although numerous studies have attempted to identify demographic and clinical factors that predict retention in treatment (Szuster et al., 1996), only sporadic and weak correlates of dropout have been found.

Generalising about any particular client's length of stay in substance abuse treatment programmes is complicated by the fact that there are many different types of programmes, client groups, and sets of predictor variables used (Bell et al., 1997). It is clear that no particular set or kind of variable can predict retention in treatment for all groups (Bell et al., 1997). Rates of dropout vary across different types of treatment programme, with maintenance pharmacotherapy programmes having by far the best retention rates, with about one third of clients dropping out in the 1st year (Bell et al., 1997). In addition, during the last decade, treatment programmes for women participating in gender-specific therapeutic programmes with specialised services for children have reported longer retention and significant improvement in post-treatment outcomes (Knight et al., 1999). Features of specialised treatment services for women and maintenance pharmacotherapy treatment among women are discussed below.

Specialist treatment services for women

In recognition of the multifaceted nature of the needs of women with substance abuse and dependence, a growing number of treatment programmes have been developed specifically for such women and their children (Chang et al., 1992; Mackie-Ramos & Rice, 1988 cited in Luthar & Walsh, 1995; Metsch et al., 1995; Schmidt & Weisner, 1995; Stevens & Arbiter, 1995 cited in Wobie et al. 1997). These services specifically aim to increase the availability, accessibility, appropriateness, and appeal of substance abuse treatment for women by recognising women's roles as mothers and the need for concurrent services for their children, as well as by addressing barriers to treatment (Luthar & Walsh, 1995).

In addition to meeting the general needs of women (see above), the Subcommittee of Women's Alcohol and Substance Abuse Treatment in the USA (1992, cited by Mejta & Lavin, 1996) advocated the inclusion of parenting training and treatment for children as basic elements in all substance abuse treatment programmes for women. Davis (1997) argues that programmes should assist mothers to create a safe, nurturing environment for their children, promote awareness of their children's emotional, cognitive and physical needs, and provide treatment that incorporates the needs of both the mothers and their children.

Outpatient treatment

A study by Marsh et al. (2000) found that women were more likely to have positive outcomes from outpatient substance abuse treatment when the programme provided transportation, outreach and child care services and when women were engaged in other interventions delivered by health and social services. Dahlgren and Willander (1989) compared the outcomes of outpatient treatment among women with early alcohol problems at a specialist women's treatment centre with that of a control group treated in a traditional mixed-sex treatment facility for people with alcohol problems. The specialised female programme included an individualised treatment programme, close contact with staff, cooperation with and support from relatives, focus on women's problems, and exchange of experiences with other women. Women treated in the specialised female programme were more likely to report abstinence at 12-and 24-month follow-ups than women who attended the traditional programme.

Residential treatment

In response to the growing evidence that it is important that children remain with their mothers in treatment and that treatment services address both substance abuse and parenting issues (e.g. Finkelstein, 1994; Harm et al., 1998), the number of residential substance abuse treatment facilities for substance dependent women and their children has grown in recent years (Knight et al., 2001). In most of these facilities, families are kept intact, childcare is provided, and women have opportunities to practice effective parenting skills while learning to overcome their addiction (Knight et al., 2001). Data suggest that these specialised residential programmes may encourage more women to enter treatment and result in higher completion rates than those obtained through programmes that do not provide safe housing or allow children to be present (Cosden & Cortez-Ison, 1999; Nunes-Dines, 1993). Szuster et al. (1996) found that women accompanied by their children stayed over twice as long in substance abuse treatment programmes, and were more than twice as likely to meet their treatment goals, than women without their children. Wobie et al. (1997) reported that women accompanied by their children in treatment tend to experience less depression and show higher self-esteem than women separated from their children.

In an evaluation of a traditional mixed sex versus specialist women's treatment service, Copeland and Hall (1992) reported better retention in the specialist service of women with dependent children, those with a history of childhood sexual assault, and lesbian women. This suggests that specialist services may fill an important gap in services offered by traditional services (see below).

While the potential benefit of specialised substance abuse treatment services for women seems clear, few empirical data are available on how women perceive the effectiveness of gender-sensitive specialised drug treatment (Nelson-Zlupko et al., 1996). Nelson-Zlupko et al. (1996) conducted in-depth interviews with 24 women who had received specialised and non-specialised drug treatment services, regarding their current and past treatment experiences. Of the 96 treatment experiences described, 25% were in residential facilities or hospitals and 75% were in outpatient settings. Services rated as "very helpful" were those aimed at meeting the particular therapeutic needs of women, included family counselling, women-only groups, individual counselling, parenting classes, and child care. The authors concluded that specialised women's services are most helpful when integrated into a treatment environment that promotes, protects, and understands women.

Clearly, specialist women's treatment services for substance abuse and dependence should have the capacity to address substance abuse and dependence issues simultaneously, and to provide child care and parenting education, and should be sensitive to issues related to roles as women and as mothers. Evidence suggests that such services may result in more women seeking and completing substance abuse treatment and better treatment outcomes for women and their children.

Women in pharmacotherapy maintenance treatment

Studies indicate that women who are dependent on heroin suffer from more general health and dental problems than do male addicts, and more than both men and women in the general population. For some women, it is the advent of such problems that leads to help-seeking. Other women addicts enter treatment because they are pregnant, and are afraid of the effect that their drug use may have on the baby. These scenarios offer an opportunity for engagement of such women in substance abuse treatment programmes, which need to be holistic but which often include pharmacological management. Thus, the main-stay of treatment for heroin addiction is substitution replacement with methadone or increasingly buprenorphine – an opiate agonist/antagonist. There is substantial evidence attesting to the efficacy of oral methadone maintenance treatment with improved outcomes in physical, social, and psychological health, reduction in criminality, illicit drug use, and improved general health. Moreover, evidence shows that the improvements are dose related and that high-dose methadone maintenance (80–120 mg/day) is more efficacious than lower doses.

There are unintended consequences of pharmacological treatment of opiate dependence. For example, when a woman first starts on methadone (or indeed any substitute medication) she may experience weight gain and return of menstruation (amenorrhoea is common amongst opiate users–related in part to poor health but also to low weight). Ovulation may restart with drug treatment before menstruation returns. It is important therefore to discuss contraception with all female drug users entering treatment.

Women with special needs

Research in the UK has shown that particular groups of women face greater difficulties when seeking help for their drug use than others (see Becker & Duffy, 2002). These women include:

- *Pregnant women and women with children*: Over 90% of female drug users presenting to services are of childbearing age. Drug use conflicts with the traditional images of women as carers, mothers, and wives. The fear of disapproval may prevent some women from admitting to their use (Hunter & Powis, 1996). Fear that their children may be taken away may prevent women from seeking help.
- *Women working within the sex industry*: In a sample of 51 sex workers who used opiates, over two thirds reported that they first used prostitution to fund their drug use (Gossop et al., 1994). Women engaged in sex-for-money or sex-for-drugs exchanges are likely to be at greater risk of both negative health and social consequences. They are also exposed to health risks due to the pressure to take part in unsafe sex and face a high risk of violence when exchanging drugs for money.

This pattern is particularly prevalent for women who use cocaine (Goldstein et al., 1991). These women are also exposed to violence and criminal activities. Women working in the sex industry may experience pressure not to take time away from their job to attend to their health needs.

- *Women involved in court proceedings*: As detailed above, there is a high rate of substance use problems associated with women entering the criminal justice system. Regrettably, there is a severe shortage of dedicated treatment services within the criminal justice system for women. Thus, women's health needs, including their addiction problems are largely ignored in many female prisons.

Heterogeneity: some women have come further than others

Recently, McPherson et al. (2004) compared women's and men's alcohol consumption patterns and alcohol-related problems in New Zealand in 1995 and 2000. They reported significant gender convergence due to women's consumption of alcohol moving towards that of men for all measures of quantity and for frequency of consumption, but with differences between age groups. The authors make the point that changes in gender roles and policy may have impacted differentially on women, particularly younger women. Hodgson and John (2004) suggest that as well as gender, researchers need to investigate the influence of gender role and cultural factors on treatment effectiveness and to determine how best to tailor messages according to different gender roles.

In addition to differences in convergence of alcohol consumption, it is important not to lose sight of individual differences in presentation and treatment response. For example, both men and women can show substantial variation in treatment response, with tailoring of treatment recommended (e.g. Swan et al., 2004).

Conclusions

To conclude, gender sensitive treatment for the growing number of women with alcohol and other drug problems is recommended, within the context of the application of evidence-based treatment strategies, allowing for individual differences in presentation and treatment response. While women have come a long way in drinking and smoking more like men, treatment services have by and large not yet met this challenge and may need significant resourcing to do so.

REFERENCES

Abel, E.L., & Sokol, R.J. (1991). A revised conservative estimate of the incidence of FAS and its economic impact. *Alcoholism: Clinical and Experimental Research*, 15, 512–524.

Andrews, G., Hall, W., Tesson, M., Henderson, S. (1999). *The mental health of Australians*. Mental Health Branch, Commonwealth Department of Health and Aged Care, Canberra.

Anthony, J.C., Warner, L.A., & Kessler, R.C. (1994). Comparative epidemiology of dependence on tobacco, alcohol, controlled substances and inhalants: Basic findings from the National Comorbidity Survey. *Experimental and Clinical Psychopharmacology, 2*, 244–268.

Bale, R.N., Van Stone, W.W., Kuldau, J.M., Engelsing, T.M.J., Elashoff, R.M., & Zarcone, V.P. (1980). Therapeutic communities vs. methadone maintenance. A prospective study of narcotic addiction treatment: Design and one year follow-up results. *Archives of General Psychiatry, 37*, 179–193.

Ballesteros, J., Gonazalez-Pinto, A., Querejeta, I., & Arino, J. (2003). Brief interventions for hazardous drinkers delivered in primary care are equally effective in men and women. *Addiction, 99*, 103–108.

Becker, J., & Duffy, C. (2002). *Women drug users and drugs service provision: Service-level responses to engagement and retention*. DPAS Paper 17. London: Home Office.

Bell, K., Cramer-Benjamin, D., & Anastas, J. (1997). Predicting length of stay of substance-using pregnant and postpartum women in day treatment. *Journal of Substance Abuse Treatment, 14*, 393–400.

Beyer, E., Cohanan, J.A. (2003). Females with dual diagnosis: Implications for specialized clinical approaches. In: O'Connell, & E Beyer (Eds.), *Managing the dually diagnosed patient: Current issues and clinical approaches* (pp. 99–151). 2nd edn.

Blume, S.B. (1992). Alcohol and other drug problems in women. In: J.H. Lowinson, P. Ruiz, R.B. Millman (Eds.), *Substance use, a comprehensive textbook* (pp. 794–807). 2nd Edn. Baltimore: Williams and Wilkins.

Blume, S.B. (1997). Women: clinical aspects. In: J.H. Lowinson, P. Ruiz, R.B. Millman, & J.G. Langrod (Eds.), *Substance abuse: A comprehensive textbook* (pp. 645–654). 3rd Edn. Baltimore: Williams & Wilkins.

Bureau of Justice. (1991). *National Update, 1986*. Washington, DC, Government Printing Office

Castle, D.J., & Solowij, N. (2004). Acute and subacute psychomimetic effects of cannabis. In: D.J. Castle, & Robin M Murray (Eds.), *Marijuana and madness* (pp. 41–53). Cambridge: Cambridge University Press.

Chander, G., & McCaul, M.E. (2003). Co-occurring psychiatric disorders in women with addictions. *Obstetric and Gynaecological Clinics of North America, 30*, 469–481.

Chang, G., Carroll, K.M., Behr, H.M., & Kosten, T.R. (1992). Improving treatment outcome in pregnant opiate-dependent women. *Journal of Substance Abuse Treatment, 9*, 327–330.

Cloninger, C.R., Bohman, M., & Sigvardsson, S. (1981). Cross-fostering analysis of adopted men. *Archives of General Psychiatry, 38*, 861–868.

Connors, G.J., Donovan, D.M., & DiClemente, C.C. (2001). *Substance abuse treatment and the stages of change: Selecting and planning interventions*. New York: Guilford Press.

Copeland, J., & Hall, W. (1992). A comparison of women seeking drug and alcohol treatment in a specialist women's and two traditional mixed-sex treatment services. *British Journal of Addiction, 87*, 1293–1302.

Cosden, M., & Cortez-Ison, E. (1999). Sexual abuse, parental bonding, social support, and program retention for women in substance abuse treatment. *Journal of Substance Abuse Treatment, 16*, 149–155.

Dahlgren, L., & Willander, A. (1989). Are special treatment facilities for female alcoholics needed? A controlled 2-year follow-up study from a specialized female unit (EWA) versus a mixed male/female treatment facility. *Alcoholism: Clinical and Experimental Research*, *13*, 499–504.

Davis, S. (1997). Comprehensive interventions for affecting the parenting effectiveness of chemically dependent women. *Journal of Obstetric, Gynaecologic and Neonatal Nursing*, *26*, 604–610.

DeLeon, G., & Schwartz, S. (1984). The therapeutic community: What are the retention rates? *American Journal of Drug and Alcohol Abuse*, *10*, 267–284.

Fillmore, K.M., Bacon, S.D., & Hyman, M. (1979). The 27-year longitudinal panel study of drinking by students in college. *Report to National Institute of Alcoholism and Alcohol Abuse*, Washington DC.

Finkelstein, N. (1994). Treatment issues for alcohol and drug-dependent pregnant and parenting women. *Health and Social Work*, *19*, 7–14.

Frezza, M., DiPadova, C., Pozzato, G., Terpin, M., Baroona, E., & Lieber, C.S. (1990). High blood alcohol levels in women: The role of decreased gastric alcohol dehydrogenase activity and first-pass metabolism. *New England Journal of Medicine*, *322*, 95–99.

Grant, B. (1997). Prevalence and correlates of alcohol use and DSM-IV alcohol dependence in the United States: Results from the National Longitudinal Alcohol Epidemiologic Survey. *Journal of Studies of Alcohol*, *58*, 464–473.

Grant, B., Harford, T., Dawson, D., et al. (1994). Prevalence of DSM-IV alcohol abuse and dependence. *Alcohol Health and Research World*, *18*, 243–348.

Greenfield, S.F., O'Leary, G. (2002). Sex differences in substance use disorders. In: F. Lewis-Hall, T.S. Williams, J.A. Panetta, and J.M. Herrera, (Eds.) *Psychiatric Illness in Women: Emerging Treatments and Research*. American Psychiatric Publishing: London, England, 467–533.

Goldstein, P., Bellucci, P., Spunt, B., & Miller, T. (1991). Volume of cocaine use and violence: A comparison between men and women. *Journal of Drug Issues*, *21*, 345–367.

Gossop, M., Powis, B., Griffiths, P., & Strang, J. (1994). Sexual behaviour and its relationship to drug taking amongst prostitutes in south London. *Addiction*, *89*, 961–970.

Harm, N.J., Thompson, P.J., & Chambers, H. (1998). The effectiveness of parent education for substance abusing women offenders. *Alcoholism Treatment Quarterly*, *16*, 63–77.

Helzer, J.E., Burnam, A., & McEvoy, L. (1991). Alcohol abuse and dependence. In: L.N. Robins & D.A. Regier (Eds.), *Psychiatric disorders in America: The epidemiological catchment area study* (pp. 81–115). New York: Free Press.

Helzer, J.E., Canino, G.J., Yeh, E.K., et al. (1990). Alcoholism – North America and Asia. A comparison of population surveys with the diagnostic interview schedule. *Archives of General Psychiatry*, *47*, 313–319.

Hill, S.Y. (2000). Alcohol and substance abuse in women. In: M. Steiner, K.A. Yonkers, & E. Eriksson. (Eds.), *Mood disorders in women* (pp. 449–468). London: Martin Dunitz.

Hodgson, R. & John, B. (2004). Gender, gender role and brief alcohol interventions. *Addiction*, *99*, 3–4.

Hubbard, R.L., Craddock, S., Flynn, P.M., Anderson, J., & Etheridge, R. (1997). Overview of 1-year follow-up outcomes in the Drug Abuse Treatment Outcome Study (DATOS). *Psychology of Addictive Behaviors*, *11*, 261–278.

Hunter, G., & Powis, B. (1995–1996). *Women drug users: Barriers to service use, and service needs.* The Centre for Research on Drugs and Health Behaviour: Executive Summary, 47.

Jenkins, R., Bebbington, P., Brugha, T.S., Farrell, M., Lewis, G., & Meltzer, H. (1998). British psychiatric morbidity survey. *British Journal of Psychiatry, 173*, 4–7.

Jones, M.C. (1971). Personality antecedents and correlates of drinking patterns in women. *Journal of Consulting and Clinical Psychology, 36*, 61–69.

Jones, B.M., & Jones, M.K. (1976). Women and alcohol. In: M. Greenblatt, & M.A. Schukit (Eds.), *Alcohol problems in women and children* (pp. 103–136). New York: Grune & Statton.

Jones, K., Smith, D., Ulleland, C., et al. (1973). Patterns of malformations of offspring of chronic alcoholic mothers. *Lancet, 1*, 1267–1271.

Kandel, D.B. (1984). Marijuana users in young adulthood. *Archives of General Psychiatry, 41*, 200–209.

Kandel, D.B., Davies, M., Karus, D., et al. (1986). The consequences in young adulthood of adolescent drug involvement. *Archives of General Psychiatry, 43*, 746–754.

Kandel, D.B., Simcha-Fagan, O., & Davies, M. (1986). Risk factors for delinquency and illicit drug use from adolescence to young adulthood. *Journal of Drug Issues, 16*, 67–90.

Kandel, D., Warner, L., Kessler, R. The epidemiology of substance use and dependence among women In: C.L. Wetherington, A.B. Roman (eds.), *Drug Addiction Research and the National Institute on Drug Abuse* (pp. 105–129).

Kantor, G.K., & Strauss, M.A. (1989). Substance abuse as a precipitant of wife abuse victimizations. *American Journal of Drug and Alcohol Abuse, 15*, 173–189.

Kavanagh, D.J., Mueser, K.T., & Baker, A. (2003). Management of comorbidity. In: M. Teesson, & H. Proudfoot (Eds.), *Comorbid mental disorders and substance use disorders: Epidemiology, prevention and treatment* (pp. 78–120). Canberra: Commonwealth of Australia.

Knight, D.K., Hood, P.E., Logan, S.M., & Chatham, L.R. (1999). Residential treatment for women with dependent children: One agency's approach. *Journal of Psychoactive Drugs, 31*, 339–351.

Knight, D.K., Logan, S.M., & Simpson, D.D. (2001). Predictors of program completion for women in residential substance abuse treatment. *American Journal of Drug and Alcohol Abuse, 27*, 1–18.

Lex, B.W. (1995). Alcohol and other psychoactive substance dependence in women and men. In: M.V. Seeman (Ed.), *Gender and psychopathology* (pp. 311–358). Washington, DC: American Psychiatric Association Press.

Lex, B.W., Goldberg, M.E., Mendelson, J.H., et al. (1994). Components of antisocial personality disorder amongst women convicted for drunk driving. *Annals of the New York Academy of Sciences, 708*, 49–58.

Lindberg, S., & Agren, G. (1988). Mortality among male and females hospitalised alcoholics in Stockholm 1962–1983. *British Journal of Addiction, 83*, 193–200.

Luthar, S.S., & Walsh, K.G. (1995). Treatment needs of drug addicted mothers: Integrated parenting psychotherapy interventions. *Journal of Substance Abuse Treatment, 12*, 341–348.

Mackie-Ramos, R., & Rice, J. (1988). Group psychotherapy with methadone maintained pregnant women. *Journal of Substance Abuse Treatment, 5*, 151–161.

Maden, A., Swinton, M., & Gunn, J. (1990). Women in prison and use of illicit drugs before arrest. *British Medical Journal, 301*, 1133.

Marsh, J.C., D'Aunno, T.A., & Smith, B.D. (2000). Increasing access and providing social services to improve drug abuse treatment for women with children. *Addiction, 95*, 1237–1247.

Marshall, J. (2000). Alcohol and drug misuse in women. In: D. Kohen (Ed.), *Women and mental health.* (pp. 189–217). London: Routledge.

McPherson, M., Casswell, S., & Pledger, M. (2004). Gender convergence in alcohol consumption and related problems: Issues and outcomes from comparisons of New Zealand survey data. *Addiction, 99*, 738–748.

Mejta, C.L., & Lavin, R. (1996). Facilitating healthy parenting among mothers with substance abuse or dependence problems: Some considerations. *Alcoholism Treatment Quarterly, 14*, 33–46.

Meltzer, H., Gill, B., Petticrew, M., & Hinds, K. (1995). OPCS surveys of psychiatric morbidity among adults living in private households. London: HMSO.

Metsch, L.R., Rivers, J.E., Miller, M., Bohs, R., McCoy, C.B., Morrow, C.J., Bandstra, E.S., Jackson, V., & Glissen, M. (1995). Implementation of a family-centered treatment program for substance-abusing women and their children: Barriers and resolutions. *Journal of Psychoactive Drugs, 27*, 73–83.

Miller, W.R., & Rollnick, S. (Eds.) (2002). *Motivational interviewing: Preparing people for change* (2nd edn). New York: Guilford.

Nelson-Zlupko, L., Dore, M.M., Kauffman, E., & Kaltenbach, K. (1996). Women in recovery: Their perceptions of treatment effectiveness. *Journal of Substance Abuse Treatment, 13*, 51–59.

Nunes-Dines, M. (1993). Drug and alcohol misuse: Treatment outcomes and services for women. In: R.P. Barth, J. Pietrzak, & M. Ramler (Eds.), *Families living with drugs and HIV: Intervention and treatment strategies* (pp. 144–176). New York: Guilford Press.

Pope, H.G., Jacobs, A., Mialet, J.-P., et al. (1997). Evidence for a sex-specific residual effect of cannabis on visuospatial memory. *Psychther Psychosom, 66*, 179–184.

Prochaska, J.O., & DiClemente, C.C. (1986). Toward a comprehensive model of change. In: W.R. Miller & N. Heather (Eds.), *Treating addictive behaviours: Processes of change.* (pp. 3–27). New York: Plenum Press.

Schmidt, L., & Weisner, C. (1995). The emergence of problem-drinking women as a special population in need of treatment. In: M. Galanter (Ed.), *Recent developments in alcoholis*m. Vol. 12: Women and alcoholism (pp. 309–334). New York: Plentum Press.

Schutte, K.K., Hearst, J., & Moos, R.H. (1997). Gender differences in the relations between depressive symptoms and drinking behavior among problem drinkers: A three-wave study. *Journal of Consulting and Clinical Psychology, 65*, 392–404.

Shand, F., Gates, J., Fawcett, J., & Mattick, R. (2003a). *The treatment of alcohol problem*s: *A review of the evidence.* Canberra: Commonwealth of Australia.

Shand, F., Gates, J., Fawcett, J., & Mattick, R. (2003b). *Guidelines for the treatment of alcohol problems.* Canberra: Commonwealth of Australia.

Simpson, D.D. (1979). The relation of time spent in drug abuse treatment to posttreatment outcome. *American Journal of Psychiatry, 136*, 1449–1453.

Simpson, D.D., Joe, G., & Brown, B. (1997). Treatment retention and follow-up outcomes in the Drug Abuse Treatment Outcome Study (DATOS). *Psychology of Addictive Behaviors, 11*, 294–307.

Smith, E.M., & Cloninger, C.R. (1981). Alcoholic females: Mortality at twelve-year follow-up. *Focus on Women*, *2*, 1–13.

Stark, M.J. (1992). Dropping out of substance abuse treatment: A clinically oriented review. *Clinical Psychology Review*, *12*, 93–116.

Stevens, S.J., & Arbiter, N. (1995). A therapeutic community for substance-abusing pregnant women and women with children: Process and outcome. *Journal of Psychoactive Drugs*, *27*, 49–56.

Swan, G.E., Javitz, H.S., Jack, L.M., Curry, S.J., & McAfee, T. (2004). Heterogeneity in 12-month outcome among female and male smokers. *Addiction*, *99*, 237–250.

Swift, W., Copeland, J., & Hall, W. (1996). Characteristics of women with alcohol and other drug problems: Findings of an Australian national survey. *Addiction*, *91*, 1141–1150.

Substance Abuse and Mental Health Services Administration. (1994). *National household survey on drug abuse: Population estimates 1993*. Rockville, MD: Office of Applied Studies.

Szuster, R.R., Rich, L.L., Chung, A., & Bisconer, S.W. (1996). Treatment retention in women's residential chemical dependency treatment: The effect of admission with children. *Substance Use and Misuse*, *31*, 1001–1013.

Thomas, H. (1996). A community survey of adverse effects of cannabis use. *Drug and Alcohol Dependence*, *42*, 201–207.

Tobin, M.B., Schmidt, M.D., & Rubinow, D.R. (1994). Reported alcohol use in women with premenstrual syndrome. *American Journal of Psychiatry*, *151*, 1503–1504.

Weismann, M., Warner, V., Wickramaratne, P., & Kandel, D. (1999). Maternal smoking during pregnancy and psychopathology in offspring followed to adulthood. *Journal of the American Academy of Child and Adolescent Psychiatry*, *38*, 892–899.

Wilsnack, S.C., & Wilsnack, R.W. (1995). Drinking and problem drinking in US women. In: M.Galanter (Ed.), *Recent developments in alcoholism*, Vol. 12. New York: Plenum Press.

Wilsnack, S.C., Wilsnack, R.W., & Klassen, A.D. (1986). Epidemiological research on women's drinking, 1978–1984. *Women and alcohol: Health-related issues. National Institute on Alcohol Abuse and Alcoholism. Research monograph no. 16*. Washington, DC: Department of Health and Human Services, pp. 1–68.

Wilsnack, S.C., Wilsnack, R.W., & Hiller-Sturmhofel, S. (1994). How women drink: Epidemiology of women's problem drinking. *Alcohol Health and Research World*, *18*, 173–184.

Winfield, I., George, L.K., Swartz, M., & Blazer, D.G. (1990). Sexual assault and psychiatric disorders among a community sample of women. *American Journal of Psychology*, *147*, 335–341.

Wobie, K., Eyler, F.D., Conlon, M., Clarke, L., & Behnke, M. (1997). Women and children in residential treatment: Outcomes for mothers and their infants. *Journal of Drug Issues*, *27*, 585–606.

Zilberman, M., Taveres, H., & el-Guebaly, N. (2003). Gender similarities and differences: The prevalence and course alcohol-and other substance-related disorders. *Journal of Addictive Disorders*, *22*, 61–74.

4

Anxiety disorders in women

Heather B. Howell[1], David Castle[2] and Kimberly A. Yonkers[3]

[1]Department of Psychiatry, Yale University School of Medicine, New Haven, CT, USA
[2]Mental Health Research Institute and University of Melbourne, Parkville, Victoria, Australia
[3]Department of Psychiatry, Yale University School of Medicine, New Haven, CT, USA

Anxiety is a common human experience, and ranges in depth and intensity. The experience is most typically in response to life stressors, and may be temporary. However, many people experience anxiety symptoms in association with a diagnosable mental illness. Individuals with an anxiety disorder are functionally impaired by the condition that is beyond a reasonable temporary response to trauma, stress or danger.

Anxiety disorders are common in that 19% of men and 31% of women will develop some type of anxiety disorder during their lifetime (Kessler et al., 1994a). The US National Comorbidity Survey (NCS), a community prevalence study, found the following risk factors to be associated with a lifetime anxiety disorder: lower income, less education, living in the northeast and female sex. The likelihood of developing an anxiety disorder was 85% higher in women than men. Although there are many characteristics that differ among the anxiety disorders, the greater risk associated with being female is consistent across the various types of pathological anxiety. In this chapter, we review sex differences in the epidemiology, clinical characteristics and illness course for the anxiety disorders. Additionally, we discuss the influence of the premenstruum as well as gestation and delivery on the expression of anxiety disorders. We do not specifically address treatment issues; the reader is referred to Chapters 5, 8 and 9 for consideration of treatment issues pertinent to women.

Panic disorder

Panic disorder is a pattern of brief but intense recurrent episodes of fear or discomfort that occur without a notable precipitant. Diagnostic criteria require at least four panic attacks in a month, or at least one panic with continuous fear of other attacks. Possible symptoms associated with panic attacks include palpitations, sweating, feeling short of breath or a choking sensation, nausea or abdominal discomfort, feeling dizzy, having a sense of unreality, numbness or tingling, chills or hot flushes, and a fear of dying or losing control (APA, 1994).

The NCS found panic attacks to have a 1-month prevalence of 3.2% (SE = 0.3) in women and 1.1% (SE = 0.2) in men. The 1-month prevalence for the full syndrome of panic disorder in women was 2% (SE = 0.3), while 0.8% (SE = 0.2) of men met full diagnostic criteria (Eaton et al., 1994). The corresponding lifetime rates for panic disorder in women and men were 5% (SE = 1.4) and 2% (SE = 0.3), respectively (Kessler et al., 1994a).

These statistics show that there are differences in the prevalence rates of panic attacks and panic disorder according to patient sex. There may also be differences in the symptoms experienced by men and women with the disorder. Data from the NCS show that, compared to men, women are more likely to endorse shortness of breath, nausea and a perception of being smothered; on the other hand, men are more likely than women to identify difficulties with sweating and stomach pain (Sheikh et al., 2002). The greater proclivity for women to develop respiratory symptoms is interesting in light of results from provocation studies. Women with panic may have greater sensitivity to panic-inducing respiratory challenge than their male counterparts (Papp & Gorman, 1988; Papp et al., 1997; Sheikh et al., 2002). Work by one group found that women have a higher resting breathing rate and lower end-tidal CO_2 that may increase anxiety sensitivity (Papp & Gorman, 1988; Papp et al., 1997).

The possibility that women may have higher anxiety sensitivity, and that this in turn enhances their risk of panic disorder, is supported by data on the clinical course of illness. The onset of pathological anxiety in both males and females is early, occurring in childhood for many individuals (Lewinsohn et al., 1998). Interestingly, the sex difference in illness risk also has an early onset and is apparent by age six (Lewinsohn et al., 1998). After this young age, the difference between males and females continues to separate further. These observations suggest some early biological differences in risk for anxiety.

Clinical course

Prospective, longitudinal data from adults also support differential anxiety sensitivity in females compared to males. In a study evaluating the course of panic disorder, men and women with uncomplicated panic were equally likely to experience improvement in their illness, but the relapse rate over 8 years of follow up was threefold higher in women compared to men (Yonkers et al., 2003). This relapsing course of illness in women may be caused by higher anxiety sensitivity, even after treatment is instituted and remission is attained. In some instances, this vulnerability may be mediated by intercurrent illness, such as depression (Hayward et al., 2000), but also by biological differences in respiratory mechanics (Sheikh et al., 2002).

Agoraphobia

Agoraphobia is the fear of being in a closed space or an area from which escape may be difficult. This typically leads to a modification of behaviour in an attempt to avoid panic attacks or the overwhelming fear. It is common for agoraphobic individuals to limit outside activities unless accompanied by a safe companion (APA, 1994). Agoraphobia can be experienced with or without panic disorder. Bekker (1996) offers a thorough review of gender and agoraphobia, finding the illness more prevalent in women than in men, across both clinical and community sample. Specifically, data from the NCS find that when panic disorder is accompanied by agoraphobia, the 1-month prevalence rate for men is 0.4% (SE = 0.2) while 1.0% (SE = 0.3) of women meet criteria (Eaton et al., 1994). Agoraphobia without panic is somewhat more common and the lifetime prevalence rate in men is 3.5% (SE = 0.4) and in women is 7% (SE = 0.6).

Women tend to adapt to their agoraphobia by limiting excursions outside of the home, especially without a companion, significantly more than men (Bourdon et al., 1988; Starcevic et al., 1998). It is notable that this is often more culturally acceptable, in that women can work inside the home while men tend to work outside the home and thus are less likely to function adequately if they are homebound. Despite this, some investigators find that women report significantly more decreased quality of life as a result of their agoraphobia than do men (Starcevic et al., 1998). This is consistent with other data showing that panic disorder with agoraphobia is a more severe condition in women than in men (Turgeon et al., 1998). Women expressed greater avoidance severity, more catastrophic fears, and more frequent comorbidity of another anxiety disorder, most notably social phobia or post-traumatic stress disorder (PTSD).

Males with agoraphobia from clinical populations are more likely than their female counterparts to suffer from alcoholism (Bibb & Chambless, 1986; Starcevic et al., 1998; Yonkers et al., 1998). Although this may reflect the overall higher rate of hazardous alcohol use in men compared to women (Kessler et al., 1994a; and see Chapter 3), some work finds a higher rate of alcohol abuse in male agoraphobics compared to male non-agoraphobics (Bibb & Chambless, 1986). In evaluating these sex differences, it is also important to consider the gender-specific social implications of agoraphobic self-disclosure. Men may be less inclined to acknowledge agoraphobic tendencies than women because it discredits male strength and bravery (Barlow, 1988). This is believed by some to contribute to the disparate rates of agoraphobia diagnoses in men and women, and it is presumed that there is a group of "hidden male agoraphobics" who tend to present with alcoholism. There is some empirical support for this. In a study of gender-specific alcohol use in agoraphobic individuals, there were significant sex differences in the ways in which each gender described the experience of the anxiety disorder (Cox et al., 1993): males consumed significantly more alcohol than females and they described their drinking as a specific coping strategy for the anxiety. Turgeon et al. (1998) did not confirm this quantitative difference and found comparable alcohol consumption in male and female samples. However, in both studies, males and not females directly reported drinking as a way to decrease agoraphobic inhibition (Cox et al., 1993; Turgeon et al., 1998).

Comorbidity

Among a group of anxiety-disordered individuals presenting in a clinical setting, 72% of whom were female, there were no significant sex differences in psychiatric comorbidity (Apfeldorf et al., 2000). Other work has found that women are more likely than males to have a co-occurring anxiety disorder, namely social phobia or PTSD (Turgeon et al., 1998). PTSD comorbidity did not predict higher agoraphobic avoidance.

Childhood/adolescence

As noted above, the gender difference in the prevalence of anxiety symptoms is evident even during childhood (Hayward et al., 2000; Lewinsohn et al., 1998; Wittchen et al., 1998). Boys and girls begin to experience the onset of pathological anxiety at about the same age (Lewinsohn et al., 1998; Wittchen et al., 1998) although phobias tend to have an earlier age of onset than does panic (Wittchen et al., 1998).

PTSD

PTSD occurs after an individual is exposed to "an extreme traumatic stressor" (APA, 1994). The individual reacts with fear, helplessness or horror in response to the event and re-experiences the event along with persistent arousal symptoms. Symptoms must be present for 1 month and must be associated with some impairment in functioning. PTSD is far more common than originally thought, with about 8% of the population afflicted (Kessler et al., 1995). According to the NCS, 5% (SE = 0.6) of men and 10.4% (SE = 0.8) of women will develop PTSD at some point in their lives. For a full discussion of PTSD in women, see Chapter 5; what follows is a brief overview of selected issues.

The NCS, like other studies, found that women are twice as likely to develop PTSD as are men. Marital status conferred different risks in that women who were previously married were at higher risk than never or currently married women, while either currently married or previously married men were at higher risk than never married men (Kessler et al., 1995). In an analysis of gender and PTSD risk, Breslau et al. (1997) used a large health maintenance organization (HMO) cohort and found that pre-existing mood or anxiety disorders modestly increased the risk of PTSD in women, but not men; further, trauma early in life showed greater gender disparity in risk than did trauma after age 15. The role of pre-existing mood disorders in enhancing risk for PTSD in women has also been noted in several other studies (Kessler et al., 1995; North et al., 1997). In the NCS database, only pre-existing anxiety disorders increased risk in men and only when the type of trauma was controlled (Bromet et al., 1998).

The types of trauma experienced by men and women in the NCS differ somewhat and may contribute to the sex differences in the prevalence of PTSD. While the overall rate of trauma exposure is higher in males than females, "high impact" traumas, that is those more likely to lead to PTSD (including sexual and physical assault) are more common in women (Kessler et al., 1995). This has been suggested as an explanation for the gender difference in risk of PTSD, but there is only partial support for this hypothesis. In the NCS, controlling for type of trauma did not entirely explain women's higher risks for PTSD since statistically controlling for the type of trauma did not diminish women's higher risk for PTSD. Some prospective follow-up studies of motor vehicle accident survivors have found sex differences in the onset of PTSD (Fullerton et al., 2001) while others have not (Freedman et al., 2002). On the other hand, a prospective follow up of survivors of a mass shooting found a higher risk of PTSD in women (North et al., 1997), and amongst emergency room trauma patients, women have higher rates of PTSD regardless of event-related factors (Holbrook et al., 2002).

Concomitants of the traumatic event may also be important in mediating the sex difference. For example, mood disorders and other anxiety disorders have been posited as possible risk factors (see above); both conditions are more common in women. Peritraumatic dissociation may also promote the development of the disorder (Fullerton et al., 2001). Similarly, women may experience negative responses to the trauma, especially if they are sexually based (Andrews et al., 2003). On the other hand, comorbid alcoholism is more common in men exposed to trauma and those with PTSD (Green, 2003; Sonne et al., 2003; Zlotnick et al., 2001). The amnestic effects of alcohol may protect against development of PTSD or decrease the severity of illness if it occurs.

Symptoms

Some work has found differences in the symptoms of PTSD expressed by men and women. One prospective study of motor vehicle accident victims found that women were more likely to experience avoidance and numbing symptoms that are part of criterion C, and the arousal symptoms that constitute criterion D (Fullerton et al., 2001). However, another study found that re-experiencing the trauma was more common in women than men (Zlotnick et al., 2001), a finding not shared by workers in the previously quoted study (Fullerton et al., 2001).

Clinical course

A number of researchers have reported that women are more likely to have a chronic course after first manifesting PTSD (Andrews et al., 2003; Breslau & Davis, 1992). Women also appear to have more impairment after developing the illness, even if the disorder itself improves (Holbrook et al., 2002). For further details, see Chapter 5.

Generalized anxiety disorder

Generalized anxiety disorder (GAD) is defined as excessive worry about a number of events or issues that is difficult to control. Worry is experienced for at least 6 months and may be accompanied by restlessness, fatigue, difficulty concentrating, irritability, muscle tension and sleep disturbance. The worry cannot be limited to a core feature of another syndrome, for example worry about having a panic attack or gaining weight because in that case, it would be supportive of the other condition and not GAD.

GAD is more common in women. In the Epidemiological Catchment Area Study (ECA), the prevalence of GAD was determined using Diagnostic and Statistical Manual of Mental Disorders (DSM-III) criteria, which stipulates only one, rather than 6 months of illness (DSM-III-R and DSM-IV) (Blazer et al., 1991). The 12-month prevalence rate in women was about twice as high as it was for men (2.4% in men and 5.0% in women). Those at greatest risk were African-American women under 30 and Hispanic women aged 45–64; the rates in both of these groups was greater than the rate in Caucasian women (Blazer et al., 1991).

According to the NCS, 3.6% (SE = 0.5) of men and 6.6% (SE = 0.5) of women will meet criteria for DSM-III-R GAD at some point in their lives (Wittchen et al., 1994). In that dataset, women were 63% more likely to develop GAD than were men (Wittchen et al., 1994).

Social stressors may have a divergent impact on the risk of depression and anxiety in men and women (Cameron & Hill, 1989). In a 3-year longitudinal study of English women, danger predicted later anxiety, while loss predicted depression (Brown et al., 1996); a combination of loss and danger led to comorbid anxiety and depression. External support did not modify the effect of these events.

Clinical course

While there is little information about the longitudinal trajectory of illness for GAD, the course appears to be similar for men and women, with a generally chronic outcome (Pigott, 1999). In a longitudinal study of anxiety disorders, women and men were roughly equally likely to experience remission (probability 0.46 in women and 0.56 in men; Log rank $\chi^2 = 1.39$ (DF $= 1$); $p = 0.24$) (Yonkers et al., 2003). Comorbidity decreased the rates of recovery, especially when the concurrent conditions were Cluster A and C personality disorders (Yonkers et al., 2000). Findings from this clinical cohort are consistent with results from the ECA study, which indicated that the majority of adult subjects with GAD are ill for more than 5 years (Blazer et al., 1991).

Comorbidity

GAD is commonly comorbid with other conditions. In their longitudinal study on the course of GAD, Yonkers et al. (1996) found that 23% of GAD subjects had two, and 16% had three or more other anxiety disorders active at initial assessment. Lifetime comorbidity of GAD with another anxiety disorder (in particular, a history of panic disorder with agoraphobia) was more likely to occur in women than men (56% versus 28%, respectively; $\chi^2 = 10.46$, $p = 0.0001$).

Cormorbidity of depression and GAD is particularly common (Angst & Vollrath, 1991). Some research suggests shared inheritance of these disorders (Kendler et al., 1992). Both men and women who have anxiety coupled with depression have a poorer outcome (Angst & Vollrath, 1991; Durham et al., 1997).

Some authors propose that the expression of anxiety in depressed women may differ from anxiety in depressed men (Katz et al., 1993; Parker et al., 1997). For example, highly anxious depressed women may express their anxious–depressive symptoms through motor retardation and vagueness, with less evident body movement, while men may show hostility and increased visible body agitation (Katz et al., 1993).

There is also some evidence that a history of GAD may predispose individuals to develop major depression (Parker et al., 1997) although this effect may not be limited to GAD amongst the anxiety disorders (Breslau et al., 1995). Another possibility is that an anxiety disorder increases the risk for a mood disorder and vice-versa (Hayward et al., 2000; Kessler et al., 2003).

Comorbidity between anxiety disorders and alcohol abuse and dependence disorders is also very common (Massion et al., 1993; Yonkers et al., 1996; and see Chapter 3). As noted above, anxious symptoms may increase the susceptibility to alcohol consumption (Fischer & Goethe, 1998). Men are overall more likely to abuse drugs and alcohol, but moderate anxiety in depressed women seems to increase their risk for alcohol abuse (Fischer & Goethe, 1998). Other work has found an association between alcoholism and anxiety disorders that is greater for phobias than for panic or generalized anxiety (Merikangas et al., 1998).

Social phobia

Social phobia (also known as social anxiety disorder) is characterized by fear of social and/or performance situations. When an individual has a fear of most social situations, he or she is given a diagnosis of generalized type of social phobia. The clinical criteria stipulate that the person has anxiety whenever exposed to the feared social situation and that they recognize the fear as excessive or unreasonable. The feared situation is either endured with difficulty or avoided altogether, and the fear and avoidance behaviours lead to disability in functioning.

In the NCS, the 1-year prevalence of social phobia was 6.6% (SE = 0.4) in men and 9.1% (SE = 0.7) in women (Kessler et al., 1994b). The lifetime risk for males was 11.1% (SE = 0.8) while for females it was 15.5% (SE = 1.0). Slightly lower lifetime rates (13.7%) were found in an epidemiological study from Ontario, Canada but a 2:1 ratio for females compared to males was noted (DeWit, 1999). A community study in Australia found that women were only slightly more likely than men to develop the illness (Lampe et al., 2003).

Possible sex differences in the expression of social phobia have been investigated in clinical cohorts. Male ($n = 108$) and female ($n = 104$) subjects with social phobia differed somewhat in the fearful situations they endorsed (Turk et al., 1998). Severity was significantly greater for women compared to men for the following tasks: talking to an authority, acting or speaking in front of an audience, being observed at work, entering into a room while others were seated, being the centre of attention, expressing disagreement, and giving a party (Turk et al., 1998). Alternatively, men had significantly more difficulty with urinating in public and returning goods to a store. An independent study also found that socially phobic women had more difficulty than men with speaking in public (Pollard & Henderson, 1988).

One small study suggests sex differences in the psychophysiological response to stress among people with social phobia (Grossman et al., 2001). Women with social phobia were more likely than men with the disorder to show an increase in heart rate and both diastolic and systolic blood pressure in response to speech stress.

Clinical course

Social phobia typically begins during adolescence (~age 16 years) with a predominance of girls over boys (Compton et al., 2000). Several studies document the chronicity associated with the condition (DeWit et al., 1999; Yonkers et al., 2001). The clinical course appears to be similar in men and women (Yonkers et al., 2001); however, those individuals with an early age of onset are less likely to recover than those with a later onset.

Comorbidity

Social phobia is commonly comorbid with other conditions, particularly panic disorder, GAD, major depressive disorder, obsessive-compulsive disorder and agoraphobia (Faravelli, 2000; Yonkers et al., 2001). In most instances, social phobia is temporally primary (Yonkers et al., 2001).

Obsessive–compulsive disorder

Obsessive–compulsive disorder (OCD) is characterized by intrusive thoughts (obsessions) and compulsive activities that attenuate (at least in the short term) the level of anxiety associated with the obsession. The condition is associated with considerable distress and impairment of daily activities, with (by definition) at least 1 h/day being expended on rituals (APA, 1994).

Increasingly, OCD is recognized as a fairly common and disabling condition, estimated to have been the 5th leading cause of disability for women aged 15–44 years, in developed countries, in 1990 (Murray & Lopez, 1996). Most epidemiological surveys suggest that the condition afflicts women at a somewhat higher rate than men. Bebbington (1990) reviewed population-based studies of OCD, and found a female:male ratio varying from 0.9:1 (Puerto-Rico) to 3.4:1 (Christchurch, New Zealand). He concluded that overall females appear somewhat more prone to the condition, with an overall relative risk of 1.5, compared to men. Clinical samples tend to show a somewhat less marked female excess, perhaps a reflection of the rather more severe illness course in men (see below) or differences in help-seeking behaviour (Castle et al., 1995; Lensi et al., 1996; Noshirvani et al., 1991).

What certainly seems consistent in the literature is that males tend to have an earlier onset of OCD than their female counterparts. For example, in a clinical series of 307 OCD patients (55% female), onset of illness for males was 21 while it was 24 years for females ($p < 0.01$)(Noshirvani et al., 1991). Similar discrepancies in onset have been reported by other researchers (Castle et al., 1995; Lensi et al., 1996; Lochner et al., 2004). What is also consistent is that early-onset samples of OCD show a preponderance of males. In a review of eight studies of child- and adolescent-onset OCD, there was a total of 174 boys and 70 girls, yielding a gender ratio of 5:2 (Noshirvani et al., 1991).

This is also reflected in case series across all ages of onset; for example, Castle et al. (1995) found males were over-represented amongst patients with an onset of illness before 16 years (26% versus 12% of females; $p = 0.01$).

In terms of symptom profile, women with OCD are generally more likely that men to manifest contamination fears and cleaning rituals, while males are more prone to aggressive and sexual obsessions, and symmetry concerns (Bogetto et al., 1999; Lensi et al., 1996).

Comorbidity

Females with OCD are more likely than their male counterparts to suffer from depression or eating disorders, but males appear more vulnerable to later hypomania (Bogetto et al., 1999; Lensi et al., 1996). Furthermore, males with OCD, and particularly those with an early-onset illness, are more likely to exhibit motor tics and neurological "soft signs" (see Blanes & McGuire, 1997).

Clinical course

Most (though not all (Lensi et al., 1996)) case series suggest a more benign longitudinal course for OCD amongst women, with a more abrupt onset and more episodic course (Bogetto et al., 1999). Women with OCD are also more likely to be married and to have less impairment of psychosocial functioning.

Whether the relatively more benign course of illness in women is due to the late mean age at onset, or is a reflection of a male vulnerability to a particularly pernicious subtype of the illness, is not clear. One hypothesis is that there is a male-predominant "neurodevelopmental" subtype of OCD, characterized by an early onset of illness, neurological soft signs, motor tics, and a poor treatment response to serotonergic antidepressants (see Blanes & McGuire, 1997).

Another interesting line of enquiry has been into the possibility that genetic factors might play a differential role between the sexes, in terms of OCD. For example, Enoch et al. (2001) reported the frequency of 5-HT2A promoter polymorphism 1438G > A to be higher in OCD women but not men, compared to controls. Of interest is that this polymorphism had been found previously to be associated with anorexia nervosa, believed by some researchers to be part of an OCD spectrum of disorders. More recently, Lochner et al. (2004) found that Caucasian females (but not males) with OCD were more likely than controls to have the high activity T allele of the EcoRV variant of the monoamine oxidase A gene. These lines of genetic enquiry need to be pursued further and to be integrated into broader explanatory models of gender differences in OCD.

Influences of the menstrual cycle on anxiety symptoms

Several researchers note high rates of anxiety disorders in their patients with Premenstrual Dysphoric Disorder (PMDD) (Facchinetti et al., 1992; Fava et al., 1992) with the most common diagnosis being panic disorder. Sexual trauma history seems prevalent in PMDD patients. In one study of 42 women (Golding et al., 2000), 95% had experienced sexual trauma at least once; upon further assessment, 65% were diagnosed with PTSD.

Worsening of panic during the premenstrual week is endorsed by many women with panic disorder. However, workers have failed to confirm worsening panic when daily calendars are used to evaluate menstrual cycle symptoms prospectively (Cameron et al., 1988; Cook et al., 1990; Stein et al., 1989). Despite this, some studies have identified anxiety as a key problematic symptom prior to the onset of menses (Stein et al., 1989). PMDD is clinically categorized as a depressive mood disorder, but further evaluation is required to understand the anxious quality of the disorder better (see also Chapter 8).

There is additional information suggesting a link between premenstrual conditions and anxiety disorders. In a study of women seeking treatment for premenstrual dysphoria ($n = 206$), women prospectively rated their daily symptoms to confirm a diagnosis of PMDD (Bailey & Cohen, 1999). According to the Structured Clinical Interview for DSM (SCID), 7.3% ($n = 15$) were diagnosed with solely an anxiety disorder. A further 8.2% ($n = 17$) had both an anxiety and a mood disorder; by far the most common diagnosis was panic disorder ($n = 18$). Furthermore, 20 undiagnosed women were already receiving treatment for a mood or anxiety disorder, possibly minimizing identification of current illness. In our own clinical sample of female patients presenting for treatment for PMDD, approximately 20% had a co-occurring Axis I anxiety disorder (Yonkers, unpublished data, 2004).

Perinatal anxiety disorders

Early studies of pregnant patients with a history of panic disorder observed an overall improvement in the illness during pregnancy (Levine et al., 2003). However, subsequent studies did not support that observation, and in fact found that the course of illness had an equal likelihood of improving, worsening or remaining unchanged during the course of pregnancy (Cohen et al., 1994, 1996; and see Chapter 8). The postpartum period offers no greater certainty of symptom abatement, and in fact is a time when some women experience the first manifestation of panic disorder. Indeed, new onset of postpartum panic disorder seems to afflict between 11 and 33% of pregnant women (Levine et al., 2003). Again, a recent review found that postpartum improvement in panic episodes was most notably due to medication treatment (Levine et al., 2003).In one cohort of patients with panic disorder, 90% were symptomatic in the immediate postpartum period (Cohen et al., 1996); the asymptomatic 10% of patients were all taking medication to treat their panic disorder.

New research has assessed rates of panic disorder and PTSD in a prenatal sample ($n = 387$) in primary care (Smith et al., 2004). The rate of panic disorder during pregnancy was 2%, and the rate of PTSD, 3%. Rates of detection by these women's obstetricians were low, although rates of treatment were high, such that at the time of the study's contact with the anxious patients, all of the women with panic disorder ($n = 9$) were currently or had previously been engaged in treatment, while 50% of the women with PTSD ($n = 5$) were currently or had previously been treated. While these sample sizes are small, the rates of participation in treatment are encouraging.

Pregnancy and the postpartum period can be times of worsening or onset of OCD (Brandes et al., 2004; Levine et al., 2003). Current data suggest that an OCD patient has little hope for symptomatic reprieve during pregnancy or postpartum (Altshuler et al., 1998; Levine et al., 2003). Of particular concern in the postpartum population are intrusive and unwanted thoughts, impulses and images of harming the infant. These thoughts could occur as symptoms of OCD and/or as indicators of postpartum depression, raising particular challenges for clinicians (see Chapter 8).

A study of self-reported anxiousness during the postpartum period (not diagnosable anxiety disorder per se) (Stuart et al., 1998) suggested a common occurrence of comorbid anxiety and depression in the postpartum period. The sample consisted of 107 community volunteers, primarily Caucasian, married and employed. Self-reported anxiety increased over time in this sample, reaching 8.7% at 14 weeks postpartum, and increasing to 16.8% at 30 weeks. One could loosely parallel this to generalized anxiety, although no formal axis I diagnoses were made. It is unknown for this sample whether their anxiety was being treated, and/or whether they had a history of anxiety or depressive disorder during pregnancy or perhaps even prior to gestation. The findings do suggest, however, a high index of suspicion amongst clinicians working with postpartum women, such that anxiety symptoms are recognized and appropriately dealt with. For a more detailed discussion of these issues, the reader is referred to Chapter 8.

Conclusions

In conclusion, anxiety disorders disproportionately affect women. The prevalence rate is higher in women compared to men for all the anxiety disorders. There is little information about the course of the various disorders and the expression of illness in men and women. Such information, as well as more data regarding gender-specific risk factors may help explain the differential risk in men and women and increase our knowledge of the pathophysiology of the various conditions. Given the early onset of illness among many males and females, studies evaluating gender and risk will need to include investigations in children and adolescents.

REFERENCES

Altshuler, L., Hendrick, V., & Cohen, L. (1998). Course of mood and anxiety disorders during pregnancy and the postpartum period. *Journal of Clinical Psychiatry, 59* (Suppl 2), 29–33.

Andrews, B., Brewin, C., & Rose, S. (2003). Gender, Social Support, and PTSD in victims of violent crime. *Journal of Traumatic Stress, 16*(4), 421–427.

Angst, J., & Vollrath, M. (1991). The natural history of anxiety disorders. *Acta Psychiatrica Scandinavica (Copenhagen), 84,* 446–452.

APA (1994). *Diagnostic and Statistical Manual of Mental Disorders-DSM-IV* (4th edn.). Washington, DC: American Psychiatric Association.

Apfeldorf, W., Spielman, L., Cloitre, M., et al. (2000). Morbidity of comorbid psychiatric diagnoses in the clinical presentation of panic disorder. *Depression and Anxiety*, *12*, 78–84.

Bailey, J., & Cohen, L. (1999). Prevalence of mood and anxiety disorders in women who seek treatment for premenstrual syndrome. *Journal of Women's Health & Gender–Based Medicine*, *8*(9), 1181–1184.

Barlow, D.H. (1988). *Anxiety and its disorders: The nature and treatment of anxiety and panic.* New York, NY: Guilford Press.

Bebbington, P. (1998) Epidemiology of obsessive-compulsive disorder. *British Journal of Psychiatry*, *173*, (Suppl. 35); 2–6.

Bekker, M.H.J. (1996). Agoraphobia and gender: A review. *Clinical Psychology Review*, *16*(2), 129–146.

Bibb, J.L., & Chambless, D.L. (1986). Alcohol use and abuse among diagnosed agoraphobics. *Behaviour Research and Therapy*, *24*(1), 49–58.

Blanes, T., & McGuire, P. (1997). Heterogeneity within obsessive-compulsive disorder: evidence for primary and neurodevelopmental subtypes. In: M.S. Keshavan, R.M. Murray (Eds.). *Neurodevelopment and adult psychopathology*, Cambridge: Cambridge University Press, pp. 206–212.

Blazer, D.G., Hughes, D., George, L.K., et al. (1991). Generalized anxiety disorder. In: L.N. Robins, & D.A. Regier (Eds.), *Psychiatric disorders in America* (pp. 181–203). 1st edn. New York, NY: Free Press.

Bogetto, F., Venturello, S., Albert, U., Maina, G., & Ravizza, L. (1999). Gender-related clinical diferences in obsessive-compulsive disorder. *European Psychiatry: The Journal of the Association of European Psychiatrists*, *14*, 434–441.

Bourdon, K.H., Boyd, J.H., Rae, D.S., et al. (1988). Gender differences in phobias: Results of the ECA community survey. *Journal of Anxiety Disorders*, *2*, 227–241.

Brandes, M., Soares, C., & Cohen, L. (2004). Postpartum onset obsessive-compulsive disorder: Diagnosis and management. *Archives of Women's Mental Health*, *7*, 99–110.

Breslau, N., & Davis, G. (1992). Posttraumatic stress disorder in an urban population of young adults: Risk factors for chronicity. *American Journal of Psychiatry*, *149*, 671–675.

Breslau, N., Schultz, L., & Peterson, E. (1995). Sex differences in depression: A role for pre-existing anxiety. *Psychiatry Research*, *58*, 1–12.

Breslau, N., Davis, G.C., Andreski, P., et al. (1997). Sex differences in posttraumatic stress disorder. *Archives of General Psychiatry*, *54*, 1044–1048.

Bromet, E., Sonnega, A., & Kessler, R.C. (1998). Risk factors for DSM-III-R posttraumatic stress disorder: Findings from the National Comorbidity Survey. *American Journal of Epidemiology*, *147*, 353–361.

Brown, G., Harris, T., & Eales, M. (1996). Social factors and comorbidity of depressive and anxiety disorders. *British Journal of Psychiatry*, *168*(Suppl. 30), 50–57.

Cameron, O.G., & Hill, E.M. (1989). Women and anxiety. *Psychiatric Clinics of North America*, *12*, 175–186.

Cameron, O.G., Kuttesch, D., McPhee, K., et al. (1988). Menstrual fluctuation in the symptoms of panic anxiety. *Journal of Affective Disorders*, *15*, 169–174.

Castle, D.J., Deale, A., & Marks, I.M. (1995). Gender differences in obsessive compulsive disorder. *Australian and New Zealand Journal of Psychiatry*, *29*, 114–117.

Cohen, L., Sichel, D., Faraone, S., et al. (1996). Course of panic disorder during pregnancy and the puerperium: A preliminary study. *Biological Psychiatry*, *39*, 950–954.

Cohen, L.S., Sichel, D.A., Dimmock, J.A., et al. (1994). Impact of pregnancy on panic disorder: A case series. *Journal of Clinical Psychiatry, 55*, 284–289.

Compton, S., Nelson, A., & March, J. (2000). Social phobia and separation anxiety symptoms in community and clinical samples of children and adolescents. *Journal of the American Academy of Child and Adolescent Psychiatry, 39*(8), 1040–1046.

Cook, B.L., Noyes, R., Garvey, M.J., et al. (1990). Anxiety and the menstrual cycle in panic disorder. *Journal of Affective Disorders, 19*, 221–226.

Cox, B.J., Swinson, R.P., Shulman, I.D., et al. (1993). Gender effects and alcohol use in panic disorder with agoraphobia. *Behaviour Research and Therapy, 31*(4), 413–416.

DeWit, D.J., Ogborne, A., Offord, D.R., et al. (1999). Antecedents of the risk of recovery from DSM-III-R social phobia. *Psychological Medicine, 29*(3), 569–582.

Durham, R.C., Allan, T., & Hackett, C.A. (1997). On predicting improvement and relapse in generalized anxiety disorder following psychotherapy. *British Journal of Clinical Psychology, 36*, 101–119.

Eaton, W.W., Kessler, R.C., Wittchen, H.U., et al. (1994). Panic and panic disorder in the United States. *American Journal of Psychiatry, 151*, 413–420.

Enoch, M.A., Greenberg, B.D., Murphy, D.L., & Goldman, D. (2001). Sexually dimorphic relationship of a 5-HT2A promoter polymorphism with obsessive-compulsive disorder. *Biological Psychiatry, 49*, 385–388.

Facchinetti, F., Romano, G., Fava, M., et al. (1992). Lactate infusion induces panic attacks in patients with premenstrual syndrome. *Psychosomatic Medicine, 54*, 288–296.

Faravelli, C., Zucchi, T., Viviani, B., Salmoria, R., Perone, A., Paionni, A., Scarpato, A., Vigliaturo, D., Rosi, S., D'adamo, D., Bartolozzi, D., Cecchi, C., & Abrardi, L. (2000). Epidemiology of social phobia: A clinical approach. *European Psychiatry: The Journal of the Association of European Psychiatrists, 15*, 17–24.

Fava, M., Pedrazzi, F., Guaraldi, G.P., et al. (1992). Comorbid anxiety and depression among patients with late luteal phase dysphoric disorder. *Journal of Anxiety Disorders, 6*, 325–335.

Fischer, E.H., & Goethe J.W. (1998). Anxiety and alcohol abuse in patients in treatment for depression. *American Journal Drug Alcohol Abuse, 24*(3), 453–463.

Freedman, S., Gluck, N., Tuval-Mashiach, R., et al. (2002). Gender differences in responses to traumatic events: A prospective study. *Journal of Traumatic Stress, 15*(5), 407–413.

Fullerton, C.S., Ursano, R.J., Epstein, R.S., et al. (2001). Gender differences in posttraumatic stress disorder after motor vehicle accidents. *American Journal Psychiatry, 158*, 1486–1491.

Golding, J., Taylor, D., Menard, L., et al. (2000). Prevalence of sexual abuse history in a sample of women seeking treatment for premenstrual syndrome. *Journal of Psychosomatic Obstetrics and Gynecology, 21*, 69–80.

Green, B. (2003). Post-traumatic stress disorder: Symptom profiles in men and women. *Current Medical Research and Opinion, 19*, P1–P5.

Grossman, P., Wilhelm, F., Kawachi, I., et al. (2001). Gender differences in psychophysiological responses to speech stress among older social phobics: Congruence and incongruence between self-evaluative and cardiovascular reactions. *Psychosomatic Medicine, 63*, 765–777.

Hayward, C., Killen, J.D., Kraemer, H.C., et al. (2000). Predictors of panic attacks in adolescents. *Journal of the American Academy of Child and Adolescent Psychiatry, 39*(2), 207–214.

Holbrook, T.L., Hoyt, D.B., Stein, M.B., et al. (2002). Gender difference in long-term post-traumatic stress disorder outcomes after major trauma: Women are at higher risk of adverse outcomes than men. *The Journal of Trauma*, *53*(5), 882–888.

Katz, M., Wetzler, S., Clioitre, M., et al. (1993). Expressive characteristics of anxiety in depressed men and women. *Journal of Affective Disorders*, *28*, 267–277.

Kendler, K., Neale, M., Kessler, R., et al. (1992). Major depression and generalized anxiety disorder: Same genes, (partly) different environments? *Arch Gen Psychiatry*, *49*, 716–722.

Kessler, R.C., McGonagle, K., Zhao, S., et al. (1994a). Lifetime and 12-month prevalence of DSM-III-R psychiatric disorders in the United States. Results from the National Comorbidity Survey. *Archives of General Psychiatry*, *51*, 8–19.

Kessler, R.C., McGonagle, K.A., Nelson, C.B., et al. (1994). Sex and depression in the National Comorbidity Survey II: Cohort effects. *Journal of Affective Disorders*, *30*, 15–26/

Kessler, R.C., Sonnega, A., Bromet, E., et al. (1995). Posttraumatic stress disorder in the National Comorbidity Survey. *Archives of General Psychiatry*, *52*, 1048–1060.

Kessler, R.C., Berglund, P., Demler, O., et al. (2003). The epidemiology of major depressive disorder. *Journal of the American Medical Association*, *289*(23), 3095–3105.

Lampe, L., Slade, T., Issakidis, C., et al. (2003). Social phobia in the Australian National Survey of Mental Health and Well-Being (NSMHWB). *Psychological Medicine*, *33*, 637–646.

Lensi, P., Cassano, G.B., Correddu, G., et al. (1996). Obsessive-compulsive disorder. Familial-developmental history, symptomatology, comorbidity and course with special reference to gender-related differences. *British Journal of Psychiatry*, *169*, 101–107.

Levine, R.E., Oandasan, A.P., Primeau, L.A., et al. (2003). Anxiety disorders during pregnancy and postpartum. *American Journal of Perinatology*, *20*(5), 239–248.

Lewinsohn, P., Lewinsohn, M., Gotlib, I., et al. (1998). Gender differences in anxiety disorders and anxiety symptoms in adolescents. *Journal of Abnormal Psychology*, *107*(1), 109–117.

Lochner, C., Hemmings, S., Kinnear, C., et al. (2004). Gender in obsessive-compulsive disorder: Clinican and genetic findings. *European Neuropsychopharmacology*, *14*, 105–113.

Massion, A., Warshaw, M., & Keller, M. (1993). Quality of life and psychiatric morbidity in panic disorder versus generalized anxiety disorder. *American Journal of Psychiatry*, *150*, 600–607.

Merikangas, K., Stevens, D., Fenton, B., et al. (1998). Co-morbidity and familial aggregation of alcoholism and anxiety disorders. *Psychological Medicine*, *28*, 773–788.

Murray, C.J., & Lopez, A.D. (Eds.). The global burden of disease: *A comprehensive assessment of mortality and disability from diseases, injuries, and risk factors in 1990 and projected to 2020. Harvard University Press, Global Burden of Disease and Injury Series*: Boston, MA.

North, C.S., Smith, E.M., & Spitznagel, E.L. (1997). One-year follow-up of a mass shooting. *American Journal of Psychiatry*, *154*, 1696–1702.

Noshirvani, H.F., Kasvikis, Y., Marks, I.M., et al. (1991). Gender-divergent aetiological factors in obsessive-compulsive disorder. *British Journal of Psychiatry*, *158*, 260–263.

Papp, L., Martinez, J., Klein, D., et al. (1997). Respiratory psychophysiology of panic disorder: Three respiratory challenges in 98 subjects. *American Journal of Psychiatry*, *154*, 1557–1565.

Papp, L.A., & Gorman, J.M. (1988). Sex differences in panic disorder. *American Journal of Psychiatry*, *145*(6), 766.

Parker, G., Wilhelm, K., & Asghari, A. (1997). Early onset depression: The relevance of anxiety. *Social Psychiatry and Psychiatric Epidemiology, 32*(1), 30–37.

Pigott, T. (1999). Gender differences in epidemiology and treatment of anxiety disorders. *Journal of Clinical Psychiatry, 60*(Suppl 18), 4–15.

Pollard, C.A., & Henderson, J.G. (1988). Four types of social phobia in a community sample. *Journal of Nervous and Mental Disease, 176*, 440–444.

Sheikh, J., Leskin, G., & Klein, D. (2002). Gender differences in panic disorder: Findings from the National Comorbidity Survey. *American Journal of Psychiatry, 159*, 55–58.

Smith, M.V., Cavaleri, M.A., Howell, H.B., et al. (2004). Screening for and detection of depression, panic disorder, and PTSD in public-sector obstetrical clinics. *Psychiatric Services, 55*(4), 407–414.

Sonne, S., Back, S., Zuniga, C., et al. (2003). Gender differences in individuals with comorbid alcohol dependence and post-traumatic stress disorder. *American Journal n Addiction, 12*, 412–423.

Starcevic, V., Djordjevic, A., Latas, M., et al. (1998). Characteristics of agoraphobia in women and men with panic disorder and agoraphobia. *Depression and Anxiety, 8*, 8–13.

Stein, M.B., Schmidt, P.J., Rubinow, D.R., et al. (1989). Panic disorder and the menstrual cycle: Panic Disorder patients, healthy control subjects, and patients with premenstrual syndrome. *American Journal of Psychiatry, 146*(10), 1299–1303.

Stuart, S., Couser, G., Schilder, K., et al. (1998). Postpartum anxiety and depression: Onset and comorbidity in a community sample. *Journal of Nervous and Mental Disease, 186*(7), 420–424.

Turgeon, L., Marchand, A., & Dupuis, G. (1998). Clinical features in panic disorder with agoraphobia: A comparison of men and women. *Journal of Anxiety Disorders, 12*(6), 539–553.

Turk, C., Heimberg, R., Orsillo, S., et al. (1998). An investigation of gender differences in social phobia. *Journal of Anxiety Disorders, 12*, 209–223.

Wittchen, H.-U., Reed, V., & Kessler, R.C. (1998). The relationship of agoraphobia and panic in a community sample of adolescents and young adults. *Archives of General Psychiatry, 55*, 1017–1024.

Wittchen, H.-U., Zhao, S., Kessler, R.C., et al. (1994). DSM-III-R generalized anxiety disorder in the National Comorbidity Survey. *Archives of General Psychiatry, 51*, 355–364.

Yonkers, K., Dyck, I., Warshaw, M., et al. (2000). Factors predicting the clinical course of generalised anxiety disorders. *British Journal of Psychiatry, 176*, 544–550.

Yonkers, K.A., Warshaw, M.G., Massion, A.O., et al. (1996). Phenomenology and course of generalised anxiety disorder. *British Journal of Psychiatry, 168*, 308–313.

Yonkers, K.A., Zlotnick, C., Allsworth, J., et al. (1998). Is the course of panic disorder the same in women and men? *American Journal of Psychiatry, 155*, 596–602.

Yonkers, K.A., Dyck, I.R., & Keller, M.B. (2001). An eight year longitudinal comparison of clinical course and characteristics of social phobia among men and women. *Psychiatric Services, 52*(5), 637–643.

Yonkers, K.A., Bruce, S., Dyck, I., et al. (2003). Chronicity, relapse and illness – course of panic disorder, social phobia, and generalized anxiety disorder: Findings in men and women from 8 years of follow-up. *Depression and Anxiety, 17*, 173–179.

Zlotnick, C., Zimmerman, M., Wolfsdorf, B.A., et al. (2001). Gender differences in patients with posttraumatic stress disorder in a general psychiatric practice. *American Journal of Psychiatry, 158*, 1923–1925.

5

Posttraumatic stress disorder in women

Mark Creamer and Jessica Carty

Australian Centre for Posttraumatic Mental Health, University of Melbourne, Melbourne, Victoria, Australia

The diagnosis of posttraumatic stress disorder (PTSD) has been the focus of considerable attention since it first appeared in the diagnostic nomenclature in 1980. Since that time, the diagnostic criteria have been refined, with both the diagnostic and statistical manual of mental disorders DSM-IV (American Psychiatric Association, 1994) and international classification of diseases (ICD-10) (World Health Organization, 1993) recognizing the condition. In recent years, a major focus of interest has been the impact of gender on the risk of developing PTSD and related conditions following traumatic exposure. Indeed, the fact that a whole book has recently been devoted to a comprehensive review of issues concerning PTSD and gender (Kimerling et al., 2002) is an indication of the importance placed on this relationship. While interested readers are referred to that volume for a more in-depth analysis of the area, the purpose of this chapter is to provide an overview of the key issues concerning women and PTSD.

The nature of PTSD

The first criterion to be met for a diagnosis of PTSD is the experience of a traumatic event (Criterion A1), usually defined as involving actual or threatened physical threat to the self or others. The person's response to the event must have involved a powerful emotional reaction, such as fear, helplessness, or horror (Criterion A2). Three broad clusters of symptoms characterize the disorder and are required in some form for a diagnosis. First, evidence of re-experiencing the trauma is required (known as the "B criteria"). This is likely to take the form of intrusive memories, images, or perceptions that invade consciousness, dreams, flashbacks, and distress on reminders. Those symptoms are very distressing and the next symptom group ("C criteria") is often conceptualized as a way of trying to prevent the return of the painful memories. The C criteria include evidence of active avoidance, often with a phobic quality (such as attempts to avoid people, places, situations, thoughts, feelings, and conversations associated with the trauma). The C criteria also include emotional numbing or "passive avoidance", with characteristic symptoms of social withdrawal, loss of interest, flattened affect, and psychogenic amnesia. Clinically, a predominance of the active C criteria tends to reflect an anxious presentation, while the passive avoidance symptoms present more of a depressive picture. The D criteria are those of persistent hyperarousal, characterized by sleep disturbance, anger and irritability, poor concentration, hypervigilance, and exaggerated startle response. The symptoms must have been present for at least 1 month before a diagnosis of PTSD can be made, and the symptoms must be associated with significant distress and/or impairment of social or occupational functioning.

While it is clear that many symptoms of PTSD overlap with other diagnoses, there is also ample evidence that PTSD is often associated with a range of comorbid conditions. Around 85–88% of men and 79–80% of women with chronic PTSD meet criteria for another Axis 1 condition (Creamer et al., 2001; Kessler et al., 1995). Thus, the clinical presentation in both men and women is often complex, with high levels of depression, anxiety, and substance use. In more chronic cases, the disorder is associated with progressively deteriorating social and occupational circumstances, often confronting the clinician with a myriad of psychosocial problems in addition to the core disorder.

Prevalence across cultures

Several epidemiological studies from the USA have indicated that, while men are more likely than women to be exposed to traumatic events, the prevalence of PTSD within the community is approximately twice as high for women. One of the most influential of those studies, the National Comorbidity Study (NCS), estimated that lifetime prevalence of trauma exposure was 51% for women and 61% for men (Kessler et al., 1995). Lifetime PTSD rates, however, were estimated at 10% for women and 5% for men. Similarly, a community survey from Detroit indicated that women were more than twice as likely to develop PTSD following trauma, with estimates of 6% and 13% for men and women respectively (Breslau et al., 1998). Again, these discrepancies were found despite the higher rates of trauma exposure reported by men.

This pattern of differential trauma response by gender has been replicated in some, but not all, other countries in which such research has been conducted. In Canada, for example, Stein et al. (1997) found that current rates of PTSD were more than twice as high for women as for men (2.7% and 1.2% respectively). Research conducted in four cities across Mexico estimated that women were twice as likely as men to be diagnosed with PTSD (lifetime rates of 15% and 7% respectively), despite the greater number of traumatic events reported by men (83% versus 71%) (Norris et al., 2003). The conditional risk for developing PTSD following trauma was over twice as high for women as for men (21% versus 9%). Conversely, employing a methodology almost identical to that used in the NCS, Creamer et al. (2001) reported on an Australian community sample of 10,641 respondents. Despite comparable patterns of trauma exposure to the US samples, the 12-month PTSD prevalence was only marginally higher in females (1.4%) than in males (1.2%). Interestingly, the overall rate of 12-month PTSD in the Australian sample was only 1.3%, considerably lower than the NCS prevalence of 3.9% (Kessler et al., 1999).

Thus, it seems likely that PTSD prevalence generally, and differential rates between men and women, may vary according to a range of cultural and environmental factors. This proposition is supported by a survey of refugees from Laos, Vietnam, and Cambodia living in the USA (Chung & Bemak, 2002). Although female gender was associated with increased rates of psychological distress, the authors noted that cultural factors appeared to mediate this risk: stress responses differed between, and within, gender groups according to their country of origin. Similarly, in a comparative study across four postconflict, low income countries, de Jong et al. (2001) found equal rates of PTSD in men and women in Ethiopia, higher rates among women in Algeria and Cambodia, and higher rates among men in Gaza. In such samples, however, gender differences may be obscured by the disproportionately high rates of posttraumatic symptomatology that characterize populations exposed to extreme prolonged trauma (Norris et al., 2002). For example, similarly elevated rates of PTSD, depression, and anxiety were reported for Armenian communities exposed to either extreme earthquake trauma or severe political violence 4 years later, regardless of gender or trauma type (Goenjian et al., 2000).

The mechanisms underlying these cultural differences remain a matter of speculation. It is reasonable to assume, however, that one aspect may be differences in the socialization of men and women reflecting cultural norms and ideals. In Western society, for example, it is generally considered more socially acceptable for women to express emotion than men, who may be discouraged from reporting such problems for fear of appearing "weak". A study of 6-month PTSD prevalence rates following hurricanes in Mexico and the USA revealed cross-cultural differences between Mexican and US respondents as a whole, as well as within the US group according to cultural background (Norris et al., 2001a). Mexican women had the highest rates of PTSD at 44%, compared with a rate of only 14% for Mexican men. The lowest rates of PTSD were found for Anglo-American men (6%), whereas there was little difference between Anglo-American women (19%), African-American men (20%), and African-American women (23%). The authors suggested that these rates may reflect differences in gender roles in Mexico and the USA: the discouragement of emotional expression in Mexican men may exacerbate gender differences in the diagnosis of PTSD and related disorders. These differences may be reduced in African-American communities which are considered to have a more egalitarian approach to gender role expectations.

In a similar vein, the process of socialization in different cultures may produce gender differences in coping style which may mediate response to stressful life events (Gavranidou & Rosner, 2003). Those authors suggest that, as a result of cultural expectations, women are more likely to practice "emotion-focused" coping whereas men are likely to exercise "problem-focused" coping; the latter tends to be associated with a better outcome. Similarly, Foster et al. (2004) suggest that gender differences in PTSD may reflect socialization processes, where women and men are taught to internalize and externalize negative emotions respectively in accordance with accepted masculine and feminine roles. Thus, males and females may respond differently to trauma, with males tending to externalize in the form of aggression and substance use, and females more inclined to internalize in the form of anxiety and depression (see also Chapter 2). The latter is more likely to result in a diagnosis of PTSD.

Taken together, the epidemiological findings suggest that, while a range of social and cultural factors may affect the incidence and expression of posttraumatic sequelae, there is a general trend across cultures indicating that women are at greater risk for such symptomatology.

The developmental context: women, trauma and PTSD across the lifespan

While few epidemiological studies have considered trauma exposure and response across the life span, preliminary evidence suggests that gender differences may be present from a relatively early age. Kessler et al. (1995) found that women were more likely than men to report adverse events specific to childhood, such as childhood parental neglect, and childhood physical abuse. Exposure to such traumatizing events at an early developmental stage potentially has serious implications for the way in which individuals deal with stress and trauma in later life. Prior trauma exposure has consistently been identified as a factor that increases the risk of both subsequent trauma exposure and the development of PTSD following such an event (Brewin et al., 2000; Ozer et al., 2003).

In addition to the possibility of higher levels of trauma exposure for girls, there is also some evidence of differential traumatic stress reactions in children exposed to trauma. Several studies have suggested that girls are likely to report higher levels of many typical traumatic stress symptoms than boys (e.g., Feiring et al., 1999; Foster et al., 2004). In a study of urban youth, Breslau et al. (1997) found that PTSD rates as a consequence of a traumatic event before the age of 15 were considerably higher for women than men. While women remained at higher risk following exposure in adulthood, the gender differences were less pronounced, suggesting that the greater vulnerability may be reduced with maturity.

Although beyond the scope of this chapter, it is important to note that the long-term effects of prolonged exposure to childhood trauma may not be best conceptualized as PTSD. The contribution of prolonged and severe childhood trauma to the development of Axis 2 personality disorders, especially the B cluster such as borderline and antisocial personality disorder, has been the subject of considerable debate in the literature (e.g., McLean & Gallop, 2003; Yen et al., 2002; and see Chapter 2). In an attempt to develop a more aetiologically useful clinical description of these effects, several authors have proposed the existence of a new diagnostic category variously known as "complex PTSD" or "disorders of extreme stress not otherwise specified" (DESNOS) (Herman, 1992; Zlotnick et al., 1996). Although not formally accepted in the DSM-IV as a diagnostic category, the construct remains the subject of considerable interest.

There is somewhat less research to inform our understanding of gender and traumatic stress at the other end of the lifespan. In a re-analysis of one of the few studies to include individuals over the age of 55 Norris et al. (2002) found that age interacted with gender to predict current PTSD. Although higher prevalence rates were apparent for women aged 18–55, rates did not differ by gender for those over 55. Interestingly, and perhaps not surprisingly, the higher levels of trauma exposure routinely reported for males only applied to the population under 30 years of age. From approximately 30 onwards, rates of trauma exposure did not differ for men or women. More recently, in a comparison of older and younger women, Acierno et al. (2002) found that women over the age of 55 reported fewer physical and sexual assaults, as well as a reduced risk of trauma-related morbidity following interpersonal violence, than women aged 18–34. Finally, while not providing a breakdown by age and gender, Creamer et al. (2001) reported comparable rates of trauma exposure among those over and under the age of 55, while rates of PTSD were significantly lower among the older sample.

In summary, it seems that gender differences in trauma exposure may begin with females at higher risk during childhood, males at higher risk during adolescence and early adulthood, and little difference between the genders from about the age of 30 onwards. With regard to psychological reactions to traumatic exposure, it appears that females may be more vulnerable from a relatively young age, with this gender difference persisting through adulthood and declining after the age of 55. As Breslau (2002) notes, however, while prior trauma exposure and response may contribute to subsequent vulnerability, it is not a sufficient explanation of gender-related differences in PTSD prevalence.

Possible explanations for gender differences in PTSD

It appears, then, that women are more vulnerable to the development of PTSD than males. While this might be influenced by cultural factors and early childhood experiences, neither explanation is sufficient to account fully for the differential rates. This section describes a number of other factors that may interact to mediate the relationship between gender, trauma exposure, culture, and PTSD vulnerability.

Assessment and phenomenology

It is conceivable that gender differences in the prevalence of PTSD may, in part, be simply an artefact of the diagnostic criteria and the assessment procedures. Several studies have reported gender-related variations in patterns of PTSD symptomatology which may increase the likelihood that women will meet criteria as currently defined. Women, for example, have been found to endorse symptoms from the C cluster (avoidance and numbing) following motor vehicle accidents (MVA) (Fullerton et al., 2001) and physical assault (Breslau et al., 1999) more often than men. Since three symptoms from this cluster are required for a diagnosis (compared with two hyperarousal and only one re-experiencing symptom), this may have a significant impact on prevalence rates. Avoidance and numbing symptoms are relatively infrequently endorsed (e.g., Foa et al., 1995; North et al., 1999) and, therefore, the presence of this symptom cluster substantially increases the likelihood of a PTSD diagnosis. In a similar vein, preliminary evidence indicates that the presence of peritraumatic dissociation predicts PTSD more accurately in women than in men (e.g., Bryant & Harvey, 2003; Fullerton et al., 2001). The mechanisms underlying this relationship require further investigation, although a range of pre- and posttrauma factors are likely to be involved. In particular, however, it is hard to disentangle this finding from the role of prior trauma: it seems likely that adverse early childhood experiences may promote the use of dissociation as a coping strategy in response to stress and trauma, thereby increasing vulnerability to subsequent PTSD.

Importantly, gender differences are not limited to PTSD rates: women are also more likely than men to be diagnosed with other anxiety and depressive disorders (Kessler et al., 1994; Korten & Henderson, 2000; and see Chapters 4 and 7). Estimates of PTSD prevalence may be complicated by the substantial overlap of symptoms between PTSD and other anxiety and depressive disorders. Thus, increased rates of PTSD may reflect a broader vulnerability to (or willingness to acknowledge) emotional distress. While elevated rates of PTSD (as well as of anxiety and depression) in females may reflect a heightened vulnerability of women to emotional disorders, they may also reflect biases in the diagnostic criteria and assessment processes.

Trauma type

A second, and highly plausible, explanation for the higher PTSD prevalence among females may be that men and women are likely to experience different types of trauma. There is a large body of evidence indicating that exposure to traumas involving interpersonal violence carries a high risk of subsequent psychological adjustment problems (e.g., Creamer et al., 2001; Kessler et al., 1995). Epidemiological studies have consistently found that women are more likely to report sexual assault and rape, whereas men are more likely to experience non-sexual physical assault, combat, accidental injury, and witnessing someone being badly injured or killed (Breslau et al., 1999; Creamer et al., 2001; Kessler et al., 1995). Sexual assault and rape, regardless of gender, are consistently associated with the highest rates of PTSD.

It is also reasonable to assume that some types of interpersonal violence (and even some types of sexual assault) are especially "psychopathogenic" (or likely to result in poorer psychological adjustment). It may be speculated that the event carries higher risk when, for example, the attacker is known to, and previously trusted by, the victim and/or when the level of perceived threat is very high. Breslau et al. (1999) argued that gender-related differences in PTSD prevalence were explained almost entirely by the fact that women are more likely than men to develop PTSD following violent assault, even when sexual assault was controlled for (32% and 6% respectively). It may be speculated that these findings result from the type of assaultive violence women experience, which is often different to that experienced by men. It may be that women are more likely to be assaulted by someone they know (and, perhaps, trust), while men are more likely to be assaulted by a stranger (e.g., in a bar room brawl). Clearly, the former event type is more likely to shatter fundamental assumptions about the self and the world, particularly those relating to trust and safety, creating greater challenges for subsequent adjustment (see Chapter 6). Furthermore, these gender differences in the nature of traumatic exposure appear to be present from a relatively early age. For example, Breslau et al. (1997) found that, while similar proportions of males and females reported a traumatic experience that occurred before the age of 15, the types of events experienced in childhood varied between the sexes. More women reported rape, assault, or ongoing physical or sexual abuse, whereas a greater number of men reported exposure to serious injury or accidents. Thus, it is possible that the higher incidence of PTSD reported by women may be, at least in part, a consequence of differential exposure to particular types of interpersonal trauma. Furthermore, exposure to such trauma at an early developmental stage has important implications for subsequent psychological function.

Such an explanation, however, cannot fully account for the gender differences in PTSD. Although studies investigating the prevalence of trauma-related symptoms following exposure to events such as natural disaster, in which males and females have been equally exposed, tend generally to confirm a greater vulnerability for women, the results are less consistent. The relevant literature has been comprehensively reviewed by Norris et al. (2002) and a detailed analysis is beyond the scope of this chapter. Briefly, however, several studies have reported similar levels of post-trauma symptomatology and rates of PTSD in men and women following disasters such as tornados and earthquakes (e.g., Greening et al., 2002; Madakasira & O'Brien,

1987). Others have reported increased rates of posttraumatic sequelae in female survivors across a range of natural disasters (e.g., Basoglu et al., 2002; Norris et al., 2001b), as well as terrorist attacks such as the Okalahoma City bombing (North et al., 1999) and the September 11 attacks in New York City (Pulcino et al., 2003). Finally, studies of the non-gender-specific trauma of MVA indicate a greater vulnerability of women to symptoms of posttraumatic stress (Bryant & Harvey, 2003; Fullerton et al., 2001; Ursano et al., 1999), although again not all studies have found this difference (e.g., Freedman et al., 2002).

Social and material support

It has been suggested that loss of resources in the aftermath of trauma, including both social and material support, may help to explain the development of PTSD and, further, that women are more vulnerable to such resource loss than men. Thus, in a sample of 714 inner city women, Hobfoll et al. (2003) found that resource loss and worsening economic circumstances had more negative impact than resource gain and improving economic circumstances had positive impact, suggesting the greater saliency of loss than gain. Perhaps the most important "resource" following trauma is that of social support, which has consistently been found to be a powerful predictor of recovery (Brewin et al., 2000; Ozer et al., 2003). Although measurement of the construct is notoriously difficult, it usually encompasses several areas such as availability, use, and perceived benefits of both practical and emotional support. Recently, however, an important distinction has been drawn between positive and negative social support. In a sample of crime victims, Andrews et al. (2003) found that perceived positive social support had a protective effect, while perceived negative response from friends and family had a detrimental effect on self-reported PTSD symptoms at 6 months. While males and females reported comparable levels of positive support and support satisfaction, females reported higher levels of negative support (even after controlling for trauma type). Furthermore, the benefits of support satisfaction and the adverse effects of negative support were far more influential on 6-month PTSD symptoms for women than men. This factor went a long way towards explaining the gender differences in symptom severity and is clearly an important direction for future research. It seems likely that social support (and particularly negative social support) interacts with acute symptom severity to influence the course of recovery following trauma.

Cognitive factors

Epidemiological studies, such as those described above, generally focus on objective trauma type and severity. It is widely recognized, however, that the individual's perception or appraisal of the threat level is a powerful predictor of subsequent adjustment (Ehlers & Clark, 2000). There is some preliminary evidence to suggest that women may perceive traumatic events as more aversive than men who experience the same event. Norris et al. (2002) note that comparable proportions of men and women meet the DSM-IV Criterion A2 (powerful emotional reactions to trauma), despite the fact that men report a higher prevalence of objective trauma exposure. Similar outcomes were reported by Goenjian et al. (2001) who found that, while Nicaraguan adolescents did not differ in their objective experience of Hurricane Mitch, girls reported significantly higher subjective levels of exposure. Thus, women may tend subjectively to experience traumatic events as more aversive, with these negative appraisals increasing vulnerability to PTSD. This is not unreasonable: women are, generally, physically weaker than men and may feel more threatened by a frightening event, particularly if the experience involves intentional harm. Thus, an assault of the same objective severity may be considerably more frightening for a woman than for a man.

This line of argument has strong theoretical support, as discussed by Tolin and Foa (2002). These authors build on the emotional processing theory described by Foa and colleagues (e.g., Foa & Rothbaum, 1998) to explore differential patterns of cognitive processing between men and women that may serve to increase PTSD vulnerability. Emotional processing theory proposes that the development of traumatic stress symptoms is dependent upon an individual's prior perception of the self and world, as well as the degree to which these views change as a consequence of trauma. Tolin and Foa (2002) reviewed the literature and found preliminary evidence to support the proposition of gender differences in patterns of cognitive processing, memory of the event, and the effect of trauma on cognitive schemas. Self-blame was more prevalent in women than men following trauma, as were negative self-beliefs and perceptions of the world as a dangerous place. It is, of course, difficult to separate the influence of trauma type from cognitive appraisals: traumas that are objectively more severe are also likely to be appraised more negatively. It was noted above, however, that trauma type accounted for only a limited amount of the variance in posttraumatic stress levels, suggesting that cognitive processing patterns may mediate vulnerability to PTSD. Again, the underlying mechanisms that explain these differential approaches to the processing of information associated with the trauma remain a matter for speculation. Presumably, the difference is accounted for by a complex interaction between environmental and genetic (or other biological) influences.

Biological factors

Few studies have investigated psychophysiological differences between men and women in acute reactions to threat that may serve as potential mediators for PTSD vulnerability. A review of the empirical data by Pierce et al. (2002) indicated little evidence for gender-specific differences in physiological responses (such as cardiovascular and skin conductance reactivity) to threat-related stimuli. They acknowledge, however, that studies are lacking and that those that exist are methodologically flawed.

Greater support has been found for the impact of hormone fluctuations across the lifespan in mediating vulnerability to anxiety disorders. Pigott (1999), in a comprehensive review of the literature, reported that oestrogen and progesterone have been associated with the regulation of neurotransmitters which mediate the anxiety response. These include the locus coeruleus-noradrenergic and serotonergic systems, as well as the gamma-aminobutyric acid (GABA) benzodiazepine receptor complex. Higher levels of oestrogen are proposed to be stress-protective while progesterone may have the reverse effect. Fluctuations in these hormones during a woman's menstrual and reproductive cycles may influence the degree of responsivity to stress cues and the course of symptomatology. No research to date has investigated timing of traumatic exposure in relation to stage of the menstrual cycle (although such research is currently being conducted by the authors). Interestingly, however, Pierce et al. (2002) note that several studies of women with current PTSD have reported high rates of dysfunctional reproductive risk factors, such as menstrual cycle irregularity, natural or induced menopause, and oral contraceptive use.

In summary, it is likely that several factors interact to explain the higher rates of PTSD among women. These include cultural and societal pressures and expectations, the types of trauma to which women are likely to be exposed, the reaction of loved ones and associates to their experience, and hormonal levels. It is likely that these factors combine to influence cognitive processing and appraisals of the trauma which, in turn, affect the course of recovery. While it is possible that the diagnostic criteria and common assessment strategies serve artificially to inflate the reported prevalence of PTSD, this seems an unlikely and unhelpful explanation. Rather than denying the existence of these elevated rates, a more productive approach is to focus upon what can be done to address the causes of this differential vulnerability and how we can best treat those affected by the condition.

Treatment

While few studies have specifically investigated gender differences in PTSD treatment outcome, the literature suggests that females may have a slightly superior response rate when compared to males (Foa et al., 2000). Comparisons between the sexes are problematic, however, since the majority of treatment studies comprise either male combat veterans or female sexual assault victims. Thus, gender differences in treatment efficacy may be obscured by several confounding variables, including trauma type.

Psychological interventions

The majority of studies investigating the efficacy of psychotherapy in the treatment of PTSD have fallen under the broad rubric of cognitive behaviour therapy (CBT). Since most of these studies have been conducted on homogeneous samples of either female rape victims or male combat veterans, little useful information can be gleaned regarding differential treatment response by gender. The only randomized-controlled trial (RCT) that has compared gender differences in treatment effect sizes was conducted by Tarrier et al. (2000). These investigators examined factors associated with response to CBT for chronic PTSD in a RCT of male and female mixed-trauma patients. Females responded better at posttreatment and at 6-month follow-up, although the latter difference was better explained by number of missed sessions, living alone, and associated general anxiety. Importantly, male gender was associated with several factors that may have contributed to poorer treatment outcome, such as poorer motivation, rating treatment as less credible, and being more likely to miss therapy appointments. Thus, it may be that males are simply "worse" patients in therapy rather than being unable to respond to treatment. In a comprehensive attempt to review the literature, Cason et al. (2002) examined the outcome of 18 PTSD treatment studies, seven of which contained both males and females. Overall, treatment effect sizes for female participants were equal to, or somewhat higher, than those for males.

Pharmacotherapy

A mounting body of empirical research has supported the efficacy of certain types of psychotropic medication in the treatment of PTSD. Few studies, however, have examined gender differences in response to pharmacotherapy. At the time of writing, the front line pharmacotherapy of choice in PTSD remains the selective serotonin reuptake inhibitors (SSRIs). They are favoured by clinicians because of their generally lower side-effect profiles and better tolerability than the older tricyclic antidepressants, as well as their perceived efficacy in all aspects of the condition. Several large-scale RCTs have indicated that both sertraline and paroxetine significantly reduce the level of symptoms across all three PTSD symptom clusters, as well as providing improvement in comorbid conditions (Brady et al., 2000; Davidson et al., 2001; Tucker et al., 2001). However, much of this research has been conducted with predominantly female samples, making it difficult to make definitive statements about efficacy with male PTSD sufferers. (Anecdotally, it is understood that this led the food and drug administration (FDA) in the USA to consider only approving these drugs for the treatment of PTSD in females. In the end, they were approved for both genders but with a warning that they had yet to demonstrate efficacy in males with PTSD.) Importantly, several RCTs have reported reduced efficacy for male veterans treated with sertraline (Zohar et al., 2002) and fluoxetine (Hertzberg et al., 2000; van der Kolk et al., 1994). It is unclear at this stage whether such findings should be interpreted on the basis of gender; it is equally plausible that the findings are better explained by something unique to the nature of combat as a traumatic event, or even the nature of military personnel.

In explaining the (apparently) differentially improved outcome in females following SSRI treatment, Brady and Back (2002) refer to the role of oestrogen in facilitating serotonin response. Although a range of other drugs have shown some promise in open trials, including newer antidepressants and antipsychotics, they are yet to prove their efficacy in multiple rigorous RCTs. When such research is published, it will be interesting to note any differential effects according to gender and to establish the efficacy of pharmacotherapy for males with PTSD.

In summary, although the data are not strong, it does appear that women may be more responsive than men to treatment for PTSD. This is despite their greater vulnerability to developing the disorder. Indeed, it may be that at least some of the factors that increase vulnerability (e.g., improved emotional expression) may be positive characteristics when it comes to treatment. Along the same lines, the type of comorbid disorders occurring with chronic PTSD may differ between men and women. For example, rates of comorbid substance abuse are higher in men with PTSD than women (Creamer et al., 2001; Kessler et al., 1995). It may be speculated that such "externalizing" comorbid conditions may be more disruptive to therapeutic efficacy. There is also evidence that women are more likely to seek treatment following traumatic exposure. For example, 77% of those who sought mental health treatment after an earthquake in Turkey were women (Livanou et al., 2002). This disproportionately high rate of women seeking treatment may, of course, simply be a function of the higher prevalence of PTSD and related reactions in females. It may also, however, be a function of the cultural influences that support emotional expression and accept vulnerability in women but not men.

Conclusions

The evidence reviewed in this chapter strongly suggests that women are at greater risk than men for the development of PTSD following exposure to a traumatic experience. Most community-based epidemiological studies attest to this risk, suggesting that women are roughly twice as likely to be diagnosed with PTSD, despite the higher rates of trauma exposure reported by men. Cross-cultural research has largely, although not always, replicated this finding in countries outside the USA. It appears that gender differences in trauma exposure may vary across the life cycle, with higher risk of exposure for females in childhood and higher risk for males in adolescence and young adulthood. Females tend to report more severe reactions throughout most of the life cycle, although this difference seems to diminish in later years, perhaps as a function of lower exposure or greater resilience acquired with age.

The mechanisms underlying this apparently increased vulnerability in females remain largely a matter of speculation. Socio-cultural factors appear to be of significance, particularly with regard to gender role socialization. These social processes may affect willingness to acknowledge distress, as well as the pattern of symptomatology expressed by men and women. They may also influence access to, and the impact of trauma on, social and material support. The nature and severity of posttraumatic morbidity is strongly influenced by the type of traumatic event. Women are more likely than men to experience interpersonal trauma, such as sexual assault, which is associated with high rates of PTSD. Cognitive appraisals are a crucial mediating factor between exposure and psychological adjustment, with research suggesting a tendency for women to experience the same trauma as more aversive than men. While evidence is lacking at this stage, gender-specific biological mechanisms, such as fluctuations in oestrogen and progesterone across a woman's menstrual and life cycle, may also be mediating factors. Finally, while women may be at greater risk for the development of psychiatric sequelae following trauma, preliminary findings from treatment outcome studies indicate that they may benefit from PTSD interventions to a greater extent than men. While further research is required, it may be speculated that many of the same gender-specific mechanisms that increase women's vulnerability to PTSD may also facilitate treatment response.

While this review has discussed a range of issues regarding the relationship between gender and PTSD, no single factor provides a sufficient explanation as to why women are more likely to be diagnosed with the disorder. Psychological adjustment following trauma is determined by a complex interaction of many factors. It is likely that these mechanisms affect both men and women, but may have differential impacts on adjustment according to gender. Future theoretical and empirical elaboration of these issues will contribute not only to our understanding of the relationship between gender and PTSD, but also to the identification of those at risk following trauma. In the long run, the goal will be to enhance early identification and intervention practices in order to reduce the debilitating effects of PTSD and related mental health sequelae of trauma.

REFERENCES

Acierno, R., Brady, K., Gray, M., Kilpatrick, D.G., Resnick, H., & Best, C.L. (2002). Psychopathology following interpersonal violence: A comparison of risk factors in older and younger adults. *Journal of Clinical Geropsychology*, 8(1), 13–23.

American Psychiatric Association (1994). *Diagnostic and statistical manual of mental disorders*, 4th edn. Washington, DC: American Psychiatric Association.

Andrews, B., Brewin, C.R., & Rose, S. (2003). Gender, social support, and PTSD in victims of violent crime. *Journal of Traumatic Stress*, 16(4), 421–427.

Basoglu, M., Salcioglu, E., & Livanou, M. (2002). Traumatic stress responses in earthquake survivors in Turkey. *Journal of Traumatic Stress*, 15(4), 269–276.

Brady, K.T., & Back, S.E. (2002). Gender and the psychopharmacological treatment of PTSD. In: R. Kimerling, P. Ouimette, & J. Wolfe (Eds.), *Gender and PTSD* (pp. 335–348). New York: Guilford Press.

Brady, K.T., Pearlstein, T., Asnis, G.M., Baker, D.G., Rothbaum, B., Sikes, C.R., et al. (2000). Efficacy and safety of sertraline treatment of posttraumatic stress disorder: A randomized controlled trial. *Journal of the American Medical Association, 283*(14), 1837–1844.

Breslau, N. (2002). Gender differences in trauma and posttraumatic stress disorder. *Journal of Gender Specific Medicine, 5*(1), 34–40.

Breslau, N., Davis, G.C., Andreski, P., Peterson, E.L., & Schultz, L.R. (1997). Sex differences in posttraumatic stress disorder. *Archives of General Psychiatry, 54*(11), 1044–1048.

Breslau, N., Kessler, R.C., Chilcoat, H.D., Schultz, L.R., Davis, G.C., & Andreski, P. (1998). Trauma and posttraumatic stress disorder in the community. *Archives of General Psychiatry, 55*, 626–632.

Breslau, N., Chilcoat, H.D., Kessler, R.C., Peterson, E.L., & Lucia, V.C. (1999). Vulnerability to assaultive violence: Further specification of the sex difference in post-traumatic stress disorder. *Psychological Medicine, 29*, 813–821.

Brewin, C.R., Andrews, B., & Valentine, J.D. (2000). Meta-analysis of risk factors for posttraumatic stress disorder in trauma-exposed adults. *Journal of Consulting and Clinical Psychology, 68*(5), 748–766.

Bryant, R.A., & Harvey, A.G. (2003). Gender differences in the relationship between acute stress disorder and posttraumatic stress disorder following motor vehicle accidents. *Australian and New Zealand Journal of Psychiatry, 37*(2), 226–229.

Cason, D., Grubaugh, A., & Resick, P. (2002). Gender and PTSD treatment: Efficacy and effectiveness. In: R. Kimerling, P. Ouimette, & J. Wolfe (Eds.), *Gender and PTSD* (pp. 305–334). New York: Guilford Press.

Chung, R.C.-Y., & Bemak, F. (2002). Revisiting the California Southeast Asian mental health needs assessment data: An examination of refugee ethnic and gender differences. *Journal of Counseling and Development, 80*(1), 111–119.

Creamer, M., Burgess, P., & McFarlane, A.C. (2001). Post-traumatic stress disorder: Findings from the Australian national survey of mental health and well-being. *Psychological Medicine, 31*(7), 1237–1247.

Davidson, J., Rothbaum, B.O., van der Kolk, B.A., Sikes, C.R., & Farfel, G.M. (2001). Multicenter, double-blind comparison of sertraline and placebo in the treatment of posttraumatic stress disorder. *Archives of General Psychiatry, 58*(5), 485–492.

de Jong, J., Komproe, I.H., Van Ommeren, M., El Masri, M., Araya, M., Khaled, N., et al. (2001). Lifetime events and posttraumatic stress disorder in 4 postconflict settings. *Journal of the American Medical Association, 286*(5), 555–562.

Ehlers, A., & Clark, D.M. (2000). A cognitive model of posttraumatic stress disorder. *Behaviour Research and Therapy, 38*(4), 319–345.

Feiring, C., Taska, L., & Lewis, M. (1999). Age and gender differences in children's and adolescents' adaptation to sexual abuse. *Child Abuse and Neglect, 23*(2), 115–128.

Foa, E.B., & Rothbaum, B.O. (1998). *Treating the trauma of rape: Cognitive-behavioral therapy for PTSD.* New York: Guilford Press.

Foa, E.B., Riggs, D.S., & Gershuny, B.S. (1995). Arousal, numbing, and intrusion: Symptom structure of PTSD following assault. *American Journal of Psychiatry, 152*(1), 116–120.

Foa, E.B., Keane, T.M., & Friedman, M.J. (2000). *Effective treatments for PTSD: Practice guidelines from the International Society for Traumatic Stress Studies.* New York: Guilford Press.

Foster, J.D., Kuperminc, G.P., & Price, A.W. (2004). Gender differences in posttraumatic stress and related symptoms among inner-city minority youth exposed to community violence. *Journal of Youth and Adolescence, 33*(1), 59–69.

Freedman, S., Gluck, N., Tuval-Mashiach, R., Brandes, D., Peri, T., & Shalev, A.Y. (2002). Gender differences in responses to traumatic events: A prospective study. *Journal of Traumatic Stress, 15*, 407–414.

Fullerton, C.S., Ursano, R.J., Epstein, R.S., Crowley, B., Vance, K., Kao, T.C., et al. (2001). Gender differences in posttraumatic stress disorder after motor vehicle accidents. *American Journal of Psychiatry, 158*(9), 1486–1491.

Gavranidou, M., & Rosner, R. (2003). The weaker sex? Gender and post-traumatic stress disorder. *Depression and Anxiety, 17*(3), 130–139.

Goenjian, A.K., Steinberg, A.M., Najarian, L.M., Fairbanks, L.A., Tashjian, M., & Pynoos, R.S. (2000). Prospective study of posttraumatic stress, anxiety, and depressive reactions after earthquake and political violence. *American Journal of Psychiatry, 157*(6), 911–916.

Goenjian, A.K., Molina, L., Steinberg, A.M., Fairbanks, L.A., Alvarez, M.L., Goenjian, H.A., et al. (2001). Posttraumatic stress and depressive reactions among Nicaraguan adolescents after hurricane mitch. *American Journal of Psychiatry, 158*(5), 788–794.

Greening, L., Stoppelbein, L., & Docter, R. (2002). The mediating effects of attributional style and event-specific attributions on postdisaster adjustment. *Cognitive Therapy and Research, 26*(2), 261–274.

Herman, J.L. (1992). *Trauma and recovery: The aftermath of violence from domestic abuse to political terror.* New York: Basic Books.

Hertzberg, M.A., Feldman, M.E., Beckham, J.C., Kudler, H.S., & Davidson, J.R.T. (2000). Lack of efficacy for fluoxetine in PTSD: A placebo controlled trial in combat veterans. *Annals of Clinical Psychiatry, 12*(2), 101–105.

Hobfoll, S.E., Johnson, R.J., Ennis, N., & Jackson, A.P. (2003). Resource loss, resource gain, and emotional outcomes among inner city women. *Journal of Personality and Social Psychology, 84*(3), 632–643.

Kessler, R.C., McGonagle, K.A., Zhao, S., Nelson, C.B., Hughes, M., Eshleman, S., et al. (1994). Lifetime and 12-month prevalence of DSM-III-R psychiatric disorders in the United States. *Archives of General Psychiatry, 51*, 8–19.

Kessler, R.C., Sonnega, A., Hughes, M., & Nelson, C.B. (1995). Posttraumatic stress disorder in the national comorbidity survey. *Archives of General Psychiatry, 52*, 1048–1060.

Kessler, R.C., Zhao, S., Katz, S.J., Kouzis, A.C., Frank, R.G., Edlund, M., et al. (1999). Past-year use of outpatient services for psychiatric problems in the National Comorbidity Survey. *American Journal of Psychiatry, 156*, 115–123.

Kimerling, R., Ouimette, P., & Wolfe, J. (Eds.). (2002). *Gender and PTSD.* New York: Guilford Press.

Korten, A., & Henderson, S. (2000). The Australian national survey of mental health and well-being. *British Journal of Psychiatry, 177*, 325–330.

Livanou, M., Baolu, M., Salciolu, E., & Kalendar, D. (2002). Traumatic stress responses in treatment-seeking earthquake survivors in Turkey. *Journal of Nervous and Mental Disease*, *190*(12), 816–823.

Madakasira, S., & O'Brien, K.F. (1987). Acute posttraumatic stress disorder in victims of a natural disaster. *Journal of Nervous and Mental Disease*, *175*(5), 286–290.

McLean, L.M., & Gallop, R. (2003). Implications of childhood sexual abuse for adult borderline personality disorder and complex posttraumatic stress disorder. *American Journal of Psychiatry*, *160*(2), 369–371.

Norris, F.H., Perilla, J.L., Ibanez, G.E., & Murphy, A.D. (2001a). Sex differences in symptoms of posttraumatic stress: Does culture play a role? *Journal of Traumatic Stress*, *14*(1), 7–28.

Norris, F.H., Perilla, J.L., & Murphy, A.D. (2001b). Postdisaster stress in the United States and Mexico: A cross-cultural test of the multicriterion conceptual model of posttraumatic stress disorder. *Journal of Abnormal Psychology*, *110*(4), 553–563.

Norris, F.H., Foster, J.D., & Weisshaar, D.L. (2002). The epidemiology of gender differences in PTSD across developmental, societal, and research contexts. In: R. Kimerling, P. Ouimette, & J. Wolfe (Eds.), *Gender and PTSD* (pp. 3–42). New York: Guilford Press.

Norris, F.H., Murphy, A.D., Baker, C.K., Perilla, J.L., Rodriguez, F.G., & Rodriguez, J.D. (2003). Epidemiology of trauma and posttraumatic stress disorder in Mexico. *Journal of Abnormal Psychology*, *112*(4), 646–656.

North, C.S., Nixon, S.J., Shariat, S., Mallonee, S., McMillen, J.C., Spitznagel, E.L., et al. (1999). Psychiatric disorders among survivors of the Oklahoma City bombing. *Journal of the American Medical Association*, *282*(8), 755–762.

Ozer, E.J., Best, S.R., Lipsey, T.L., & Weiss, D.S. (2003). Predictors of posttraumatic stress disorder and symptoms in adults: A meta-analysis. *Psychological Bulletin*, *129*(1), 52–73.

Pierce, J.M., Newton, T.L., Buckley, T.C., & Keane, T.M. (2002). Gender and psychophysiology of PTSD. In: R. Kimerling, P. Ouimette, & J. Wolfe (Eds.), *Gender and PTSD* (pp. 177–204). New York: Guilford Press.

Pigott, T.A. (1999). Gender differences in the epidemiology and treatment of anxiety disorders. *Journal of Clinical Psychiatry*, *60*(Suppl 18), 4–15.

Pulcino, T., Galea, S., Ahern, J., Resnick, H., Foley, M., & Vlahov, D. (2003). Posttraumatic stress in women after the September 11 terrorist attacks in New York City. *Journal of Womens Health*, *12*(8), 809–820.

Stein, M.B., Walker, J.R., Hazen, A.L., & Forde, D.R. (1997). Full and partial posttraumatic stress disorder: Findings from a community survey. *American Journal of Psychiatry*, *154*, 1114–1119.

Tarrier, N., Sommerfield, C., Pilgrim, H., & Faragher, B. (2000). Factors associated with outcome of cognitive-behavioural treatment of chronic post-traumatic stress disorder. *Behaviour Research and Therapy*, *38*(2), 191–202.

Tolin, D.F., & Foa, E.B. (2002). Gender and PTSD: A cognitive model. In: R. Kimerling, P. Ouimette, & J. Wolfe (Eds.), *Gender and PTSD* (pp. 76–97). New York: Guilford Press.

Tucker, P., Zaninelli, R., Yehuda, R., Ruggiero, L., Dillingham, K., & Pitts, C.D. (2001). Paroxetine in the treatment of chronic posttraumatic stress disorder: Results of a placebo-controlled, flexible-dosage trial. *Journal of Clinical Psychiatry*, *62*(11), 860–868.

Ursano, R.J., Fullerton, C.S., Epstein, R.S., Crowley, B., Kao, T.-C., Vance, K., et al. (1999). Acute and chronic posttraumatic stress disorder in motor vehicle accident victims. *American Journal of Psychiatry, 156*(4), 589–595.

van der Kolk, B.A., Dreyfuss, D., Michaels, M., Shera, D., et al. (1994). Fluoxetine in post-traumatic stress disorder. *Journal of Clinical Psychiatry, 55*(12), 517–522.

World Health Organization (1993). *The ICD-10 classification of mental and behavioural disorders: Diagnostic criteria for research*. Geneva: World Health Organization.

Yen, S., Shea, M.T., Battle, C.L., Johnson, D.M., Zlotnick, C., Dolan-Sewell, R., et al. (2002). Traumatic exposure and posttraumatic stress disorder in borderline, schizotypal, avoidant, and obsessive-compulsive personality disorders: Findings from the collaborative longitudinal personality disorders study. *Journal of Nervous and Mental Disease, 190*(8), 510–518.

Zlotnick, C., Zakriski, A.L., Shea, M.T., & Costello, E. (1996). The long-term sequelae of sexual abuse: Support for a complex posttraumatic stress disorder. *Journal of Traumatic Stress, 9*(2), 195–205.

Zohar, J., Amital, D., Miodownik, C., Kotler, M., Bleich, A., Lane, R.M., et al. (2002). Double-blind placebo-controlled pilot study of sertraline in military veterans with posttraumatic stress disorder. *Journal of Clinical Psychopharmacology, 22*(2), 190–195.

6

Domestic violence and its impact on mood disorder in women: Implications for mental health workers

Alison L. Warburton and Kathryn M. Abel

Centre for Women's Mental Health Research, Division of Psychiatry, University of Manchester, Williamson Building, Manchester, UK

Physical, emotional, and sexual abuse of women by an intimate partner is strongly associated with depression, anxiety and anxiety disorders, and a variety of other psychiatric problems, including substance abuse, dissociation and dissociative disorders, and post-traumatic stress disorder (PTSD). Intimate partner violence, or domestic violence, affects an estimated one in four women and, along with depression, has been recognised by the World Health Organisation (1998) to be a significant public health concern. Domestic violence also affects children, who may themselves be subject to abuse and/or witness the violence. Both girl and boy child victims of abuse have significantly higher rates of childhood mental disorders, anxiety disorders, personality disorders and major affective disorders, and witnessing violence as a child has particularly been associated with anxiety in girls (Spataro et al., 2004). Despite the recognition that domestic violence is a major risk factor for depression and that depression adds significantly to the global burden of disease for women (Ustun et al., 2004), to date detailed exploration of possible causes and systematic studies of interventions are lacking. Depression is commonly treated without knowledge of the context of violence in which it might occur. If mental health professionals placed more emphasis on the experience of violence as a cause of depression and anxiety, some of this burden might be reduced. In this chapter we (1) define domestic violence, (2) consider its mental health outcomes, (3) highlight barriers that might prevent health professionals' adequate assessment of the problem, and (4) suggest possible solutions.

Defining the problem

What is domestic violence?

"Domestic violence" (often referred to as intimate partner violence/spouse abuse) has been defined as a pattern of coercive control consisting of a physical, sexual and/or psychological assault against a current or former intimate partner (Flitcraft et al.,

1992). Whilst in the UK there is currently no legal definition of domestic violence, generally it is considered to be an act carried out with the intention or perceived intention of physically injuring another person (Straus et al., 1980). It encompasses a wide range of behaviours including threats, physical, sexual, emotional, verbal, and financial abuse.

Domestic violence usually refers to violence between adults, although it is recognised to affect children who may live within a violent relationship. Worldwide, women and children are most often the victims and are especially vulnerable to physical aggression, violence and abuse by family members, caretakers and intimate partners (WHO, 1998). In the majority of cases, the abuser is a man (Stanko, 2000; Williamson, 2000). Compared with men, women are more likely to experience domestic violence at some point in their lives (Home Office, 2000) and are twice as likely to be injured by a partner (Mirrlees-Black, 1999): 74% (560,000) of victims of domestic violence in the UK are women (Kershaw et al., 2000). Men may also experience abuse within their relationships, but are less likely to report being hurt, frightened, or upset and are also less likely to be subjected to repeated abuse (Mirrlees-Black, 1999).

Incidence and prevalence

Ten to fifty per cent of women experience domestic violence at some point in their lives (Watts & Zimmerman, 2002; WHO, 1998) and annual prevalence estimates range from under 1% (Kershaw et al., 2000) to roughly one in nine of the adult female population (Stanko et al., 1998). In the UK, it is estimated that one incident of domestic violence occurs every 6–20 s (Stanko, 2000), that 70% of incidents result in injury (Kershaw et al., 2000) and that approximately every 3 days a woman dies as a result of domestic violence (Home Office, 2000). For a number of reasons these figures are likely to be underestimates: women feel ashamed of living in an abusive relationship; they suppose the abuse is their own fault; and they often are unwilling to disclose abuse (Baird, 2002). Reporting rates tend to be higher in clinical populations, such as those accessing obstetric services (Bacchus et al., 2002) and amongst women psychiatric patients (in-patients and out-patients), than in community samples (Carlile, 1991; Carmen et al., 1984; Dienemann et al., 2000; Post et al., 1980). Incidence and prevalence rates from community samples of women range from 1% to 20% (e.g., Straus & Gelles, 1986; Tjaden & Thoennes, 2000) whilst estimates from clinical samples tend to be even higher at 6–23% of women (McCauley et al., 1998).

Pattern of abuse

Domestic violence involves a pattern of abusive and controlling behaviour that tends to increase in severity and frequency over time and to continue beyond the ending of the relationship. It typically occurs on several occasions: in 1999, 57% of sufferers of violence had been re-victimised, not necessarily by the same perpetrator (Kershaw et al., 2000), and a third of those abused by partners had reportedly been abused by another person (Porcellini et al., 2003). The abuse can begin at any time – in the first year or after many years in a relationship. It may begin, continue, or escalate after a couple have separated and may happen not only in the home but also in public settings (Kershaw et al., 2000). People experience domestic violence regardless of their social group, class, age, race, disability, sexuality, and lifestyle, although some studies have shown that risk of exposure to violence in the home is greater in families of lower socio-economic status (Wright & Kariya, 1997). Violence is often aimed at reinforcing the perpetrator's authority and control (Jewkes, 2002), particularly with the physically and mentally ill (Home Office, 2000).

Predictors of risk of domestic violence

Being a woman is the single most important risk factor for experiencing domestic violence (Walker et al., 1999). Women are also more likely to be raped, assaulted, or murdered by intimate partners than by strangers (Mahoney et al., 2001). Generally, however, risk factors relate to male perpetrators of violence, with studies suggesting that women at greatest risk of injury from domestic violence are those with male partners who abuse alcohol/drugs, are unemployed, poorly educated, and carry ex-partner status (Kyriacou et al., 1999). Risk of violence against women is increased in separating couples, women are at greatest risk as they attempt to leave (Kurtz, 1996), in poor households and in situations where women lack their own economic resources and depend on their partners (Home Office, 2000). Women under 25 (Ratner, 1993) with higher educational levels than their partners are also at greater risk (Kyriacou et al., 1999).

Features associated with an elevated risk of domestic violence include depression (Saunders & Hamberger, 1993), pregnancy (Richardson et al., 2001) and previous childhood sexual abuse (Bifulco & Moran, 1998; Calam et al., 1998; McCauley et al., 1997). Depressed women are significantly more likely to have experienced severe combined (physical, emotional, and sexual) abuse than women who are not depressed, even after adjusting for other significant sociodemographic variables such as being unmarried, poor education, low income, being unemployed or receiving a pension, or being abused as a child (Hegarty et al., 2004). Some have suggested that women who suffer from depression and anxiety disorders may be drawn to or attract dominant or aggressive partners, and/or partners with some degree of emotional problems, unstable personality, substance misuse, or psychosis (Royal College of Psychiatrists, 2002), thus increasing their vulnerability to and likelihood of experiencing abuse.

Domestic violence and pregnancy

One of the times of highest risk for women experiencing domestic violence is during pregnancy. Studies outside the UK have estimated that between 5% (Torres et al.,

2000) and 22% (Purwar et al., 1999; Renker, 1999) of pregnant women are abused by their partners, whilst a recent UK study reported the prevalence as 2.5% (Mezey et al., 2003). Overall, prevalence rates of violence during pregnancy of up to 34% have been reported. The variations in reported rates are attributable to differences in definitions of violence and in the populations studied, as well as differences in the frequency and timing of the interviews with the subjects (Bacchus et al., 2004; Gazmararian et al., 1996; Huth-Bocks, 2002; Johnson et al., 2003).

In a study of 290 pregnant women randomly selected from public and private pre-natal clinics, almost 30% of cases of abuse reported that the first episode occurred during pregnancy (Helton et al., 1987). If a pregnancy is unintended or unwanted, the risk of abuse increases fourfold (Heise, 1993). A common explanation for the increased risk of violence during pregnancy is that the father/male partner feels threatened by the impending birth, which is manifest as frustration and directed back at the perceived source: the mother and her unborn child. The underlying causes of the stress experienced by the father are unclear (Moore, 1999).

Whilst there appears to be an association between pregnancy and the postpartum period and the initiation of violence within a relationship or an increase in the sever-ity or frequency of abuse (e.g., McFarlane et al., 1999; Mezey & Bewley, 1997), some researchers (e.g., Gazmararian et al., 1996) have suggested that physical violence does not seem to be initiated or increase during pregnancy for most abused women. In a study of 199 abused pregnant women, 30% of the women were abused the year before but not during pregnancy (McFarlane et al., 1999). It could be that most women are already in a pattern of violence and only some experience abuse for the first time during pregnancy (Moore, 1999). Regardless, violence during pregnancy poses a threat to health and at its extreme can result in the death of the mother and her unborn child (NICE, 2001).

Physical abuse during pregnancy has been associated with substance abuse, depres-sion and other mental health symptoms (Martin et al., 1998; Newberger et al., 1992). In a study of 85 prenatal care patients the links between women's experiences of domestic violence and their use of substances became stronger during pregnancy (Martin et al., 2003). Women who experience domestic violence are also more likely to begin their antenatal care late and/or to describe their pregnancy as unwanted or unplanned (Lipsky et al., 2004; Taggart & Mattson, 1996). Inadequate care during pregnancy may lead to physical complications or an exacerbation of pre-existing problems, which can result in admission to hospital. In a retrospective cohort study of women with a police-reported incident of domestic violence during pregnancy (Lipsky, 2004), those reporting any domestic violence during pregnancy were twice as likely as unexposed women to experience an antenatal hospitalisation not associ-ated with delivery; they were also more likely to have been hospitalised with a sub-stance abuse-related diagnosis (adjusted OR 2.70; 95% CI 1.52, 4.78) or a mental health-related diagnosis (adjusted OR 1.93; 95% CI 0.96, 3.91). Physical abuse was more strongly associated with antenatal hospitalisation than non-physical abuse or abuse overall. Also, in a cross-sectional survey of 200 women receiving antenatal/postnatal care, higher levels of depressive symptoms were significantly associated with a history of domestic violence and both a history of domestic violence and increased depression scores were significantly associated with obstetric complications (Bacchus et al., 2004).

Adverse pregnancy outcomes could also be the result of associated factors such as smoking, illicit drug use, alcohol use, and anxiety and depression (Bacchus et al., 2001). There is an association between psychological well-being and physical health during pregnancy. Symptoms of depression and anxiety may be associated with poor self-care and with adverse physical health outcomes (Campbell et al., 1997; Schulberg et al., 1987).

Domestic violence and child abuse

Having been the victim of childhood sexual abuse, or having witnessed family violence as a child also enhances the risk of domestic violence as an adult (McCauley et al., 1997; Walker et al., 1999). From a sample of 153 women attending a community counselling service, Briere (1984) reported that, compared with women with no history of childhood sexual abuse, women with such a history were significantly more likely to report a fear of men, anxiety attacks, and problems with anger: 49% of these women had also been abused in an adult relationship. The severity of previous abuse also predicts the severity of mental health symptoms (Golding, 1999; McCauley et al., 1997). Lifetime and current prevalence of major depression is also higher amongst women with a history of childhood sexual abuse (Stein et al., 1988). Furthermore, where the abuse involved penetrative sexual intercourse, the likelihood of psychiatric admissions following domestic violence has been reported as sixteen times greater than for women subject to lesser forms of childhood abuse (Mullen et al., 1993).

The mental health outcomes of domestic violence

It has been suggested that most mental health-care providers will treat victims of domestic violence, although many will be unaware that their patients have formerly or recently been abused (National Advisory Council, 2001). Women suffer long-term adverse health consequences even after abuse has ended (Campbell & Lewandowski, 1997) and these effects can manifest as poor health status, high use of health and mental health services and poor quality of life (Wisner et al., 1999). Domestic violence may also precipitate psychiatric admission (Carlile, 1991). However, abused women do not generally present with obvious trauma (Dearwater et al., 1998).

Fear of violence as well as the actual experiences of violence are both stressful, and as high levels of stress may be associated with mental disorders (Coyne & Downey,

1991), it is anticipated that violence is an important determinant of risk for a number of adverse mental health outcomes. In a survey of 200 women who had experienced domestic violence and sought help from the Women's Aid Federation (England), 69% reported fearing for their emotional well being and 60% for their mental health. Sixty-eight per cent had had contact with health services in relation to the violence; recurring themes were admission to psychiatric wards and descriptions of mental health breakdowns (Humphreys & Thiara, 2002). Additionally, 93% of women experiencing chronic domestic violence reported emotional distress, whilst 75% of women experiencing intermittent violence reported being "very upset". Women were also fearful: according to the British Crime Survey (BCS)[1], 80% of women exposed to chronic abuse and 52% of those exposed to intermittent violence reported being very frightened during the incident and remaining fearful around the incident (Mirrlees-Black, 1999).

Depression and suicide

Although to some extent the rates of mood disorders associated with domestic violence depend on the sample studied, it is likely that domestic violence and fear of domestic violence are important among the causes of mood disorder in women worldwide. Depression and PTSD, which have substantial co-morbidity, are the most prevalent mental health sequelae of domestic violence (Cascardi et al., 1999; Golding, 2002; Ratner, 1993; and see also Chapter 5). In one study, 42.9% of cases of current (past 30 days) domestic-violence-related PTSD also had major depressive disorder (MDD) and most cases of current MDD occurred in women who also had current domestic-violence-related PTSD (Stein & Kennedy, 2001). Compared with non-abused women, abused women are up to three times more likely to be diagnosed with depression (Stark & Flitcraft, 1996), with the highest rates found amongst women using domestic violence shelter services. Here, estimated rates of depression vary from 38% to 83% (Cascardi et al., 1999). There is also evidence that domestic violence triggers first episodes of depression (Campbell & Soeken, 1999), and severity of depressive and PTSD symptoms have been shown to be highly correlated (Stein & Kennedy, 2001).

The experience of physical abuse may be important in the aetiology of depression in battered women. Campbell et al. (1997) found, in a sample of 164 battered women recruited through newspaper and bulletin board advertisements, that 28% were moderately to severely depressed and 11% severely depressed, with physical abuse by a partner, and childhood physical abuse being amongst the significant predictors of the depression. A woman's capacity to take care of herself is seen as a protective

---

[1] The British Crime Survey (BCS) asks adults in private households about their experience of victimisation in the previous 12 months and moved to an annual cycle from 2001/02, with 40,000 interviews of people aged 16 or over taking place per year.

factor mitigating the development of depression (Campbell et al., 1997). However, because of the difficulties in accessing a representative and large enough sample of women, no systematic determinants of outcome studies have yet addressed these questions adequately.

Stark & Flitcraft (1996) estimate that an abused woman is five times more likely to attempt suicide than a non-abused woman. One review of 13 different studies reported prevalence rates of suicide or suicidality ranging from 4.6% to 77% among abused women – a weighted mean prevalence of 17.9% (Golding, 1999). Furthermore, alcohol and substance misuse is also associated with domestic violence (see Chapter 3), and this may further increase suicide risk in women (McCloud et al., 2004). Suicidal tendencies/suicidality (actual attempts at suicide, and/or suicidal thoughts) have been associated with domestic violence, especially in women experiencing sexual assault (Housekamp & Foy, 1991).

As mentioned above, women with a history of childhood sexual abuse are at increased risk of experiencing abuse as an adult. Furthermore, Gladstone et al. (2004) reported such women were more likely to have attempted suicide and/or engaged in deliberate self-harm, to have become depressed earlier in life, as well as being more likely to have panic disorder, and to report a recent assault (Gladstone et al., 2004). The severity of childhood sexual abuse is associated with higher rates of depression in adulthood (Cheasty et al., 1998) and often predicts a chronic course of depression in women (Zlotnick et al., 1995). There have been several studies that have investigated the association between sexual abuse in childhood and subsequent incidents of deliberate self-harm in women (e.g., Boudewyn & Liem, 1995; Gratz et al., 2002; Peleikis et al., 2004). Romans et al. (1995), in a random community sample of 252 women who had been sexually abused as children, found a clear statistical association between sexual abuse in childhood and later self-harm; the effect was mostly marked in those subjected to frequent intrusive abuse. Sexual abuse in childhood was found to be associated with later incidents of deliberate self-harm, and self-harm was associated with becoming involved in further abusive relationships as an adult. Similarly, interview data from 126 women with depressive disorders consecutively referred to a Mood Disorders Unit found that women with a history of childhood sexual abuse reported more childhood physical abuse, childhood emotional abuse, and parental conflict in the home, compared to women without such a history (Gladstone et al., 2004).

PTSD and anxiety disorders

Estimated rates of PTSD in abused women vary from 31% to 84%, with the highest rates reported in women using shelter services (Cascardi et al., 1999): 84% of battered women in shelters met criteria for PTSD (Kemp et al., 1991). Compared with non-abused women, the prevalence of PTSD is much higher in abused women (weighted mean odds ratio 3.74). Severity of abuse, previous trauma and partner dominance have all been identified as important precursors of abuse-related PTSD (Campbell et al., 1995; Silva et al., 1997). In one study, a convenience sample of 160 abused, post-abused, and non-abused women, the rate of PTSD was elevated in those who had been abused, and even women who had been out of the abusive relationship an average of 9 years continued to experience PTSD symptoms (Woods, 2000).

"Battered woman syndrome" has been described as a mental health problem arising from chronic and persistent domestic violence and characterised by psychological, emotional and behavioural deficits (British Medical Association (BMA), 1998; Chambliss, 1997). The central features include "learned helplessness", passivity and paralysis (BMA, 1998). It commonly manifests as denial of the abusive situation and defence of the relationship by the woman (Curnow, 1997) and may, in part, explain why women may be reluctant to leave such relationships.

In a population-based survey in Canada, Ratner (1993) found that, compared to non-abused women, those who had been abused experienced higher levels of insomnia and social dysfunction. Abused women are also more likely to suffer from anxiety, psychosomatic symptoms and eating disorders (Campbell, 2002). In a general population survey, 46% of 366 women who had experienced domestic-violence experienced symptoms of an anxiety disorder (Gelles & Harrop, 1989); the effects were stronger in those experiencing physical violence than those experiencing only psychological violence. However, anxiety disorders such as panic and generalised anxiety disorder appear to be less common than MDD in the setting of domestic violence (Stein & Kennedy, 2001).

Domestic violence and substance misuse

Alcohol and drug use have been associated with both the perpetration and experience of violence and increase the risk of harm, both physical and psychological, to partners and children of the household (Masten et al., 1990; Mirrlees-Black, 1999; Mullender & Morley, 1994; Stanko et al., 1998; and see Chapter 3). Causal mechanisms are varied and difficult to establish, and it may be that the substance abuse leads to the violence, or conversely that the violence leads to the substance abuse. Women are more likely to be exposed to violence if their partner misuses substances, which may, in turn, be associated with substance misuse in the woman either in response to the trauma or not. Those who misuse substances and alcohol are also more likely to perpetrate domestic violence (Royal College of Psychiatrists, 2002) and to have a co-morbid mental illness (Glass & Jackson, 1988; Hall & Farrell, 1997; Marsden et al., 2000). The mechanism by which a woman's misuse of substances makes her more likely to be exposed to violence can be separated into direct and social effects (Royal College of Psychiatrists, 2002). Direct effects include: disinhibition, which may reduce the threshold for violent behaviour; intoxication, which may contribute to violence through increased irritability; and paranoia, which increases the likelihood of violence. Social effect mechanisms include interpersonal strife that acts as a trigger for violence, and addiction that confers a dependence on the abusive partner for funds (Royal College of Psychiatrists, 2002).

Abused women frequently develop addictions to alcohol, illicit drugs and tranquillisers in response to the trauma (Gerbert et al., 1996; Stark & Flitcraft, 1996). Women who have experienced physical or psychological violence are fifteen times more likely to abuse alcohol and nine times more likely to abuse drugs than nonabused women (Stark & Flitcraft, 1996). In the review of Golding (1999), the prevalence of alcohol abuse or dependence among abused women ranged from 6.6% to 44% (weighted mean 18.5%) and rates of drug abuse or dependence ranged from 7% to 25% (weighted mean 8.9%). Furthermore, drug use has been shown to increase the risk of victimisation (Kilpatrick et al., 1997) and both alcohol and/or drug dependency may further increase the woman's reliance on her partner and reduce her capacity to initiate change (Royal College of Psychiatrists, 2002). A cycle of substance abuse and victimisation may therefore be likely to ensue (Campbell, 2002) and the woman may find herself in a situation of "learned helplessness" as she becomes passive, accepting and paralysed by the unremitting violence (Walker, 1979). It is thus important to understand and address the complex interrelationships between domestic violence, and substance abuse problems (Campbell, 2002).

Abused women frequently present with co-morbid substance abuse and depression and anxiety disorders (Haver & Dahlgram, 1995; Helzer & Pryzbeck, 1998; O'Connor et al., 1994), both of which are linked to experience of abuse trauma. Unfortunately, however, women co-presenting with both depression and substance misuse problems have less access to appropriate health-care services than those presenting with only a single problem (Glover-Reed & Mowbray, 1999). Similarly, abused women with substance misuse problems have increased difficulties accessing support services, such as women's refuges.

Effects of domestic violence on children

In 90% of domestic violence incidents occurring within families, children are in the same or next room (Home Office, 2000). Children who are either present at or hear incidents of domestic violence can be deeply affected and may suffer longterm behavioural, physical and psychological consequences (see NICHD, 2002). In 1998/99, an estimated 8% of children aged four to seven were reported to have seen violent behaviour at home and witnessing violence was concurrently associated with overt aggression for girls and boys; furthermore, anxiety among the girls was predictive of overt aggression 2 and 4 years later (Moss, 2003). The precise nature of a child's reaction will, of course, vary according to their age and stage of development; for example, infants and toddlers may experience problems with trust, whilst pre-school children may react through behaviours such as aggression, clinging, or cruelty to animals (Wolfe et al., 2003).

The development of unborn children may also be affected. A woman abused during pregnancy is more likely to respond to the abuse with self-destructive behaviour, for example alcohol/drug abuse (Baird, 2002; Bhatt, 1998) and there is a weak but significant association between abuse during pregnancy and low-birthweight infants (Silva et al., 1997). Women abused during pregnancy also show higher rates of miscarriage (Stewart & Cecutti, 1993), and are more likely to suffer postnatal depression (Zeitlin et al., 1999). Studies have also associated abuse during pregnancy with antepartum haemorrhage, premature labour, pre-eclampsia, and foetal distress (Gazmararian et al., 2000; Stewart & Cecutti, 1993; Webster et al., 1996). Domestic violence also impacts on maternal–foetal bonding; mothers abused during pregnancy may be less likely to bond well with their foetus and subsequently their child (Zeitlin et al., 1999). This is turn may have detrimental effects on the child's social, cognitive, emotional and behavioural development (Wolfe et al., 2003) and may also lead to subsequent depression and other mental health problems in the child (Spataro et al., 2004).

Barriers to change

Detecting domestic violence

Many women who experience domestic violence go undetected in health-care settings (BMA, 1998) and health professionals are only likely to enquire about domestic violence if there is a physical injury – but, even then, women frequently receive treatment for their injuries without being asked about the cause (Plichta, 1992). Several communication barriers prevent women from speaking to health professionals: fear of reprisal, fear of losing custody of children, shame, self-blame, humiliation, denial of the situation, and a lack of understanding by others (Gerbert et al., 1996; Gremillion & Kanof, 1996). A woman may also be reluctant to disclose abuse if she feels her provider is rushed and does not have adequate time to listen or is only interested in discussing her medical or physical complaints (Mayer & Coulter, 2002). Thus, communication is key, and improved communication between service user/provider, health professionals, and other key agencies is needed (Mayer & Coulter, 2002). Domestic violence is a common cause of injury in women, and although such injuries are usually not severe enough to require treatment (Plichta, 1992), it is the consequences of the violence, for example depression, that cause the most problems. Many health-care professions, for example psychiatric services, will have repeated opportunities to observe a situation or ask about domestic violence.

There are many reasons for the low rates of detection of domestic violence in health-care settings. These include fear and apprehension by staff, alongside lack of

---

BOX 6.1 Reasons cited by the BMA (1998) for the non-identification of domestic violence victims in a health-care setting

- Doctors' fears/experiences of exploring domestic violence.
- Lack of knowledge of community resources.
- Fear of offending the woman.
- Fear of jeopardising the doctor–patient relationship.
- Lack of time; training and/or control.
- Infrequent patient visits.
- Unresponsiveness of patients to questions.
- Feeling of powerlessness; not being able to fix the situation.

BOX 6.2 Predictors of domestic violence include (see Department of Health, 2000)

- Frequently missed appointments.
- Injuries inconsistent with explanations of accidental causation.
- Evidence of multiple injuries.
- The woman appearing frightened, excessively anxious and depressed or distressed.

---

awareness, lack of training, lack of time and a feeling of powerlessness because there is no quick fix solution. Many solutions are complex and need to be enacted over long periods (Box 6.1). Health-care professionals may also have encountered domestic violence themselves and may not feel able to offer support to others – a problem which is only beginning to be recognised (Mezey et al., 2003).

Misconceptions by health professionals and the general public about domestic violence may also help explain the lack of effective health-care responses. These include the notion that domestic violence incidence is low; that it is the domain of the individual, and not society, and therefore a private matter between adults (Stanko, 2000); that people experiencing domestic violence prefer to keep it hidden; and that the needs of those who seek help are adequately met within current service provision. These misconceptions pose an important problem for both women and children exposed to violence and attitudes of those working in key agencies, and the public as a whole, need to be changed.

Identification of domestic violence

The identification of individuals experiencing domestic violence is the first step towards ensuring appropriate care. All health-care professionals in contact with patients should be aware of the risks of domestic violence and alert to the possible indicators (Department of Health, 2000). A history of psychiatric illness and/or alcohol/drug dependency is particularly relevant to mental health professionals. Other indicators are shown in Box 6.2.

Early identification can reduce the consequences of domestic violence and decrease the likelihood of further victimisation (Garcia-Moreno, 2002). Without identification, abused women are denied documentation for future court reference and denied education on prevention, safety planning, options for leaving the abuse and referrals to resources in the community (Campbell & Parker, 1996). The children of abused women, who may also be experiencing violence, are also left unprotected.

Introducing protocols or validated screening tools increases rates of identification and documentation of domestic violence (Covington et al., 1997) and professional health-care organisations have called for the routine screening of women for domestic violence (e.g., Heath, 1998; Royal College of Midwives, 1997). Some practitioners, though, have argued that this approach may not be feasible in certain settings and that only selected "at risk" groups of women should be screened (Garcia-Moreno, 2002, Taket et al., 2003). Despite these uncertainties, the Department of Health (UK) and the WHO agree that health services have an important role in tackling domestic violence, and that, in general, asking about abuse is a good thing. However, psychiatric patients, or patients with a psychiatric history, while being at higher risk of having experienced domestic violence, are significantly less likely to be screened by health professionals than non-psychiatric patients (Larkin et al., 2000). Given that a history of psychiatric illness is an indicator of domestic violence, careful screening of women presenting to mental health-care facilities should be a priority in service development.

Unfortunately, there is a lack of evidence of the effectiveness of physician screening (and counselling, and referral) for domestic violence (Rhodes & Levinson, 2003) and a lack of formal assessment of such interventions – in particular from the perspective of the women themselves (Garcia-Moreno, 2002). In a recent review (Wathen & MacMillan, 2003) no studies were identified that examined the effectiveness of screening in terms of improved outcomes for women (as opposed to identification of abuse). Furthermore, some advocates of women's rights have challenged the assumption that disclosure of domestic violence is always beneficial to the woman (O'Connor, 2002).

Disclosing domestic violence

Women experiencing domestic violence are often reluctant to disclose their experiences to others and it has been estimated that only 30% of women seek help after the first or subsequent episode (BMA, 1998). They may be afraid of the situation and fear talking about it to others. They are also likely to feel depressed, insecure and lacking in self-esteem and confidence (Department of Health, 2000). On average, 35 incidents will occur before a woman seeks help (Bewley et al., 1997). Asking for help can be a decisive moment in a woman's life, and may be a first step in a process of leaving a violent relationship (Garcia-Moreno, 2002). However, it is also a time of risk: for example, the woman is at risk of retaliation from her violent partner and of being made

> **BOX 6.3 How mental health-care systems can make a difference**
> - Raise awareness: educate mental health professionals about domestic violence: prevention, detection and treatment.
> - Develop training modules and protocols.
> - Explore underlying problems from which the presenting problem may have arisen.
> - Improve detection of domestic violence: routine or selective screening.
> - Establish health-care outcome measures for evaluating mental health status improvement as response to domestic violence is enhanced.
> - Protect victim health records.
> - Conduct public health campaigns: establish domestic violence as a serious mental health issue.
> - Create protocol and documentation guidelines and disseminate widely.

homeless, which may also affect her children. After close friends and family, women will often turn to health-care professionals for help and support (Baird, 2002), and health professionals should then prioritise a woman's safety and security in any subsequent intervention.

Providing the right environment can be an important incentive to disclosure of domestic violence: confidentiality, privacy, sensitive questioning, and a nonjudgmental attitude are required. Abused women may leave and return to the abuser many times before making the final decision to break (Landenburger, 1998) and it is important that health-care providers try to understand the numerous reasons why women return to their abusers. For example, although the woman may want the violence to end, she may not want the relationship to end: if the perpetrator then demonstrates remorse she will want to believe it is genuine (Williamson, 2000).

Questioning is essential and unless asked directly, very few women voluntarily disclose violence (Bacchus et al., 2003). However, women are mostly willing to be asked about their experiences by health professionals (Mezey et al., 2003), and cite not being asked as a reason for non-disclosure of domestic violence (Mullender & Hague, 2000; Williamson, 2000). In one US study, only 6 out of 476 consecutive women seen by a family practice clinic reported having ever been asked about domestic violence by their general practitioner (GP) (Hamberger et al., 1992).

Clinical and service recommendations

Ways in which services might respond to the issue of domestic violence more effectively include (see also Box 6.3):
- *Raising awareness*: Mental health professionals must work together to develop and deliver public health campaigns that raise public awareness about domestic violence and its health, and mental health, consequences. Such campaigns should

challenge misconceptions, advocate the unacceptability of violence and prioritise domestic violence as a mental health concern. Mental health-care professionals should inform themselves about domestic violence and its impact on health and familiarise themselves with local appropriate support services available to abused women. Mental health professionals must be able to recognise that many mental health problems and their sequelae are more often the result of, rather than the cause of violence (Stark & Flitcraft, 1996).

- *Training*: Health-care workers often lack the fundamental knowledge about domestic violence as well as the necessary skills to identify and discuss violence with women (Cann et al., 2001). Inadequate training prevents professionals from identifying and responding appropriately to domestic violence and more importantly, questioning by untrained staff can be damaging and leave the woman vulnerable to further abuse (Department of Health, 2000). Some countries have recommended that modules on domestic violence and its health consequences are included in the core curricula of all courses taken en-route to becoming a health professional (Department of Health, 1995). This implies that the health outcomes associated with the experience of violence should be introduced at undergraduate level in medical schools, nursing colleges and other health-practitioner-related courses (e.g., health visitor training). At postgraduate/professional level, more practical aspects of health-care responses to domestic violence should be incorporated in training. This should involve working alongside key voluntary sector agencies who have experience in dealing with women exposed to domestic violence and who have developed expertise in training, as well as different professional groups involved in responding to violence, such as the police (Department of Health, 2000). Graduate medical education and training programmes must also address the negative feelings that many physicians associate with helping women experiencing domestic violence – that it is "significant work," difficult and stressful (Garimella et al., 2002). In a postal questionnaire survey of 150 practicing general hospital physicians, Garimella et al. (2002) found that the majority of the 76 respondents (89%) had negative feelings about assisting domestic violence victims.

  For training to be effective and to enable staff to respond appropriately to the needs of women (and children), it must address concerns of power and abuse in the lives of those being trained, at work, and in society and must help providers address their values and attitudes towards violence against women (Garcia-Moreno, 2002). Training that can increase effectiveness of health care and have long-term effects has to be carefully balanced with realities of limited time for participation in training, high-staff turnover, affordability, and sustainability (Garcia-Moreno, 2002).

- *Intervention*: Intervention in the context of domestic violence has several roles: improving detection; reducing rates of abuse/re-abuse; helping the woman validate the violence as inherent in the relationship/acknowledge its occurrence; providing medical treatment, information and support; and facilitating referral. However, it is important to emphasise that the nature of domestic violence means that health professionals assist in a gradual process of empowerment and self-management by the woman of her situation, and a considerable time may elapse before the woman is ready to take definitive action (Stevens, 1997). Therefore, an apparently unsuccessful interaction between a health service provider and an abused woman may actually have been more successful than supposed. Domestic violence interventions are unlikely to provide easily identified outcomes. Rather, if an intervention/interaction empowers a woman to face her situation and/or reduces the number of incidents before she takes definitive action, it may be considered successful. The precise nature of "successful" interventions in domestic violence needs to be defined, and requires further research.

A first step is to develop appropriate screening protocols, and to target high-risk groups of women, including those with a mental illness. These protocols should also include appropriate guidance for the care of screen-positive women and should include, for example, referral to support groups. The benefits of intervention strategies in treating both women and men need to be evaluated and the potential harms assessed. For example, no high-quality evidence exists to evaluate the effectiveness of shelter stays to reduce violence. Among women who spent at least one night in a shelter, there was some evidence that those who received a specific program of advocacy and counselling services experienced a decreased rate of re-abuse and an improved quality of life (Wathen & MacMillan, 2003).

- *Inter-agency collaboration*: Domestic violence is not the sole responsibility of a single agency and it is now accepted that inter-agency strategies need to be developed as part of a multi-agency effort (BMA, 1998; Department of Health, 2002). Health sector professionals remain largely unaware of appropriate agencies that can offer help to abused women (Cann et al., 2001). To date, the voluntary sector has been the main provider of services and support to women. Voluntary organisations have been particularly successful in engaging women in the development of such services; a so-called consumer-led, "bottom-up" approach – increasingly recognised as essential strategy (Hague et al., 2002). In a recent study that explored the extent of consumer participation in inter-agency initiatives, the statutory sector was reported to have no appropriate consultation mechanisms in place, and domestic violence forums overestimated their own effectiveness (Hague et al., 2002). Furthermore, the majority of women interviewed felt their views were overlooked and silenced by service providers and that their needs were inadequately met. Whilst 54% of the women felt that the response of police services to domestic violence had improved following recent attempts to change policy and practice, 75% considered the response of health services to have shown no improvement (Hague et al., 2002).

Mental health-care professionals should develop formal partnerships with other agencies – especially the voluntary sector – and build strategies for intervention in consultation with women. These strategies should determine appropriate methods of training professionals, detecting violence and responding to disclosure, for example by counselling or referral. The identification and modification of factors that will improve the psychological well being of abused women should be considered a high priority for any mental health promotion programme.

Conclusions

Domestic violence affects at least 25% of women and has wide-reaching, long-term physical and mental health consequences. Depression and anxiety disorders, including PTSD, commonly arise. The detection of domestic violence in health-care settings is inadequate. As a result, abused women are denied appropriate support, and their health and that of their children is compromised. A lack of awareness about domestic violence amongst the public, health-care organisations and individual mental health professionals, and a lack of training in how to identify and respond to abused women is an important barrier to change. As a first step to improving mental health service responses to women exposed to domestic violence, health-care organisations and individual mental health-care professionals must develop training to improve their knowledge and understanding of domestic violence and its impact upon women. They will then be in a better position to improve detection rates by developing and implementing screening protocols. Appropriate interventions that improve the health and well being of screen-positive women (and their children) might then be instigated. Evaluation of such interventions is a key research priority.

REFERENCES

Bacchus, L., Bewley, S., & Mezey, G. (2001). Domestic violence in pregnancy. *Fetal Maternal Medical Review*, *12*, 249–271.

Bacchus, L., Mezey, G.C., & Bewley, S. (2002). Women's perceptions and experiences of routine enquiry for domestic violence in a maternity service. *British Journal of Obstetrics and Gynaecology*, *109*, 9–16.

Bacchus, L., Mezey, G., & Bewley, S. (2003). Experiences of seeking help from health professionals in a sample of women who experienced domestic violence. *Health Social Care Community*, *1*, 10–8.

Bacchus, L., Mezey, G., & Bewley, S. (2004). Domestic violence: Prevalence in pregnant women and associations with physical and psychological health. *European Journal of Obstetrics & Gynecology and Reproductive Biology*, *113*, 6–11.

Baird, K. (2002). Domestic violence in pregnancy: A public health concern. *Midwifery Digest*, *12*(1), S12–S15.

Bewley, S., Friend, J., Mezey, G. (Eds.) (1997). *Violence against women*. London: Royal College of Obstetricians and Gynaecologists Press.

Bhatt, R.V. (1998). Domestic violence and substance abuse. *International Journal of Gynecology & Obstetrics*, *63*, S25–S31.

Bifulco, A., & Moran, P. (1998). Wednesday's child: research into women's experience of neglect and abuse. In: *Childhood, and adult depression*. London: Routledge.

Boudewyn, A.C., & Liem, J.H. (1995). Childhood sexual abuse as a precursor to depression and self-destructive behavior in adulthood. *Journal of Trauma Stress*, *8*(3), 445–459.

Briere, J. (1984). The effects of childhood sexual abuse on later psychological functioning: defining a post-sexual abuse syndrome. Paper presented at the *Third National Conference on Sexual Victimisation of Children*, Washington, DC.

British Medical Association (1998). *Domestic violence: A healthcare issue*. London: BMJ books.

Calam, R., Horne, L., Glasgow, D., & Cox, A. (1998). Psychological disturbance and child sexual abuse: a follow-up study. *Child Abuse Neglect*, *22*, 901–913.

Campbell, J.C. (2002). Health consequences of intimate partner violence. *The Lancet*, *359*, 1331–1336.

Campbell, J.C., & Lewandowski, L. (1997). Mental and physical health effects of intimate partner violence on women and children. *Psychiatric Clinics North America*, *20*, 353–374.

Campbell, J.C., & Parker, B. (1996). Battered women and their children: a review and policy recommendations. In: J. Fitzpatrick, B.J. McElmurry, & R. Parker (Eds.), *Annual Review of Women's Health* (pp. 259–81). New York, NY: National league for nursing press.

Campbell, J.C., & Soeken, K. (1999). Women's responses to battering over time: an analysis of change. *Journal of Interpersonal Violence*, *14*, 21–40.

Campbell, J.C., Sullivan, C.M., & Davidson, W.S. (1995). Women who use domestic violence shelters: Changes in depression over time. *Psychiatric Women Quarterly*, *19*, 237–255.

Campbell, J.C., Kub, J., Belknap, R.A., & Templin, T.N. (1997). Predictors of depression in battered women. *Violence Against Women*, *3*, 271–293.

Cann, K., Withnell, S., Shakespeare, J., Doll, H., & Thomas, J. (2001). Domestic violence: A comparative survey of levels of detection, knowledge, and attitudes in healthcare workers. *Public Health*, *115*, 89–95.

Carlile, J.B. (1991). Spouse assault on mentally disordered wives. *Canadian Journal of Psychiatry*, *36*, 265–269.

Carmen, E.H., Rieker, P.P., & Mills, T. (1984). Victims of violence and psychiatric illness. *American Journal of Psychiatry*, *141*, 378–383.

Cascardi, M., O'leary, K.D., & Schlee, K.A. (1999). Co-occurrence and correlates of posttraumatic stress disorder and major depression in physically abused women. *Journal of Family Violence*, *14*, 227–250.

Chambliss, L.R. (1997). Domestic violence: A public health crisis. *Clinical Obstetrics and Gynaecology*, *40*, 630–638.

Cheasty, M., Clare, A.W., & Collins, C. (1998). Relation between sexual abuse in childhood and adult depression: Case-control study. *British Medical Journal*, *316*, 198–201.

Covington, D.L., Dalton, V.K., Diehl, S.J., Wright, B.D., & Piner, M.H. (1997). Improving detection of violence among pregnant adolescents. *Journal of Adolescent Health, 21*, 18–24.

Coyne, J.C., & Downey, G. (1991). Social factors and psychopathology: Stress, social support, and coping processes. *Annual Review of Psychology, 42*, 401–425.

Curnow, S.A. (1997). The open window phase: Helpseeking and reality behaviours by battered women. *Applied Nursing Research, 10*, 128–135.

Dearwater, S.R., Coben, J.H., Campbell, J.C., Nah, G., Glass, N., McLoughlin, E., & Bekemeier, B. (1998). Prevalence of domestic violence in women treated at community hospital emergency department. *Journal of the American Medical Association, 280*, 433–438.

Department of Health (2000). Domestic violence: A resource manual for health care professionals. London: DoH. www.doh.gov.uk

Department of Health (2002). Women's mental health: Into the mainstream. Strategic development of mental health care for women. www.doh.gov.uk/mentalhealth

Department of Health, Social Services Inspectorate (1995). Domestic violence and social care: A report on two conferences held by the SSI, p. 37.

Dienemann, J., Boyle, E., Baker, D., Resnick, W., Wiederhorn, N., & Campbell, J. (2000). Intimate partner abuse among women diagnosed with depression. *Issues in Mental Health Nursing, 21*, 499–513.

Flitcraft, A.H., Hadley, S.M., Hendricks-Matthews, M.K., McLeer, S.V., & Warshaw, C. (1992). *Diagnostic and treatment guidelines on domestic violence*. Chicago: American Medical Association.

Garcia-Moreno, C. (2002). Dilemmas and opportunities for an appropriate health-service response to violence against women. *Lancet, 359*, 1509–1514.

Garimella, R.N., Plichta, S.B., Houseman, C., & Garzon, L. (2002). How physicians feel about assisting female victims of intimate-partner violence. *Academic Medicine, 77*, 1262–1265.

Gazmararian, J.A., Lazorick, A., Spitz, A.M., Ballard, T.J., Saltzman, L., & Marks, J.S. (1996). Prevalence of violence against pregnant women. *Journal of the American Medical Association, 275*, 1915–1920.

Gazmararian, J.A., Petersen, R., Spitz, A.M., Goodwin, M.M., Saltzman, L.E., & Marks, J.S. (2000). Violence and reproductive health: Current knowledge and future research directions. *Maternal Child Health Journal, 4*, 79–84.

Gelles, R.J., & Harrop, J.W. (1989). Violence, battering, and psychological distress among women. *Journal of Interpersonal Violence, 4*(1), 400–420.

Gerbert, B., Johnston, K., Caspers, N., Bleecker, T., Woods, A., & Rosenbaum, A. (1996). Experiences of battered women in health care settings: a qualitative study. *Womens Health, 24*, 1–17.

Gladstone, G.L., Parker, G.B., Mitchell, P.B., Malhi, G.S., Wilhelm, K., & Austin, M.-P. (2004). Implications of childhood trauma for depressed women: An analysis of pathways from childhood sexual abuse to deliberate self-harm and revictimization. *American Journal of Psychiatry, 161*, 1417–1425.

Glass, I., & Jackson, P. (1988). Maudsley Hospital survey: prevalence of alcohol problems and other psychiatric disorders in a hospital population. *British Journal of Addiction, 83*, 1105–1111.

Glover-Reed, B., & Mowbray, C.T. (1999). Mental illness and substance abuse: Implications for women's health and health care access. *Journal of the American Medical Womens Association, 54*, 71–78.

Golding, J.M. (1999). Intimate partner violence as a risk factor for mental disorders: A meta analysis. *Journal of Family Violence, 14,* 99–132.

Golding, J.M. (2002). Intimate partner violence as a risk factor for mental disorders: a meta-analysis. *Journal of Family Violence, 14,* 99–132.

Gratz, K.L., Conrad, S.D., & Roemer, L. (2002). Risk factors for deliberate self-harm among college students. *American Journal of Orthopsychiatry, 72*(1), 128–140.

Gremillion, D.H., & Kanop, E.P. (1996). Overcoming barriers to physician involvement in identifying and referring victims of domestic violence. *Annals of Emergency Medicine, 27,* 769–773.

Hague, G., Mullender, A., Aris, R., et al. (2002). Abused women's perspectives: The responsiveness of domestic violence provision and inter-agency initiatives. *Economic and Social Research Council: Research Findings from the Violence Research Programme.*

Hall, W., & Farrell, M. (1997). Co-morbidity of mental disorders with substance misuse. *British Journal of Psychiatry, 171,* 4–5.

Hamberger, L.K., Saunders, D.G., & Hovey, M. (1992). Prevalence of domestic violence in community practice and rate of physician inquiry. *Family Medicine, 24*(4), 283–287.

Haver, B., & Dahlgram, L. (1995). Early treatment of women with alcohol addiction (EWA): a comprehensive evaluation and outcome study. 1. patterns of psychiatric co-morbidity at intake. *Addiction, 90,* 101–109.

Heath, I. (1998). *Domestic violence: The General Practitioner's role.* London: Royal College of General Practitioners.

Hegarty, K., Gunn, J., Chondros, P., & Small, R. (2004). Association between depression and abuse by partners of women attending general practice: Descriptive, cross sectional survey. *British Medical Journal, 328*(7440), 621–624.

Heise, L. (1993). Reproductive freedom and violence against women: What are the intersections? *The Journal of Law, Medicine and Ethics, 21,* 206–216.

Helton, A., McFarlane, A., & Anderson, E. (1987). Battered and pregnant: A prevalence study. *American Journal of Public Health, 77,* 1337–1339.

Helzer, J.E., & Pryzbeck, T.R. (1998). The co-occurrence of alcoholism with other psychiatric disorders in the general population and its impact on treatment. *Journal of Studies on Alcohol, 49,* 219–224.

Home Office (2000). Domestic violence: Break the chain. Multi-agency guidance for addressing domestic violence. http://www.homeoffice.gov.uk/docs/mag.html

Housekamp, B.M., & Foy, D. (1991). The assessment of posttraumatic stress disorder in battered women. *Journal of Interpersonal Violence, 6*(3), 367–375.

Humphreys, C., & Thiara, R. (2002). Routes to safety: protection issues facing abused women and children and the role of outreach services. Bristol: Women's Aid Federation of England, www.womensaid.org.uk

Huth-Bocks, A.C., Levendosky, A.A., & Bogat, G.A. (2002). The effects of violence during pregnancy on maternal and infant health. *Violence and Victims, 17,* 169–185.

Jewkes, R. (2002). Violence against women III. Intimate partner violence: Causes and prevention. *Lancet, 359,* 1423–1429.

Johnson, J.K., Haider, F., Ellis, K., Hay, D.M., & Lindow, S.W. (2003). The prevalence of dv in pregnant women. *British Journal of Obstetrics and Gynaecology, 110,* 272–275.

Kemp, A., Rawlings, E.I., & Green, B.I. (1991). Post-traumatic stress disorder (PTSD) in battered women: A shelter sample. *Journal of Traumatic Stress, 4,* 137–147.

Kershaw, C., Budd, T., Kinshott, G., Mattinson, J., Mayhew, P., & Myhill, A. (2000). *The British Crime Survey 2000.* London Home Office Statistical Bulletin 18/00.

Kilpatrick, D.G., Acierno, R., Resnick, H.S., Saunders, B.E., & Best, C.L. (1997). A 2 year longitudinal analysis of the relationships between violent assault and substance abuse in women. *Journal of Consulting and Clinical Psychology, 65,* 834–847.

Kurtz, D. (1996). Separation, divorce and woman abuse. *Violence Against Women, 2,* 63–81.

Kyriacou, D.N., Anglin, D., Taliaferro, E., Stone, S., Tubb, T., Linden, J.A., Muelleman, R., Barton, E., & Kraus, J.F. (1999). Risk factors for injury to women from domestic violence. *New England Journal of Medicine, 16,* 1892–1898.

Landenburger, K.M. (1998). The dynamics of leaving and recovering from an abusive relationship. *Journal of Obstetric, Gynaecology and Neonatal Nursing, 27,* 700–706.

Larkin, G.L., Rolniak, S., Hyman, K., MacLeod, B.A., & Savage, R. (2000). Effect of an administrative intervention on rates of screening for domestic violence in an urban emergency department. *American Journal Public Health, 90,* 1444–1448.

Lipsky, S., Holt, V.L., Easterling, T.R., & Critchlow, C.W. (2004). Police-reported intimate partner violence during pregnancy and the risk of antenatal hospitalization. *Maternal Child Health Journal, 8,* 55–63.

Mahoney, P., Willliams, L.M., & West, C.M. (2001). Violence against women by intimate relationship partners. In: C.M. Renzetti, J.L. Edleson, & R.K. Bergen (Eds.), *Sourcebook on violence against women* (pp. 143–178). Thousand Oaks, CA: Sage.

Marsden, J., Gossop, M., Stewart, D., Rolfe, A., & Farrell, M. (2000). Psychiatric symptoms among clients seeking treatment for drug dependence. Intake data from the National Treatment Outcome Research Study. *British Journal of Psychiatry, 176,* 285–289.

Martin, S.L., Kilgallen, B., Dee, D.L., Dawson, S., & Campbell, J.C. (1998). Women in a prenatal care/substance abuse treatment program: Links between domestic violence and mental health. *Maternal Child Health Journal, 2,* 85–94.

Martin, S.L., Beaumont, J.L., & Kupper, L.L. (2003). Substance use before and during pregnancy: Links to intimate partner violence. *American Journal of Drug Alcohol Abuse, 29*(3), 599–617.

Masten, A., Best, K.M., & Garmezey, N. (1990). Resilience and development: Contributions from the study of children who overcome adversity. *Development and Psychopathology, 2,* 425–444.

Mayer, B.W., & Coulter, M. (2002). Psychosocial aspects of partner abuse. *American Journal of Nursing, 102,* 24–33.

McCauley, J., Kern, D.E., Kolodner, K., Dill, L., Schroeder, A.F., DeChant, H.K., Ryden, J., Derogatis, L.R., & Bass, E.B. (1997). Clinical characteristics of women with a history of childhood abuse: Unhealed wounds. *Journal of the American Medical Association, 277,* 1362–1368.

McCauley, J., Kern, D.E., Kolodner, K., Derogatis, L.R., & Bass, E.B. (1998). Relation of low-severity violence to women's health. *Journal of General Internal Medicine, 13,* 687–691.

McCloud, A., Barnaby, B., Omu, N., Drummond, C., & Aboud, A. (2004). Relationship between alcohol use disorders and suicidality in a psychiatric population. *British Journal of Psychiatry, 184,* 439–445.

McFarlane, J., Parker, B., Soeken, K., Silva, C., & Reed, S. (1999). Severity of abuse before and during pregnancy for African, American and Anglo women. *Journal of Nurse–Midwifery*, *44*, 139–144.

Mezey, G., & Bewley, S. (1997). Domestic violence in pregnancy. *British Journal of Obstetrics and Gynaecology*, *104*, 528–531.

Mezey, G., Bacchus, L., Haworth, A., & Bewley, S. (2003). Midwives' perceptions and experiences of routine enquiry for domestic violence. *British Journal of Obstetrics and Gynaecology*, *110*, 744–752.

Mirrlees-Black (1999). Domestic Violence: findings from a new British Crime Survey self-completion questionnaire. Home Office Research Study 191. London: Home Office.

Moore, M. (1999). Reproductive health and intimate partner violence. *Family Planning Perspectives*, *31*, 302–306.

Moss, K. (2003). Witnessing violence–aggression and anxiety in young children. *Health Report*, *14*, 53–66.

Mullen, P.E., Martin, J.L., Anderson, J.C., Romans, S.E., & Herbison, G.P. (1993). Childhood sexual abuse and mental health in adult life. *British Journal Psychiatry*, *163*, 721–732.

Mullender, A., & Hague, G. (2000). Reducing domestic violence … What works? Women survivors views. Crime reduction series, briefing note. London: Home Office.

Mullender, A., & Morley, R. (Eds.) (1994). *Children living with domestic violence*. London: Whiting and Birch.

National Advisory Council on Violence Against Women and the Violence Against Women Office (2001). Toolkit to end violence against women. chapter 2. Improving the health and Mental Health Care Systems' Responses to violence against women. What the health and Mental Health Care Systems can do to make a difference. http://toolkit.ncjrs.org/vawo_2.html

National Institute of Child Health and Human Development (NICHD) (2002). Workshop on children exposed to violence: Current status, gaps and research priorities. Washington DC: July 24–26. http://www.nichd.nih.gov/crmc/cdb/Workshop_on_ChildrenViolence.pdf

National Institute of Clinical Excellence (NICE) (2001). Scottish Executive Health Department, Department of Health, Social Service and Public Safety Northern Ireland (2001). Why mother die, 1997–1999. The confidential enquiries into maternal deaths in the United Kingdom. (pp. 241–251). London: RCOG Press.

Newberger, E.H., Barkan, S.E., Lieberman, E.S., McCormick, M.C., Yllo, K., Gary, L.T., & Schechter, S. (1992). Abuse of pregnant women and adverse birth outcome. *Journal of the American Medical Association*, *267*, 2370–2372.

O'Connor, M. (2002). Consequences and outcomes of disclosure for abused women. *International Journal Obstetrics Gynaecology*, *73*, 583–589.

O'Connor, L.E., Berry, J., Inaba, D., Weiss, J., & Morrison, A. (1994). Shame, guilt and depression in men and women in recovery from addiction. *Journal of Substance Abuse Treatment*, *11*(6), 503–510.

Peleikis, D.E., Mykletun, A., & Dahl, A.A. (2004). The relative influence of childhood sexual abuse and other family background risk factors on adult adversities in female outpatients treated for anxiety disorders and depression. *Child Abuse & Neglect*, *28*(1), 61–76.

Plichta, S.B. (1992). The effects of woman abuse on health care utilization and health status: a literature review. *Women's Health Issues*, *2*, 154–163.

Porcellini, J.H., Cogan, R., West, P.P., et al. (2003). Violent victimization of women and men: Physical and psychiatric symptoms. *Journal of the American Board of Family Practice, 16*, 32–39.

Post, R.D., Willett, A.B., Franks, R.D., House, R.M., Back, S.M., & Weissberg, M.P. (1980). A preliminary report on the prevalence of domestic violence among psychiatric inpatients. *American Journal of Psychiatry, 137*, 974–975.

Purwar, M.B., Jeyaseelan, L., Varhadpande, U., Motghare, V., & Pimplakute, S. (1999). Survey of physical abuse during pregnancy GMCH, Nagpur, India. *Journal of Obstetrics & Gynecology Research, 25*, 165–171.

Ratner, P.A. (1993). The incidence of wife abuse and mental health status in abused wives in Edmonton. *Canadian Journal of Public Health, 84*, 246–249.

Renker, P.R. (1999). Physical abuse, social support, self-care and pregnancy outcomes of older adolescents. *Journal of Obstetrics & Gynecological Neonatal Nursing, 28*, 377–388.

Rhodes, K.V., & Levinson, W. (2003). Interventions for intimate partner violence against women. *Journal of the American Medical Association, 289*, 601–605.

Richardson, J., Feder, G., Eldridge, S., Chung, W.S., Coid, J., & Moorey, S. (2001). Women who experience domestic violence and women survivors of childhood sexual abuse: A survey of health professionals' attitudes and clinical practice. *British Journal of General Practice, 51*, 468–470.

Romans, S.E., Martin, J.L., Anderson, J.C., Herbison, G.P., & Mullen, P.E. (1995). Sexual abuse in childhood and deliberate self-harm. *American Journal of Psychiatry, 152*(9), 1336–1342.

Royal College of Midwives (1997). *Domestic abuse in pregnancy*. Position Paper 19, London: Royal College of Midwives.

Royal College of Psychiatrists (2002). *Domestic violence*. Council Report April 2002. London.

Saunders, D.G., & Hamberger, K. (1993). Indicators of woman abuse based on chart review at a family practice centre. *Archives of Family Medicine, 2*, 537–543.

Schulberg, W.C., McClelland, M., & Burns, B.Y. (1987). Depression and physical illness: The prevalence. *Clinical Psychology Review, 7*, 145–167.

Silva, C., McFarlane, J., Soeken, K., Parker, B., & Reel, S. (1997). Symptoms of post-traumatic stress disorder in abused women in a primary care setting. *Journal of Women's Health, 6*, 543–552.

Spataro, J., Mullen, P.E., Burgess, P.M., Wells, D.L., & Moss, S.A. (2004). Impact of child sexual abuse on mental health: Prospective study in males and females. *British Journal of Psychiatry, 184*, 416–421.

Stanko, E. (2000). The Day to Count. The National Domestic Violence Snapshot, undertaken by Elizabeth on September 28th 2000, (Stanko, "*Enough is enough*" *Conference*, October 2000; Women's Aid Newsletter, December 2000). http://www.domesticviolencedata.org

Stanko, E., Crisp, D., Hale, C., et al. (1998). Counting the costs: Estimating the impact of domestic violence in the London Borough of Hackney. Swindon, Crime Concern.

Stark, E., & Flitcraft, A. (1996). Women at risk: Domestic violence and women's health. London: Sage.

Stein, M.B., & Kennedy, C. (2001). Major depressive and post-traumatic stress disorder comorbidity in female victims of intimate partner violence. *Journal of Affective Disorder, 66*(2–3), 133–138.

Stein, J.A., Golding, J.M., Siegel, J.M., Burnam, M.A., & Sorenson, S.B. (1988). Long-term psychological sequelae of child sexual abuse: The Los Angeles epidemiologic catchment area study. In: G.E. Wyatt, & G.J. Powell (Eds.), Lasting effects of child sexual abuse (pp. 135–154). Newbury Park, CA: Sage.

Stevens, K.L. (1997). The role of accident and emergency department. In: S. Bewley, J. Friend, & G. Mezey (Eds.), *Violence against women* (pp. 168–178). London: Royal College of Obstetricians and Gynaecologists Press.

Stewart, D.E., & Cecutti, T. (1993). Physical abuse in pregnancy. *Canadian Medical Association Journal, 149*, 1257–1268.

Straus, M.A., & Gelles, R.J. (1986). Societal change and change in family violence from 1975–1985 as revealed by two national surveys. *Journal of Marriage and the Family, 48*, 465–478.

Straus, M.A., Gelles, R.J., & Steinmetz, S.K. (1980). Behind closed doors: Violence in the American family. New York: Doubleday.

Taggart, L., & Mattson, S. (1996). Delay in prenatal care as a result of battering in the pregnancy: Cross-cultural implications. *Health Care Women International, 17*, 25–34.

Taket, A., Nurse, J., Smith, K., Watson, J., Shakespeare, J., Lavis, V., Cosgrove, K., Mulley, K., & Feder, G. (2003). Routinely asking women about domestic violence in health settings. *British Medical Journal, 327*, 673–676.

Tjaden, P., & Thoennes, N. (2000). Resilience factors associated with female survivors of childhood sexual abuse. *Violence Against Women, 6*, 142–161.

Torres, S., Campbell, J., Campbell, D.W., Ryan, J., King, C., Price, P., Stallings, R.Y., Fuchs, S.C., & Laude, M. (2000). Abuse during and before pregnancy: Prevalence and cultural correlates. *Violence Victims, 15*, 303–321.

Ustun, T.B., Ayuso-mateos, J.L., Chatteri, S., Mathers, C., & Murray, C.J.L. (2004). Global burden of depressive disorders in the year 2000+. *British Journal of Psychiatry, 184*, 386–392.

Walker, L.E. (1979). *The battered woman.* New York: Harper & Row.

Walker, E.A., Gelfand, A., Katon, W., Koss, M.P., Von Korff, M., Bernstein, D., & Russo, J. (1999). Adult health status of women with histories of childhood abuse and neglect. *American Journal of Medicine, 107*(4), 332–339.

Wathen, & MacMillan (2003). Interventions for violence against women. *Journal of the American Medical Association, 289*, 589–600.

Watts, C., & Zimmerman, C. (2002). Violence against women: Global scope and magnitude. *Lancet, 359*, 1232–1237.

Webster, J., Chandler, J., & Battistutta, D. (1996). Pregnancy outcomes and health care use: Effects of abuse. *American Journal of Obstetrics & Gynaecology, 174*, 760–769.

Williamson, E. (2000). *Domestic violence and health: the response of the medical profession.* Bristol: The Policy Press.

Wisner, C.L., Gilmer, T.P., Saltzman, L.E., et al. (1999). Intimate partner violence against women: do victims cost health plans more? *Journal of Family Practice, 48*, 439–443.

Wolfe, D.A., Crooks, C.V., Lee, V., McIntyre-Smith, A., & Jaffe, P.G. (2003). The effects of children's exposure to domestic violence: a meta-analysis and critique. *Clinical Child and Family Psychology Reviews, 6*, 171–187.

Woods, S.J. (2000). Prevalence and patterns of posttraumatic stress disorder in abused and postabused women. *Issues Mental Health Nursing, 21*, 309–324.

World Health Organisation (1998). Violence against women information pack: A priority health issue. Geneva: WHO. http://www.int/frh-whd/VAW/infopack/English/VAW_infopack.html

Wright, J., & Kariya, A. (1997). Aetiology of assault with respect to alcohol, unemployment and social deprivation: A Scottish accident and emergency department case-control study. *Injury, 28,* 369–372.

Zeitlin, D., Dhanjal, T., & Colmsee, M. (1999). Maternal-foetal bonding: The impact of domestic violence on the bonding process between a mother and a child. *Archives of Women's Mental Health, 2,* 183–189.

Zlotnick, C., Ryan, C.E., Miller, I.W., & Keitner, G.I. (1995). Childhood abuse and recovery from major depression. *Child Abuse & Neglect, 19,* 1513–1516.

7

Depression in women: Hormonal influences

Kathryn M. Abel[1] and Jayashri Kulkarni[2]

[1]Senior Lecturer and Honourary Consultant, Centre for Women's Mental Health Research, Division of Psychiatry, University of Manchester, Manchester, UK
[2]Professor of Psychiatry, The Alfred, Melbourne, Australia; Professor Monash University, Faculty of Medicine, Melbourne, Australia

By 2020, the World Health Organisation (WHO, 1997) has predicted that depression will be the "second leading cause of global disability burden" and that as many as one in four women will suffer from a mood disorder during their lifetime.

Women have an increased vulnerability to depressive disorders during their child-bearing years. During this time, they are also more likely to experience sexual and domestic violence, social and financial inequities, and often to undertake many different roles with attendant responsibilities. The child-bearing years are associated with specific hormonal changes related to menstrual cycle variations, contraception, pregnancy and the postpartum period and the menopause. Increasingly there are also the iatrogenic hormonal manipulations associated with contraception and assisted reproductive technologies.

Clearly, these sex-specific factors deserve special consideration in the understanding and management of depression in women. The reader is also referred to Chapter 1 for an overview of depression in adolescence, Chapter 9 for a more detailed discussion of mood disorders in pregnancy and postpartum and Chapter 11 for a review of mood in the menopausal period.

Epidemiology

Worldwide, major depression is at least twice as common in women as men (Weissman et al., 1993), accounting for 41.9% of the disability from neuropsychiatric disorders among women compared to 29.3% among men; these data appear consistent with current UK figures (Office for National Statistics (ONS), 2001). Atypical depression and somatisation are three times more common in women than men, as is comorbidity: women are more likely than men to present with mixed anxiety and depression; and alcohol dependence is preceded by depression in up to 65% of women in alcohol treatment (Dixit & Crum, 2000; see also Chapter 3).

Some suggest that the preponderance of unipolar depression in women may be accounted for by recurrent major depression rather than single episodes of depression, which tend towards an equal sex ratio (see WHO, 1997, p. 4–14). Others suggest that atypical depression alone may account for the female excess (Angst & Dobler-Mikola, 1984). Point prevalence is affected by age: before puberty, the sex ratio for major depression is 1:1 (Angold et al., 1998; and see Chapter 1), but females are more vulnerable during their entire reproductive period, and into the menopause (see Chapter 11); older groups tend to show less marked gender differences in rates of depression (see Chapter 12), such that the most emphatic difference is seen during the reproductive years (Bebbington et al., 1998; WHO, 1997). Middle age proves the most vulnerable time for both women and men: only 10% of 65–69-year-old women and 9% of those aged 70–74 years report mood symptoms, compared with almost 20% of women from the 40 to 54 years age group (although older age groups tend to report fewer symptoms).

Despite convincing statistics, some argue that the rates of mood disorder in women are falsely inflated by greater help seeking, symptom reporting and a tendency for professionals to be more likely to diagnose depression in women. However, studies have not generally shown clinicians more likely to diagnose depression in women in primary care settings. Women are likely to seek help more than men, but often do so indirectly through their children. More importantly, only approximately half of mood disorders in general, and depression in particular, remain diagnosed world-wide (Gater et al., 1998); in the UK, it is estimated that less than a quarter of patients with neurotic disorder receive treatment (ONS, 2001). Added to this, longer term follow-up studies of large epidemiological samples suggest that mood disorders (both unipolar and bipolar) are chronic and disabling diseases with particular risk of recurrence in women, especially women with young age at first episode. Furthermore, repeated episodes of illness further increase the risk of recurrence of both unipolar and bipolar disorder (Kessing et al., 2000).

For women, then, the problem appears less one of over-diagnosis and over-treatment of mood disorder, and more one of vulnerability to a chronic and disabling disease with major health consequences: an increased risk of cardiovascular disease and physical illness in general, worse outcome from cardiovascular illness and breast cancer and increased mortality rates (Wulsin et al., 1999).

In premenopausal women, depression has also been associated with disturbances of the hypothalamic gonadal axis, hypooestrogenaemia and amenorrhoea.

Thus, we turn now to a consideration of hormonal influences on depression, beginning with an overview of the actions of the gonadal steroids.

Gonadal hormonal influences and depression

The impact of gonadal steroids on the limbic system and neurotransmitter activity is well-recognised (Huttner & Shepherd, 2003). Traditionally gonadal steroid effects are classified into organisational or activational, depending on the duration and timing of the effect (Phoenix et al., 1959). Organisational effects happen early in life, especially during prenatal brain development. Structural changes in the brain and other long-term metabolic effects are brought about largely by the hormonal milieu (Arnold & Breedlove, 1985). Activational effects are not associated with a critical period of development and result in relatively transient changes in neurophysiology and behaviour (Moffat & Resnick, 2002). Activational effects often depend on earlier organisational effects of gonadal steroids (Breedlove, 1992). In humans, systems involved in regulating sexual and maternal behaviours appear to be the most sensitive to gonadal hormones. Overall activity levels, including motor behaviour, aggression, feeding and taste preferences and avoidance learning are all influenced by gonadal steroids (Beatty, 1992).

Cortisol and thyroid hormones are also important in mood disorders, but their specific impact in the aetiology or treatment of depression in women is less well defined and are not the focus of this chapter. Here we shall consider how oestrogen, progesterone and androgens impinge on female risk and illness course.

Oestrogen

Levels of oestradiol are characterised by cyclical fluctuations in the adult premenopausal woman. Under pituitary gonadotrophin control by luteinising hormone (LH) and follicle stimulating hormone (FSH), oestrogen has many potent effects in the central nervous system (CNS) as well as peripherally. It also acts as a powerful neurosteroid, with organisational and activational effects.

Specific receptors for oestrogens are found in the amygdala, hippocampus, cortex, locus coeruleus, mid-brain raphe nuclei, glial cells and central grey matter. This suggests extensive involvement by oestrogen in the control of the psychophysiology of mood, cognition and memory (Genazzani & Bernardi, 2003). The action of oestrogen on neurons can be categorised by its rate of effect. Short term, rapid effects of oestrogen, such as activation of ligand-gated ion channels and G protein-coupled second messenger systems, may occur over minutes or hours (Alson-Solis, 2002), and can modulate synaptic functioning and neuronal morphological features (Genazzani & Bernardi, 2003). In contrast, oestrogen exerts long-term action by stimulating specific intracellular receptors responsible for modulating protein

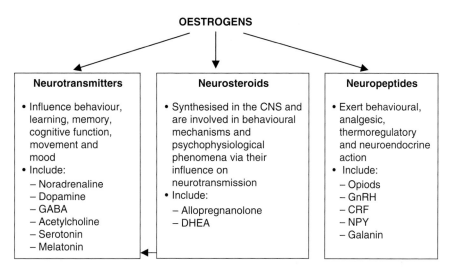

Figure 7.1   Oestrogen effects in the brain (CRF: corticotrophin-releasing factor; NPY: neuropeptide Y)

synthesis and the transcription of genes. This latter process is governed by the classical genomic mechanism of steroids, while the former is modulated by non-genomic procedures. As indicated by Genazzani and Bernardi (2003), short- and long-term effects of oestrogen interact to facilitate broad and diverse modulation of cerebral function. There exists a complex interplay between oestrogen and neurotransmitters, neurosteroids and neuropeptides through which oestrogen exerts some of its actions. A detailed discussion of such relationships is beyond the scope of the present text; interested readers are referred elsewhere (Genazzani & Bernardi, 2003) for further detail. A summary of these effects of oestrogen in the brain are shown in Figure 7.1.

Our understanding of the influences of oestrogen upon mood and the mechanisms underpinning them, has benefited greatly from the work of Manji and Lenox (1999). Their work examining the pharmacological stabilisation of mood led to their conclusion that "the PKC (Protein Kinase C) signalling pathway is clearly a target for the actions of two structurally dissimilar antimanic agents, lithium and valproate" (Manji & Lenox, 1999, p. 1338). The administration of such pharmacotherapies is proposed to decrease levels of myoinositol, which initiates a cascade of secondary alterations in the PKC signalling pathway and gene expression in the CNS. It is these secondary processes of inhibiting PKC to which Manji and Lenox attribute the therapeutic efficacy of lithium. The authors tested their conclusion in a sample of acutely manic participants by administering a PKC inhibitor known as tamoxifen, which is also a type of anti-oestrogen. Tamoxifen significantly reduced manic symptoms, and Manji and Lenox (1999) acknowledged "… the relative contribution of oestrogen receptor blockage" (p. 1338).

Progesterone

Progesterone is vital for the establishment and maintenance of pregnancy, through its effect on the endometrium and myometrium (Croxatto, 2003). Chronic progesterone administration in humans leads to inhibition of endometrial growth, in spite of high oestrogen levels (Chwalisz et al., 2000) which may also be a consequence of modulation of progesterone action through isoform binding. Progestins are progesterone analogues that bind agonistically to progesterone receptors. More recently, there has been recognition of three classes of progesterone analogues – called "progesterone receptor modulators" (PRMs) that include agonists (progestins), mixed agonist and antagonists (mesoprogestins) and antagonists (antiprogestins) (Croxatto, 2003). All of the PRMs bind to the same receptor, but with complex outcomes.

The recent discovery of two isoforms (A and B) of the progesterone receptor gene expression allows some unravelling of their complex actions. For example, isoform A is more potent than B for mediating antiprogestational actions (Horwitz et al., 1997). The impact of progesterone administration on the CNS requires further study, but the identification of the receptor isoforms and their impact on gene transcription under oestradiol control strongly suggests that PRMs have great diversity of action on many target organs.

Androgens

The concept that testosterone is exclusively a male hormone, is a widely held myth. Testosterone in women has a number of important functions including maintenance of libido, muscle mass, decrease of fat mass, increase of bone mineral density, increase in haematocrit, as well as effects on cognition (Morley, 2003).

Between ages 20 and 45 years, serum androgen concentrations decrease in women as observed by decline in testosterone and dehydroepiandrosterone sulphate (DHEA). Burger et al. (2000) reported no change in serum testosterone in the menopause transition, but a decrease in sex hormone-binding globulin, leading to an overall increase in free testosterone index around the menopause. The impact of this on mood, cognition and memory involves a complex interplay of androgens and other sex hormones in the CNS in both reproductive age and menopausal women and requires much further research (see also Chapter 11). Certainly there is no consistent relationship between androgen levels and mood; for example, women with high circulating androgens as part of a polycystic ovarian syndrome are not uniformly depressed, whilst administration of androgens to ovariectomised or menopausal women is generally associated with, if anything, enhanced mood (see Eriksson et al., 2000).

Specific life cycle related depressive disorders in women

Premenstrual dysphoric disorder

Premenstrual mood disturbance is extremely common, particularly in women under 25 (Wittchen et al., 2002). Severe, functionally incapacitating mood disorder affording a diagnosis of premenstrual dysphoric disorder (PMDD) occurs in anything from 3% to 8% of women in Europe and the USA. Around a third of these women suffer from major depression in their lifetimes, and they are also more likely to suffer postpartum depression. The Diagnostic and Statistical Manual of Mental Disorders, Edition IV (DSM-IV) criteria for diagnosing PMDD include marked depressed mood, anxiety, affective lability, anger, anhedonia, anergia, appetite changes, sleep changes and feeling out of control for the last week of the luteal phase in most menstrual cycles. Symptoms usually remit within a few days of menses. PMDD includes physical symptoms such as breast soreness and headaches. It is likely that dysregulation of hypothalamic–pituitary–adrenal (HPA) and other key systems (β-endorphin, cholinergic, serotonergic, adrenergic), possibly from genetic susceptibility, make PMDD women vulnerable to physiological fluctuations of gonadal steroids.

Abnormal levels of almost every hormone have been implicated in the aetiology of PMDD including oestrogen, progesterone, FSH, LH, cortisol, dihydrotestosterone, thyroid hormones and serotonin. However, the only clear relationship between physiology and symptoms is cyclical menstrual phase change, specifically ovulation; PMDD symptoms do not occur before puberty or after menopause (Burt & Hendrick, 1997a), nor during anovulatory cycles or after oophorectomy (see Backstrom et al., 2000).

Managing patients with PMDD involves screening out other psychiatric and medical disorders. A nutritional assessment may also be useful since high levels of caffeine, salt and alcohol may worsen PMDD. Some types of contraception may also worsen PMDD – hence a full contraceptive history should be taken.

Treatment strategies include validating women's experiences. Often, the patient has attended many doctors and may have been told that her symptoms are normal or minor. A patient-kept diary over 2–3 consecutive months is essential to make a diagnosis of PMDD.

Several non-pharmacological treatments may assist with the milder symptoms. Thus adequate sleep, relaxation and a healthy diet may all benefit women. In terms of specific non-pharmacological approaches, Blake et al. (1998) described success with cognitive behavioural therapy (CBT) in PMDD. Some reports suggest that light therapy may also be effective in PMDD.

In terms of medication trials, we are aware of at least 15 randomised controlled trials of selective serotonin reuptake inhibitors (SSRIs) for severe premenstrual syndrome (PMS) or PMDD that show superiority over placebo at treating psychological and physical symptoms; it should be noted, though, that the placebo response is high (20–40%) in this group (Dimmock et al., 2000). There is some evidence that SSRIs are more effective in PMDD than tricyclic antidepressants (TCAs) (apart from clomipramine, which is highly serotonergic), suggesting a serotonergic perturbation underpinning the disorder. Whilst all SSRIs studied thus far have shown efficacy in PMDD, fluoxetine and sertraline are the best-studied compounds. Fluoxetine at 20 or 60 mg daily or sertraline at 50–150 mg daily are effective, although drop out rates are high for the higher doses. Women with PMDD appear to respond to SSRIs rapidly (within a week), but withdrawal due to side effects is 2–3 times than that with placebo (Dimmock et al., 2000). The commonest side effect of long-term treatment is sexual dysfunction. Intermittent dosing may be more acceptable for women who are likely to require long-term treatment, but there is no convincing evidence that this approach is better tolerated than continuous therapy. Since tolerance to the common unwanted effects of SSRIs often develops during continuous treatment, intermittent therapy might, in theory, have disadvantages and some women may not prefer continuous treatment. We are aware of no controlled studies of long-term maintenance treatment with any SSRI in PMDD, but women tend to relapse within two months of stopping treatment. Few studies have compared SSRIs with other relevant treatments for PMDD.

Hormonal treatments for PMDD have encompassed both oestrogen and progesterone. In two studies, transdermal oestradiol was more effective than placebo for symptoms of PMS/PMDD, but a further (small) study of conjugated oestrogens was negative (see Yonkers et al., 2000). Progesterone has been investigated in 10 double-blind studies of over 400 women with PMS/PMDD, with only one study being positive (reviewed by Yonkers et al., 2000). In sum, oestradiol might have a place in the treatment of PMS/PMDD, but further work is required, whilst progesterone does not appear to be effective.

Calcium carbonate has been shown to decrease symptom scores in PMS/PMDD by 48% compared with 30% for placebo; pyridoxine or vitamin B6 is twice as effective as placebo in PMS; and evening primrose oil has also been shown to improve symptoms. Other pharmacological treatments without controlled trial evidence include the use of diuretics during symptomatic days; prostaglandin inhibitors (e.g., ibuprofen, naproxen sodium) during symptomatic days; and vitamin E and magnesium throughout the cycle.

Depression related to hormonal contraception

Since the 1960s, exogenous gonadal steroid hormones have been in widespread use globally as oral contraceptives (OCs). The high efficacy rates and ease of use make them very popular. Physical risks associated with "the pill" are well described, and include increased risk of thromboembolism (especially in smokers), hypertension, cerebrovascular accidents and gallstones. However, there are very few controlled studies exploring the relationship to depression, especially of the newer, low-dose hormonal contraceptives. This is despite the commonly reported, anecdotal evidence from women describing mood changes on certain types of "the pill"; indeed, Goldzieher (1994) reported that change in mood, specifically depression, is one of the most common reasons given for discontinuing usage.

Current types of hormonal contraception include the combination OCs, with both oestrogen and progesterone. Most include one week off-active hormone supplementation, to allow simulated menstrual bleeding. Within this group are monophasic OCs – in which both the oestrogen and progestin levels remain steady throughout the active pill cycle; and triphasic OCs – in which the hormone levels vary across the pill cycle to simulate a normal cycle.

Progesterone-only OCs should be taken at approximately the same time each day and are often chosen for breast feeding patients or where oestrogenic complications may be problematic. Depot-Provera or medroxyprogesterone acetate injections every month enhance treatment adherence. More recently subcutaneous progesterone implants (implanon/norplant) have become more popular.

The effects of the different types of OCs on mood have not been consistently reported. A recent review of 13 studies (Oinonen & Mazmanian, 2002) comparing the daily ratings of affect in both OC users and non-users, showed differences between the groups, but the direction of the differences were not consistent. Individual variation, mediated by factors such as a personal or family history of depression, or predisposition to vitamin B6 deficiency, greatly influence the effect of OCs on mood. More studies examining such variables are required. The Canadian Pharmaceutical Association (2000) has reported that some women continue to experience negative mood while taking OCs. The lower oestrogen dose OCs appear to be associated with more negative mood changes (Akerlund et al., 1993). In general, the monophasic OCs appear to stabilise the affect across the cycle. This may occur through a reduction in the cyclical fluctuations of oestrogen and progesterone, which in turn stabilises the central neurotransmitters – especially serotonin (Felthous & Robinson, 1981).

Mechanisms cited for a possible link between exogenous steroid use and mood disturbance include (Oinonen & Mazmanian, 2002):
(a) Pyridoxine (vitamin B6 component) deficiency (see McCarty, 2000).
(b) Progesterone- and oestrogen-mediated augmentation of gamma-aminobutyric acid (GABA)-induced inhibition of glutamate transmission (Smith et al., 1997).
(c) Progesterone-mediated increase in monoamine oxidase (MAO) activity, resulting in lower serotonin levels (Sherwin, 1996).

(d) Potentiation of progesterone-mediated mood effects, by oestrogen (Fink et al., 1998).

Clear guidelines are needed to assist the practitioner working with women with a history of depression, who wish to take an OC. At the very least, the patient's subjective description of lowered mood on an OC should prompt the clinician to review this carefully with the woman, and possibly change the particular OC.

Abortion and miscarriage and depression

Few data are available on the psychological effects of pregnancy termination or loss. Shame, secrecy and thought suppression are all associated with greater post-abortion depression, anxiety and hostility (Dagg, 1991). A recent large US study reported that married women were at significantly higher risk of a depressive episode following termination, compared to single women. This was thought to reflect the release of burden for single women of not rearing a child on their own (Reardon & Cougle, 2002). Others have reported that most women who abort an unintended pregnancy in the first trimester do not suffer any adverse outcomes at two years, unless there is a past history of depression (Major et al., 2000). For most women, negative emotional effects are transient (Butler, 1996), but it should also be noted that psychological sequelae may impact upon other family members, including partners and surviving children (Frost & Condon, 1996).

Several studies have now reported that unintentional foetal loss is associated with subsequent risk of depression, post traumatic stress disorder (PTSD) or an exacerbation of obsessive compulsive symptoms (Boyce et al., 2002). In case-control studies of women who have experienced a spontaneous abortion, rates of major depression approximate around 11%, compared to 4% in controls. It is also the case that subsequent pregnancies and puerperia may be complicated by an increase in anxiety compared to the same period in women who have never experienced foetal loss.

A prospective follow-up of 144 women after miscarriage (see Klier et al., 2002) found that at 8 months, non-pregnant women were at increased risk of emotional distress, and were three times more likely than age-matched controls to be using psychotropic medication. By 18 months, those women who had not conceived still reported high rates of emotional problems and were more likely to have sought health care for a depressive disorder, than those who had conceived. There were no consistent associations between the psychological status of the women after the miscarriage, and the experience and outcome of a subsequent pregnancy.

Women who experience pregnancy loss increasingly value supportive non-medical interventions (DOH Women into the Mainstream, 2001). Psychological interventions such as bereavement counselling are becoming more widely available. However, for women following miscarriage or abortion, clinicians may still fail to recognise the need for such interventions or indeed the risk of psychological distress. Although few interventions have been formally evaluated, both parents (and both partners in homosexual couples) should be offered support and follow-up (see Klier et al., 2002). Future development of modern health services should take these needs into account (Dagg, 1991).

Pregnancy and depression

As discussed in Chapter 8, some 10–20% of women suffer a depressive episode during pregnancy. Antenatal depression is a powerful predictor of postnatal depression (PND) and is likely to be under-diagnosed during pregnancy as many symptoms overlap (e.g., loss of energy, fatigue and sleep disturbance) and symptoms coincide with peaks of physical discomfort (i.e., first and third trimesters). Antenatal depression may adversely affect the foetus (Teixeira et al., 1999), and women at risk should be closely monitored.

The treatment of depression in pregnancy presents very specific issues pertinent to women only. It is generally presumed that it is best to refrain from medications in pregnancy if possible but there are serious risks associated with severe depression during pregnancy. A detailed discussion of such factors is provided in Chapter 9.

Prophylaxis against postpartum relapse may be achieved through re-introduction of an antidepressant (AD) late in the third trimester or early puerperium (see below). Women at high risk of relapse who wish to conceive, should be given the option to have their AD dose reduced, with regular monitoring by the psychiatric team and/or may switch to a "safe" AD (for details see Chapter 9).

AD levels decline steadily during gestation, and during the second trimester dosing requirements of ADs increase to an average of 1.6 times the pre-pregnancy dose (range 1.3–2.0). If a plasma level has been measured pre-conception, or early in the first trimester, it can be used to titrate an increased dose as pregnancy proceeds. A postpartum "withdrawal syndrome" has been described in neonates following tricyclic and SSRI use near term. It occurs within a few days of birth and can last up to 1 month. Symptoms include irritability, constant crying, restlessness, shivering, hypothermia, increased tonus, eating and sleeping difficulties and convulsions. Monitoring maternal AD drug concentration and careful observation of the neonate for signs of toxicity are suggested. The reader is referred to Chapter 9 for a more detailed discussion of AD use during pregnancy, and for references.

PND

As reviewed in Chapter 8, anything from 25% to 85% (depending on diagnostic criteria) of women experience "postpartum blues" – the mildest form of postpartum mood disturbance (Stein et al., 1981). The symptoms begin with the 1st week following childbirth and resolve by day 12 postpartum. There are no specific treatment needs for blues, but severe blues may serve as a harbinger of PND.

In a woman's lifetime, the first five weeks postpartum represent the period of greatest risk of de novo depression, with rates estimated at 10–20% (see Chapter 8). The adverse impact of maternal depression on child development is well described (Cooper, 1997). Most depressive episodes occur within four weeks of birth, and risk of new episodes appears to fall off after eight weeks. In women with a past history of depression, the risk of a postpartum relapse is estimated to be as high as 30%, whilst in those with a past episode of PND, the risk after subsequent pregnancies is as high as 60% (Cooper & Murray, 1995). The risk of PND is also increased in women with a history of PMDD, while women undergoing traumatic deliveries (instrumental deliveries or emergency caesarean section) show more symptoms of depression and feel less healthy 1–3 months postpartum (see Wijma et al., 2002). Whether PND is nosologically distinct from depression at other times remains controversial (see Chapter 8). Cooper and Murray (1995) reported that for women whose first ever episode of depression occurred postnatally, recurrence was significantly more likely to occur postnatally (41%), compared to women with previous non-puerperal episodes (18%). Women with first onset postnatally were also less likely to suffer recurrence of depression at times other than postpartum, than were women with previous non-puerperal episodes.

The factors contributing to PND include a personal or family history of mood disorder (Stowe et al., 1998), a previous episode of PND (Cooper & Murray, 1995; O'Hara, 1991) and a number of psychosocial factors including marital discord, unplanned or unwanted pregnancies, lack of support and stressful life events (O'Hara, 1991). No consistent biological associations have been reported in PND. However, both increased plasma cortisol levels (Okano & Nomura, 1992) and abnormalities of HPA axis functioning following childbirth have been reported. One group suggest that the HPA axis of women with PND may be relatively slow to recover from the effects of pregnancy-related steroid changes causing prolongation of the HPA axis blunting, and transient suppression of hypothalamic corticotrophin-releasing hormone (CRH) which normally occurs in healthy women during pregnancy and postpartum (Chrousos et al., 1998; Magiakou et al., 1996). Some suggest that transient thyroid dysfunction following childbirth is associated with PND (Pederson et al., 1993). Harris et al. (1992) reported that in some women, depressive symptoms are associated with positive thyroid antibody status during the postpartum period. Around 1% of all postpartum women will show a mood disorder associated with transient thyroid dysfunction and treatment of the thyroid condition must be part of the management (Steiner et al., 2003).

Although the rapid fall of circulating oestrogen after delivery has been associated with the onset of postpartum *psychosis* (Wieck et al., 1991), no differences in absolute steroid levels have been found in PND. Of interest here, however, are those studies suggesting potential therapeutic benefit from postpartum administration of oestrogens in women at risk for PND (see Chapter 8). Fluctuation in steroid levels may trigger key changes in central and peripheral monoamine systems resulting in serious postpartum mental illness in vulnerable women. Changes in serotonin receptor sensitivities have also been reported in women with PND (Hannah et al., 1992). Abnormality of serotonergic responses to gonadal steroids may occur in some women with particular genetic susceptibility (see Manji & Lenox, 1999). This may explain the impressive overlap between various mood syndromes and physiological steroid fluctuations (e.g., Yonkers, 1997).

Systematic randomised controlled trials of the efficacy of preventive AD treatment versus placebo in women at risk of postpartum depression are limited. Wisner et al. (2001, 2004) reported that sertraline, but not nortripyline, conferred additional preventative efficacy beyond that of placebo. Further studies are required to replicate these initial findings. SSRIs directly alter the activity of neurosteroidogenic enzymes in the brain, which may be an important mechanism related to their superior AD response in this group. These data point to the recommendation that mothers with a history of severe or recurrent PND, or previous severe depression not associated with childbirth, should be considered for pharmacological prophylaxis immediately postpartum if this has not occurred previously (see Chapters 8 and 9). Women who have been treated with ADs antenatally may have required an increased dose of medication to compensate for the pharmacodynamic changes of pregnancy. These changes return to the non-gravid state approximately 48 h postpartum. To minimise neonatal exposure to ADs in breast milk the dose should be reduced, if possible, postnatally and titrated against symptoms (Altshuler et al., 1996).

Controlled trials show that established PND responds to treatment with SSRIs, up to 12 sessions of CBT (Appleby et al., 1997) or interpersonal therapy (O'Hara et al., 2000) and that these treatments are superior to spontaneous remission in the short term. However, if women are asked about treatments, they consistently state a preference for locally delivered, non-medical or "talking" treatments with an emphasis on practical help and support, and are often reluctant to take any form of drug. Whilst these approaches appear effective in the short term, a recent controlled trial following women for five years after early intervention with CBT, non-directive counselling and psychodynamic psychotherapy showed no benefit on maternal mood beyond nine months and no reduction in subsequent rates of PND (Murray et al., 2003). This group also reported that psychological treatments delivered to mothers with PND within the first five months postpartum had limited benefit on cognitive or behavioural outcomes of the children as assessed at 18 months and five years (Cooper & Murray, 1997; Murray et al., 2003). St John's Wort is effective in mild to moderate depression, but contraindicated during breastfeeding. There are no convincing data that progesterone is more effective than placebo.

As reviewed in Chapter 9, special attention needs to be given to the medications used in breastfeeding mothers with PND. Established guidelines on AD safety in breastfeeding infants now exist (American Academy of Paediatrics, 1991). Antenatal doses of ADs should be reduced to pre-partum doses 48 h after delivery to minimise neonatal exposure in breast milk. Generally, sertraline in 50–100 mg doses is recommended as treatment of choice and women may be allowed to continue breast-feeding (Stowe et al., 1995, 2003). Once the mother's medication serum levels are at a steady state, breast milk levels of medication and infant serum levels can be assayed to establish safety. The field of available ADs is a rapidly changing one and current local guidelines should be consulted. At present, it appears that sertraline is the safest of SSRIs for use in breastfeeding mothers (American Academy of Paediatrics, 1991). Other aspects of the comprehensive treatment of PND are provided in Chapter 8.

Infertility and depression in women

Up to 15% of couples suffer with infertility (Speroff et al., 1994). Postponed childbearing and decreasing sperm quality add to the increasing number of people in Western societies requesting assisted reproductive technologies. Traditionally, infertility was blamed solely on the woman and still today, infertile women feel frustrated, less feminine and have poor self-esteems (Facchinetti et al., 1992). Women in an infertile couple appear more likely than men to report psychiatric symptoms in association with a couple's infertility; such symptoms include distress, anger, anxiety, low self-esteem and depression (Burt & Hendrick, 1997b; Wright et al., 1991). As many as 25% of women compared to 12% men have been reported to suffer mild depression following repeated failed fertility treatments (Newton et al., 1990).

Treatments for ovulatory failure, luteal phase deficiency and unknown causes of infertility include the administration of clomiphene citrate, pulsatile Gonadotrophin-releasing hormone (GnRH) and pump administration of injectable GnRH agonists. All of these agents may be associated with instability of mood, although assessment is confounded by the psychosocial strain of long-term infertility. Surgical procedures for tubal damage or endometriosis can also add to the woman's sense of poor self-esteem and exacerbate depression. Some endometriosis treatments such as danocrine/danazol or nafarelin acetate may also cause mood disturbance (Burt & Hendrick, 1997b).

Assisted reproduction (e.g. in vitro fertilisation (IVF), gamete intrafallopian transfer (GIFT) or zygote intrafallopian transfer (ZIFT)) are all very expensive and generally have success rates of less than 25% (McCartney & Downey, 1993). When infertility is due to an untreatable male factor, artificial insemination with donor sperm (AID) is highly successful. Few attempts have been made to assess the impact of anonymous donor egg or sperm on the family and even successful pregnancy may be fraught with anxiety after a prolonged wait (Kovacs et al., 1993). Couple psychotherapy, supportive individual psychotherapy for the woman are useful treatments for depression in women (and couples) undergoing assessment and treatment for infertility.

Perimenopause, menopause and depression

As detailed in Chapter 11, the transition to menopause is a major hormonal event and many women experience a range of normal but unpleasant physical and psychosocial effects. However, large epidemiological surveys do not support the notion of a nosologically distinct "involutional melancholia" (Avis et al., 1994; Woods & Mitchell, 1996). In the Massachusetts Women's Health Study, a prospective, 5-year observational trial, investigators sought to ascertain whether a change in menopausal status had an effect on mood in a cohort of 2565 women aged 45–55 years at baseline (Avis et al., 1994). No link was found between the onset of natural menopause and an increased risk of depression. However, women experiencing a lengthy perimenopause (27 months) did have a moderately increased rate of depressive symptoms, although this was mostly transient.

Perimenopause may be associated with depressive symptoms, although not necessarily depressive disorder. The most prevalent mood symptoms during the perimenopause include anxiety, tearfulness, irritability, depressed mood, lability of mood, poor concentration, worsening of memory, interrupted sleep, lack of motivation and decreased energy (Prior, 1998). The most common, disabling symptoms described are vasomotor symptoms of hot flushes, night sweats, urogenital dryness and atrophy causing dyspareunia.

Oestrogen and testosterone depletion is the physiological hallmark of the menopause. As suggested above, some women appear exquisitely vulnerable to physiological fluctuation in gonadal steroids (e.g., women with a past history of depression, PND or PMDD). As outlined above, oestrogen has a range of important effects on CNS function (McEwen, 2001 for review). It regulates synaptogenesis; has significant 5-hydroxytryptamine (5HT) 2A ($5HT_{2A}$) agonist effects by increasing the $5HT_{2A}$ receptor binding sites in areas that regulate mood and cognition; increases 5HT synthesis and uptake as well as increasing [3_H] imipramine binding; and has a trophic effect on cholinergic neurons (Fink et al., 1996; McEwen, 2001; Steiner et al., 2003). In addition, oestrogen regulates pathways traditionally associated with the control of mood (see Manji & Lenox, 1999). These actions suggest that oestrogen has AD activity, possibly reflected in a positive effect on mood states in some women following oestrogen replacement therapy (ERT) (Zweifel & O'Brien, 1997). Indeed, clinical studies of perimenopausal women with depressive symptoms given oestrogen therapy have found their symptoms improved (Schmidt et al., 2000; Soares et al., 2001). And Sherwin and Suranyi-Cadotte (1990) found that young, surgically menopausal women experienced improvements in mood and cognition with ERT.

The use of ERT is still controversial, particularly with the recent publication of the results of the Women's Mental Health Initiative Randomised Controlled Trial studies (Rossouw *et al.*, 2002; and see Chapter 11). However, each woman's particular situation need to be individually assessed. ERT is a useful short-term treatment for women with troubling psychological or physical symptoms. It is not a "fountain of youth" to be used for cosmetic reasons over a long period of time. The risks in terms of thromboembolism, breast and endometrial cancers associated with ERT need to be weighed against the benefits for some women on mood, cognition and vasomotor symptoms. Clinicians treating depressive illness in a perimenopausal woman need to understand these factors in deciding to use ERT rather than conventional AD medication – or combining both types of treatment. Women should be given the opportunity to be fully involved in the decision-making process. If ERT is considered, clinicians need to familiarise themselves with the numerous types, doses, delivery systems and combinations. Women with intact uteri run a great risk of endometrial cancer if unopposed ERT is used. This risk is significantly decreased by adding progestin (Grady et al., 1992). Again, there are many different types of progestin preparations including different classes, doses and delivery systems. Some women may experience depressive symptoms related to progestins; OC-induced dysphoria may be a useful indicator of this vulnerability.

The place for ERT in managing depression in perimenopausal/menopausal women remains controversial. Nonetheless, it remains an important treatment option for some women. Psychosocial therapies and physical monitoring are also vital accompaniments to physical therapies. Further consideration of the treatment of mood disorders in the menopause is provided in Chapter 11.

Conclusion

Women experience very different physiological changes in gonadal steroids and psychosocial stressors compared to men. The impact of normal reproductive events on mood, cognition and function may be profound. Accumulating evidence implicates oestrogen as a key regulator of mood and many other non-reproductive CNS functions. We are only just beginning to explore the complexities of the relationship between such potent neurosteroids and mental illnesses such as depression in women. Studying the integration of body and mind through the effect of gonadal hormones in the brain offers great potential for a better understanding and improved management of depression in women.

REFERENCES

American Academy of Paediatrics, Committee on Drugs (1991). Transfer of drugs and other chemicals into human milk. *Paediatrics, 93*, 137–150.

Akerlund, M., Rode, A., & Westergaard, J. (1993). Comparative profiles of reliability, cycle control and side-effects of two oral contraceptive formulations containing 150 micrograms desogesterel and either 30 micrograms or 20 micrograms ethynyl estradiol. *British Journal of Obstetrics & Gynaecology, 100*, 832–838.

Altshuler, L.L., Cohen, L., & Szuba, M.P. (1996). Pharmacologic management of psychiatric illness during pregnancy: Dilemmas and guidelines. *American Journal of Psychiatry, 153*, 592–606.

Angold, A., Costello, E.J., & Worthman, C.M. (1998). Puberty and depression: The roles of age, pubertal status and pubertal timing. *Psychological Medicine, 28*, 1–61.

Angst, J., & Dobler-Mikola, A. (1984). Do the diagnostic criteria determine the sex ratio in depression? *Journal of Affective Disorders, 7*, 189–198.

Appleby, L., Warner, R., Whitton, A., & Faragher, B. (1997). A controlled study of fluoxetine and cognitive-behavioural counselling in the treatment of postnatal depression. *British Medical Journal, 134*, 932–936.

Arnold, A.P., & Breedlove, S.M. (1985). Organizational and activational effects of sex steroids on brain and behaviour: A re-analysis. *Hormonal Behavior, 19*, 469–498.

Avis, N.E., Brambilla, D., McKinlay, S.M., & Vass, K. (1994). A longitudinal analysis of the association between menopause and depression: Results from the Massachusetts Women's Health Study. *Annals of Epidemiology, 4*, 214–220.

Backstrom, T., Appelblad, P., Bixo, M., Haage, D., Johansoon, S., Landgren, S., Seippel, L., Sundstrom, I., Wang, M., & Wahlstrom, G. (2000). Female sex steroids, the brain and behaviour. In: M. Steiner, K.A. Yonkers, & E. Eriksson (Eds.), *Mood disorders in women,* Washington, DC: pp. 189–206, Martin Dunitz.

Beatty, W.W. (1992). Gonadal hormones and sex differences in noreproductive behaviours. In: A.A. Gerall, H. Moltz, & I.L. Ward (Eds.), *Handbook of behavioural neurology Vol. II: Sexual differentiation* (pp. 85–128), New York: Plenum.

Boyce, P.M., Condon, J.T., & Ellwood, D.A. (2002). Pregnancy loss: A major life event affecting emotional health and well-being. *Medical Journal of Australia, 176*, 250–251.

Breedlove, S.M. (1992). Sexual dimorphism in the vertebrae nervous system. *Journal of Neuroscience, 12*, 4133–4142.

Burger, H.G., Dudley, E.C., Cui, J., et al. (2000). A prospective longitudinal study of serum testosterone dehydroepiandrosterone sulphate and sex hormone binding globuline levels through the menopause transition. *Journal of Clinical Endocrinology and Metabolism, 85*, 2832–2838.

Burt, V.K., & Hendrick, V.C. (1997a). *Concise guide to women's mental health* (pp. 11–24), Washington: American Psychiatric Press.

Burt, V.K., & Hendrick, V.C. (1997b). Infertility: Psychological implications of diagnosis and treatment. In: Burt, & Hendrick (Eds.), *Women's mental health*, 1st edn. Washington, DC: American Psychiatric Publishing, pp. 89–102.

Canadian Pharmaceutical Association (2000). *CPS: Compendium of pharmaceuticals and specialties.* 35th edn. Ottawa, Ontario. *CMAJ*, 2000, *162*, 1405.

Chrousos, G.P., Torpy, D.J., & Gold, P.W. (1998). Interactions between the hypothalamic-pituitary adrenal axis and the female reproductive system: Clinical implications. *Annals of Internal Medicine, 129,* 229–240.

Chwalisz, K., Brenner, R.M., Fuhrmann, U.U., Hess-Stumpp, H., & Elger, W. (2000). Antiproliferative effects of progesterone antagonists and progesterone receptor modulators on the endometrium. *Steroids, 65,* 741–751.

Cooper, P.J. (1997). Postpartum depression and child development. *Psychological Medicine, 27,* 253–260.

Cooper, P.J., & Murray, L. (1995). Course and Recurrence of Postnatal Depression: Evidence for the specificity of the diagnostic concept. *British Journal of Psychiatry, 166,* 191–195.

Croxatto, H.B. (2003). Clinical prospects of progesterone receptor modulators. In: H.P.G. Schneider (Ed.), *Menopause the state of the art – in research and management* (pp. 43–46), UK: The Parthenon Publishing Group.

Dagg, P.K.B. (1991). The Psychological sequence of therapeutic abortion – denied and completed. *American Journal of Psychiatry, 148,* 578–585.

Department of Health (UK) (2002). *Women's mental health: Into the mainstream: Strategic development of mental health care for women.* London, UK: HMSO Publications.

Department of Health (2003). *Mainstreaming Gender and Women's mental health.* London: Department of Health.

Eriksson, E., Sundblad, C., Landen, M., & Steiner, M. (2000). Behavioural effects of androgens in women. In: M. Steiner, K.A. Yonkers, & E. Eriksson (Eds.), *Mood disorders in women* (pp. 233–246), Martin Dunitz, London.

Facchinetti, F., Demyttenaere, K., & Floroni, L. (1992). Psychosomatic disorders related to gynaecology. *Psychotherapy Psychosom, 58,* 137–154.

Felthous, A.R., & Robinson, D.B. (1981). Oral contraceptive medication in prevention of psychotic exacerbations associated with phases of the menstrual cycle. *Journal of Preventive Psychiatry, 1,* 5–15.

Fink, G., Sumner, B.E., Rosie, R., Grace, O., & Quinn, J.P. (1996). Estrogen control of central neurotransmission: Effect on mood, mental state, and memory. *Cellular and Molecular Neurobiology, 16,* 325–344.

Fink, G., et al. (1998). Sex steroid control of mood, mental state and memory. *Clinical and Experimental Pharmacol Physiology, 25,* 764–775.

Frost, M., & Condon, J.T. (1996). The psychological sequelae of miscarriage: A critical review of the literature. *Australian and New Zealand Journal of Psychiatry, 30,* 54–62.

Gater, R., Tansella, M., Korten, A., Tiemens, B.G., Mavreas, V.G., & Olataura, M.O. (1998). Sex differences in the prevalence and detection of depressive and anxiety disorders in general health care settings: report from WHO collaborative study on psychological problems in general health care. *Archives of General Psychiatry, 55,* 405–413.

Genazzani, A.R., & Bernardi, F. (2003). Estrogen effects on neuroendocrine function: The new challenge of pulsed therapy. In: H.P.G. Schneider (Ed.), *Menopause the state of the art – in research and management* (pp. 465–470), UK: The Parthenon Publishing Group.

Goldzieher, J. (1994). *Hormonal contraception: Pills, injections and implants.* 3rd edn, London/Ontario: Emis-Canada.

Grady, D., Rubin, S.M., & Petitti, D.B. (1992). Hormone therapy to prevent disease and prolong life in post-menopausal women. *Annals of Internal Medicine, 117,* 1016–1037.

Hannah, P., Adams, D., Glover, V., & Sandler, M. (1992). Abnormal platelet 5-hydroxytryptamine uptake and imipramine binding in postnatal dysphoria. *Journal Psychiatric Research, 26,* 69–75.

Harris, B., Othman, S., Davies, J., Weppner, G., Richards, C., Newcombe, R., Lazarus, J., Parkes, A., Hall, R., & Phillips, D. (1992). Association between postpartum thyroid function and thyroid antibodies and depression. *British Medical Journal, 305,* 152–156.

Horwitz, K.B., Tung, L., & Takimoto, G.S. (1997). The molecular biology of progesterone receptors: Why are there two isofroms? In: H.M. Beier, M.J.K. Harper, & K. Chwalisz (Eds.), *The endometrium as a target for contraception* (pp. 1–49), Ernst Schering Research Foundation Workshop 18, Berlin: Springer-Verlag.

Huttner, R.P., & Shepherd, J.E. (2003). Gonadal steroids, selective serotonin re-uptake inhibitors and mood disorders in women. *Medical Clinics of North America, 87*(5), 1065–1076.

Kessing, L.V., Andersen, E.W., & Andersen, P.K. (2000). Predictors of recurrence in affective disorder-analyses accounting for individual heterogeneity. *Journal of Affective Disorders, 57,* 139–145.

Klier, C.M., Geller, P.A., & Ritscher, J.B. (2002). Affective disorders in the aftermath of miscarriage: A comprehensive review. *Archives of Women's Mental Health, 5,* 129–149.

Kovacs, G.T., Mushin, D., Kane, H., et al. (1993). A controlled study of the psychosocial development of children conceived following insemination with donor semen. *Human Reproduction, 8,* 788–790.

Magiakou, M.A., Mastorakos, G., Rabin, D., Dubbert, B., Gold, P.W., & Chrouses, G.P. (1996). Hypothalamic corticotropin-releasing hormone suppression during the post-partum period: Implications for the increase of psychiatric manifestations at this time. *Journal of Clinical Endocrinology and Metabolism, 81,* 1912–1917.

Major, M., Cozzarelli, C., Cooper, M.L., Zubeck, J., Richards, C., Wilhite, M., & Granzow, R.H. (2000). Psychological responses of women to first-trimester abortion. *Archives of General Psychiatry, 57,* 777–784.

Manji, H.K., & Lenox, R.H. (1999). Protein kinase C signalling in the brain: Molecular transduction of mood stabilization in the treatment of manic depressive illness. *Biological Psychiatry, 46,* 1328–1351.

McCartney, C.F., & Downey, J. (1993). New reproductive technologies. In: A. Stouduire, & P.S. Fogel (Eds.), *Medical psychiatric practice* (pp. 302), Washington: American Psychiatric Press.

McCarty, M.F. (2000). High-dose pyridoxine as an "anti-stress" strategy. *Medical Hypotheses, 54,* 803–807.

McEwen, B.S. (2001). Invited Review: Estrogens' effects on the brain: Multiple sites and molecular mechanisms. *Journal of Applied Physiology, 91,* 2785–2801.

Moffat, S.D., & Resnick, S.M. (2002). Gonadal steroid influences on Adult Neuropsychological function. In: M.D. Lewis-Hall, T.S. Williams, J.A. Panetta, & J.M. Herrera (Eds.), *Psychiatric illness in women. emerging treatments and research* (pp. 404–405), Washington: American Psychiatric Publishing Inc.

Morley, J.E. (2003). Androgens and ageing: The dawning of a new age. In: H.P.G. Schneider (Ed.), *Menopause the state of the art – in research and management* (pp. 47–51), UK: The Parthenon Publishing Group.

Murray, L., Cooper, P.J., et al. (2003). Controlled trial of the short- and long-term effect of psychological treatment of post-partum depression 2. Impact on the mother–child relationship and child outcome. *The British Journal of Psychiatry, 182,* 420–427.

Newton, C.R., Hearn, M.T., & Yuzpe, A.A. (1990). Psychological assessment and follow-up after in vitro fertilization: Assessing the impact of failure. *Fertility and Sterility*, *54*, 879–886.

O'Hara, M.W. (1991). Postpartum mental disorders. In: J.J. Sciarra (Ed.), *Gynecology and Obstetrics*. Vol. 6, Chapter 84. Philadelphia: Harper & Row. (Reproduced by the American of Physician Assistants, CD-ROM, Education 2000: Mood Disorders Across the Life Cycle in Women, 1996.)

O'Hara, M.W., Stuart, S., Gorman, L.L., & Wenzel, A. (2000). Efficacy of interpersonal psychotherapy for postpartum depression. *Archives of General Psychiatry*, *57*, 1039–1045.

Oinonen, K.A., & Mazmanian, D. (2002). To what extent do oral contraceptives influence mood and affect? *Journal of Affective Disorders*, *70*, 229–240.

Okano, T., & Nomura, J. (1992). Endrocine study of maternity blues. *Progress in Neuro-psychopharmacology and Biological Psychiatry*, *16*, 921–932.

ONS Office of National Statistics (2001). Available at "http://www.statistics.gov.uk".

Pederson, C.A., Stern, R.A., Pate, J., Sergers, M.A., Bowes, W.A., & Mason, G.A. (1993). Thyroid and adrenal measures during late pregnancy and the puerperium in women who have been depressed or who become dysphoric postpartum. *Journal of Affective Disorders*, *29*, 201–211.

Phoenix, C.H., Goy, R.W., & Gerall, A.A. (1959). Organising action of prenatally administered testosterone papionate on the tissues mediating mating behaviour in the female guinea pig. *Endocrinology*, *65*, 369–382.

Prior, J.C. (1998). Perimenopause: The complex endocrinology of the menopausal transition. *Endocrine Review*, *19*, 397–428.

Reardon, D., & Cougle, J. (2002). Depression and unintended pregnancy in the National Longitudinal Survey of Youth: A cohort study. *British Medical Journal*, *324*, 151–152.

Rossouw, JE., Anderson, G.L., Prentice, R.L., LaCroix, A.Z., Kooperberg, C., Stefanick, M.L., Jackson, R.D., Beresford, S.A., Howard, B.V., Johnson, K.C., Kotchen, J.M., Ockene, J. Writing Group for the Women's Health Initiative Investigators (2002). Risks and benefits of estrogen plus progestin in healthy postmenopausal women: principal results from the Women's Health Initiative randomized controlled trial. *JAMA*, *288*: 321–33.

Schmidt, P.J., Neiman, L., Danaceau, M.A., Tobin, M.B., Roca, C.A., Murphy, J.H., & Rubinow, D.R. (2000). Estrogen replacement in perimenopause-related depression: A preliminary report. *American Journal of Obstetrics and Gynaecology*, *183*, 414–420.

Sherwin, B. (1996). Hormones, mood and cognitive functioning in postmenopausal women. *Obstetrics and Gynaecology*, *82* (Suppl), 20s–26s.

Sherwin, B.B., & Suranyi-Cadotte, B.E. (1990). Up-regulatory effect of estrogen on platelet 3H-imipramine binding sites in surgically menopausal women. *Biological Psychiatry*, *28*, 339–348.

Smith, S., Waterhouse, B.D., Chapin, J.K., & Woodward, D.J. (1997). Progesterone alters GABA and glutamate responsiveness: A possible mechanism for its anxiolytic action. *Brain Research*, *400*, 353–359.

Soares, C., Almeida, O.P., Joffe, H., & Cohen, L.S. (2001). Efficacy of estradiol for the treatment of depressive disorders in perimenopausal women: A double blind, randomized, placebo-controlled trial. *Archives of General Psychiatry*, *58*, 529–534.

Speroff, L., Galss, R.H., & Kase, N.G. (1994). *Clinical and gynaecologic endocrinology and infertility*. Baltimore, MD: Williams & Wilkins.

Stein, G., Marsh, A., & Morton, J. (1981). Mental symptoms, weight changes and electrolyte excretion in the first postpartum week. *Journal of Psychosomatic Research*, *25*, 395–408.

Steiner, M., Yonkers, K.A. & Eriksson, E. (Eds) (2000). *Mood Disorders in Women*. London: Martin Dunitz Ltd.

Steiner, M., Dunn, E.T., BW & Born, L. (2003). Hormones and mood: From menarche to menopause and beyond. *Journal of Affective Disorders, 74,* 67–83.

Stowe, Z.N., Cassarella, J., Landry, J., & Nemeroff, C.B. (1995). Sertraline in the treatment of women with postpartum major depression. *Depression 3,* 49–55.

Stowe, Z.N., Strader, J.R., & Nemeroff, C.B. (1998). Psychopharmacology during pregnancy and lactation. In: *Textbook of psychopharmacology* (pp. 979–996), 2nd edn. Washington, DC: The American Psychiatric Press.

Stowe, Z.N., Hostetter, A.L., Owens, M.J., Ritchie, J.C., Sternberg, K., Cohen, L.S., & Nemeroff, C.B. (2003). The pharmacokinetics of sertraline excretion into human breast milk: Determinants of infant serum concentrations. *Journal of Clinical Psychiatry, 64,* 73–80.

Teixeira, J.M.A., Fisk, N.M., & Glover, V. (1999). Association between maternal anxiety in pregnancy and increased uterine artery resistance index: Cohort based study. *British Medical Journal, 318,* 153–157.

Wieck, A., Kumar, R., Hirst, A.D., Marks, M.M., Campbell, I.C., & Checkley, S.A. (1991). Increased sensitivity of dopamine receptors and recurrence of affective psychosis after childbirth. *British Medical Journal, 303,* 613–616.

Wisner, K.L., Perel, J.M., Peindl, K.S., Hanusa, B.H., Findling, R.L., & Rapport, D. (2001). Prevention of recurrent postpartum depression: A randomized clinical trial. *Journal of Clinical Psychiatry, 62,* 82–86.

Wisner, K.L., Perel, J.M., Peindl, K.S., Hanusa, B.H., Piontek, C.M., & Findling, R.L. (2004). Prevention of postpartum depression: A pilot randomized clinical trial. *American Journal of Psychiatry, 161,* 1290–1292.

Wittchen, H.-V., et al. (2002). Prevalence, incidence and stability of premenstrual dysphoric disorder in the community. *Psychological medicine, 32,* 119–132.

Woods, N.F., & Mitchell, E.S. (1996). Patterns of depressed mood in midlife women: Observations from the seattle midlife women's health study. *Research in Nursing and Health, 19,* 111–123.

World Health Organization (1997). Pincelli, M., & Homen, F.G. *Gender differences in the epidemiology of affective disorders and schizophrenia*. WHO.

World Health Organization (2002). *The world health report: The global burden of disease*. Geneva: WHO.

Wright, J., Duchensne, C., Sabourin, S., et al. (1991). Psychosocial distress and infertility: Men and women respond differently. *Fertility and Sterility, 55,* 100–108.

Wulsin, L.R., Vaillant, G.E., & Wells, V.E. (1999). A systematic review of the mortality of depression. *Psychosomatic Medicine, 61,* 6–17.

Yonkers, K. (1997). The association between premenstrual dysphoric disorder and other mood disorders. *Journal of Clinical Psychiatry, 58* (Suppl), 19–25.

Yonkers, K.A., Bradshaw, K.D., & Halbreich, U. (2000). Oestrogens, progestins and mood. In: M. Steiner, K.A. Yonkers, E. Eriksson (Eds.), *Mood disorders in women* (pp. 207–232), Martin Dunitz, London.

Zweifel, J.E., & O'Brien, W.H. (1997). A meta-analysis of the effect of hormone replacement therapy upon depressed mood. *Psychoneuroendocrinology, 22,* 189–212.

8

Anxiety and mood disorders in pregnancy and the postpartum period

Anne Buist[1], Lori E. Ross[2] and Meir Steiner[3]

[1]Austin Health, Repatriation Campus, Department of Psychiatry, West Heidelberg, Vic., Australia
[2]Women's Mental Health & Addiction Research Section, Centre for Addiction & Mental Health, Toronto, Ont., Canada
[3]Department of Psychiatry Behavioural Neurosciences and Obstetrics & Gynecology, McMasters University,
 St Joseph's Healthcare, Hamilton, Ont., Canada

Mental illness either in pregnancy or postpartum has significant and potentially serious long-term deleterious outcomes, not just for the woman but also for her entire family, and in particular, for her infant.

The immediate effects of depression, anxiety and stress during pregnancy include an increase in the rate of pre-term delivery, lower APGAR scores, lower birth weights and smaller head circumference (Dayan et al., 2002; Hedegaard et al., 1996; Lou et al., 1994; Orr & Miller, 1995; Orr et al., 2002; Steer et al., 1992; Wichers et al., 2002). It is as yet unclear whether these effects are related directly to physiological changes occurring in the depressed mother, in particular those associated with stress responses along the hypothalamic-pituitary-adrenal axis (Dieter et al., 2001; Gitau et al., 2001; Lockwood, 1999; Sandman et al., 1997; Weinstock, 1997); or indirectly as a result of poor health behaviours (Lindgren, 2001; Zuckerman et al., 1989).

The long-term adverse effects of prenatal depression, anxiety and stress on the offspring have been known for some time and are well documented. For example, newborns of depressed mothers consistently show behavioural differences and developmental problems when compared to infants born to non-depressed mothers (Grace et al., 2003; Jones et al., 1998; Lundy & Field, 1996; Lundy et al., 1999; Martins & Gasffan, 2000; Weinberg & Tronick, 1998). Children of depressed mothers have also been shown to exhibit ineffective emotional regulation, poor social skills, and delays in cognitive development; they are also more likely to experience emotional instability later in life (Galler et al., 2000; Newport et al., 2002; Nonacs & Cohen, 2003). Data from research on animal parenting reinforce the notion that maternal mental illness can be viewed as the first adverse life event for a child (Newport et al., 2002).

Recent literature suggests that perinatal mood and anxiety disorders are not culturally bound: they affect women in every society and from every socioeconomic background. Many of these women either fail to recognize that the symptoms are not "normal" for postpartum women, or else neglect to seek help out of shame or fear of having their children apprehended. Health care providers fail to diagnose a great many cases of perinatal depression (Buist et al., 2002).

This chapter provides an overview of these problems; outlines ways of identifying women at risk and/or women who already show signs and symptoms of depression/anxiety associated with childbearing; and suggests treatment options and preventive measures. The reader is referred to Chapter 9 for a more detailed consideration of pharmacological treatments of depression and anxiety in pregnancy and during breastfeeding.

Anxiety disorders in the perinatal period

Anxiety disorders are common, and are more prevalent in women. Recognized disorders include panic disorder, social anxiety disorder, generalized anxiety disorder, posttraumatic stress disorder and obsessive–compulsive disorder (OCD). Pregnancy is a time of great change and uncertainty. Demographic changes in the first world may contribute to increased sub-syndromal levels of anxiety. Thus, the majority of pregnancies in the first world currently are either a first or second birth. The total percentage of primigravid births as a proportion is rising and many women experience more anxiety during their first pregnancy. Additionally, there has been an increase in the availability and active recommendation of screening-for-abnormalities in early pregnancy. This enhances maternal choice, but the screening process itself has been shown to increase anxiety, which abates if a normal result ensues (Kowalcek, 2002).

Both quantitative and qualitative studies have identified anxiety as one of the primary features of perinatal depression (Beck, 2002; Matthey et al., 2003; Ross et al., 2003; Stuart et al., 1998). This anxiety often relates to the welfare of the infant, insecurity about one's parenting abilities, or being alone, and may meet criteria for a diagnosis of an anxiety disorder. Anxiety disorders per se during the perinatal period have been much less studied than depressive disorders, and little is known about their prevalence (Steiner & Born, 2002).

Panic disorder during the perinatal period can have a significant impact on functioning, including being confined to the home and subsequently feeling that one is a burden to one's family (Beck, 1998; Metz et al., 1983). Many women with pre-existing panic disorder (approximately 40%) have a reduction in panic and phobic avoidance symptoms during pregnancy (Hertzberg & Wahlbeck, 1999; Northcott & Stein, 1994; Villeponteaux et al., 1992). A smaller but clinically significant sub-group (20–30%) report more severe panic symptoms during pregnancy (Cohen et al., 1994; Northcott & Stein, 1994). In a review of 278 pregnancies described in eight studies on this topic, 38% of patients exhibited either postpartum onset or worsening of symptoms (Hertzberg & Wahlbeck, 1999). The most common outcome of pregnancy on existing panic disorder, however, is no change in symptoms (Wisner et al., 1996). The postpartum period is associated with first lifetime onset of panic disorder in some women (Wisner et al., 1996).

The prevalence of *OCD* in the perinatal period has not been systematically studied, though it has been suggested that the postpartum period in particular may be a time of increased vulnerability to OCD symptoms (Arnold, 1999; Williams & Koran, 1997). Obsessions and/or ruminative thoughts, particularly related to harming the infant, are relatively common features of postpartum depression (Wisner et al., 1999). A recent study of a community sample determined that 65% of new parents (including both mothers and fathers) reported obsessional intrusive thoughts, suggesting that symptoms associated with OCD may be common in the perinatal period, even in the absence of other psychopathology (Abramowitz et al., 2003).

Mood in pregnancy

Depression during pregnancy is not uncommon, with reports suggesting that approximately 10–20% of pregnant women meet criteria for a major or minor depressive disorder (Gotlib et al., 1989; Kelly et al., 2001; Kitamura et al., 1993; Kumar & Robson, 1984; Murray & Cox, 1990; O'Hara et al., 1984). The highest rates of clinical depression have been reported during the first trimester of pregnancy, with a second peak during the third trimester (Kitamura et al., 1993; Kumar & Robson, 1984).

The prevalence rates for clinical depression in perinatal populations are comparable to those seen in non-childbearing groups (O'Hara et al., 1991); however, higher than expected rates of sub-clinical symptoms of depression are reported at this time. During pregnancy in particular, as many as 25% of women report depressive symptoms (Gotlib et al., 1989; Johanson et al., 2000; Marcus et al., 2003; Morse et al., 2000). Higher rates have been reported during pregnancy than during the postpartum period (Elliott et al., 1983; Evans et al., 2001; Gotlib et al., 1989; Josefsson et al., 2002; O'Hara et al., 1991). This may reflect an overestimation of the prevalence of depression as a result of screening tools capturing the "normal" concerns about labour, delivery, and the health of the foetus that is typically associated with the late stages of pregnancy. On the other hand, antenatal depression can go unrecognized due to the overlap between the normal physical consequences of pregnancy and the somatic symptoms of depression. Decreases in libido, appetite and sleep disturbances, fatigue, and general aches and pains are particularly problematic in this regard (Coverdale et al., 1996; Elliott et al., 1983). Thus, careful history-taking, eliciting the core features of depression such as low mood and loss of interest in things in general, is required.

Postpartum mood disorders

"*The Blues*" is by far the most common of the mood changes related to the postpartum period, occurring usually on day 3–5 and lasting hours or at most a few days. Given it is so common, self limiting, and does not require any treatment other than reassurance and support, it should not be considered a disorder, but is mentioned because of a possible biological link between it and more significant mood changes (Bergant et al., 1999). Research at a hormonal level has as yet been inconclusive (Nappi et al., 2001; Parry et al., 2003; Pearson Murphy et al., 2001).

Perinatal Depression is more severe and enduring than the "blues". Anything between 10% and 20% of women exhibit depressive symptoms in the weeks before or following delivery. In a meta-analysis of 12,810 women, the average prevalence rate for non-psychotic postpartum depression (assessed after at least two weeks postpartum) was 13% (O'Hara & Swain, 1996). Prevalence rates vary by assessment method, with higher rates (14%) recorded when self-report measures such as the Edinburgh Postnatal Depression Scale (EPDS; Cox et al., 1987) or Centre for Epidemiological Studies-Depression (CES-D) (Radloff, 1977) are used, and lower rates when diagnostic criteria are applied by a clinician using set diagnostic criteria (10.5% for Research Diagnostic Criteria and 7.2% for Diagnostic and Statistical Manual III or III-R Criteria) (O'Hara & Swain, 1996).

The difficulty in differentiating normal emotional responses to the events associated with childbirth, from symptoms of perinatal depression per se, is reflected in the fact that there are no universally applied criteria for the diagnosis of perinatal depressive disorder. In particular, there are inconsistencies with respect to the number of weeks or months within which postpartum symptoms must emerge in order to be considered part of a postnatal episode (as opposed to a depressive episode that occurs independent of childbirth). According to the 4th edition of the Diagnostic and Statistical Manual of Mental Disorders (DSM) (American Psychiatric Association, 1994), symptoms must have their onset within four weeks postpartum in order for the episode to qualify for the "postpartum onset" specifier. Most clinicians and researchers prefer less stringent criteria, using a time frame of anything up to three months (Wisner et al., 2002).

According to DSM-IV criteria, postnatal depression (PND) is not qualitatively different from other depressive illnesses, with mood symptoms, low energy, loss of interest, and sleep and appetite disturbance commonly present. Although many women with PND do report these symptoms, the context of pregnancy or the postnatal period is often apparent in the manner in which the symptoms are manifested. There are themes common to women's experiences of childbirth and motherhood that separate PND from depression at other times. These themes may aid the clinician in better understanding the illness. For example, in Beck's metasynthesis of 18 qualitative studies on PND (Beck, 2002), four common themes arose, namely:

1 incongruence between the type of postpartum experience that was expected and that which occurred;

2 spiraling downward (feelings of anxiety and anger, feeling overwhelmed, obsessive thinking and cognitive impairment);

3 pervasive loss (notably loss of former identities); and

4 making gains through acceptance of help.

While these symptoms are common components of any depressive illness, in PND they occurred in response to specific triggers that occur very predictably for many women after childbirth.

Another feature which differentiates PND from other depressive illness is that while self-harm and suicidal thoughts do occur (Beck, 2002), suicide itself is relatively uncommon (Appleby et al., 1998). The postpartum context is thought to be protective, in that the mother recognizes the infant's dependency upon her.

Postpartum psychosis

Approximately one in 600 women will develop a postpartum psychosis. It appears that postpartum psychosis is most likely to be a variant of bipolar disorder rather than a discrete subtype of psychotic illness (Kendall et al., 1987): women with a history of bipolar disorder have a high chance of relapse in the early postpartum period. Evidence, though limited, suggests that there is an increased risk of postpartum relapse in women with schizoaffective disorder, but not women with schizophrenia, providing treatment is maintained (Meltzer & Kumar, 1985). However, risk of a postpartum psychosis is increased in any woman with a previously existing psychotic illness if medication is stopped during pregnancy or the early postpartum period; some clinicians do this due to fears of teratogenicity, side effects in the newborn, or for illness related reasons (see Chapter 9). Puerperal psychosis tends to have a more rapid onset than PND: usually within the first week or at the latest, the first month, postpartum. "Weaning" psychosis when breastfeeding ceases has been described and may be a related, though less common, phenomenon.

Postpartum psychosis may have any of the features of acute schizophreniform disorder, but most frequently resembles an episode of bipolar disorder, with an early manic phase and later depressive swing (Brockington et al., 1981). Many women who develop postpartum psychosis have no previous psychiatric history, though a family history of bipolar disorder is not uncommon. All women who have a postpartum psychosis will be at higher risk for developing bipolar disorder at any future time, though the risk is greatest for episodes related to future pregnancies (Llewellyn et al., 1998). Postpartum psychosis carries a significant suicide risk, with the peak incidence occurring in the first month postpartum (Appleby, 1991). A recent review of maternal deaths in the UK concluded that suicide was the leading cause (Oates, 2003).

Confusion and clouding of consciousness are also considered to be classic features of postpartum psychosis (Brockington et al., 1981; Prothoroe, 1969). These characteristics, together with the rapidity of onset, have provoked research into a potential hormonal or biological aetiology (see below). The symptoms of postpartum psychosis represent a striking change from a woman's usual personality, and are therefore easily detected in most cases. However, the early discharge policy of most Western obstetric services has placed the onus of detection on families and community services.

Risk factors/aetiology

Biological variables

Genetic

Family psychiatric history is an important predictor of both prenatal (Kumar & Robson, 1984) and postpartum depression, leading some to suggest a genetic component to its aetiology. Women with postpartum depression have a higher than expected proportion of first-degree relatives with history of a mood disorder (Johnstone et al., 2001; Steiner & Born, 2002; Steiner & Tam, 1999). However, there is no clear evidence from twin or sibling analyses for a strong genetic risk for perinatal depression apart from genetic risk for major depression more generally. Without data from twin studies to separate the effects of heritability and environmental factors, it cannot be determined whether the risk associated with family history of depression is attributable to a genetic vulnerability to depression or, rather, to the effects of growing up in close proximity to relatives suffering from mental illness. Regardless of the exact mechanism, however, it is clear that personal and family psychiatric history, and in particular a history of major depression, are useful in prospectively identifying women at high risk for developing perinatal depression and/or anxiety (Steiner & Born, 2002).

Hormonal factors

From the earliest writings on perinatal mood and anxiety disorders, hormonal fluctuations associated with pregnancy and the postpartum period have been postulated to play a causal role (see also Chapter 7). During pregnancy, significant changes are observed in several steroid and peptide hormones, including oestrogen, progesterone, corticotrophin-releasing hormone, prolactin, and oxytocin (Russell et al., 2001). Attempts to identify a consistent relationship between one or more of these hormones and symptoms of depression and anxiety have met with limited success. Though some evidence suggests either high prenatal progesterone concentrations (Buckwalter et al., 1999) or the magnitude of the postpartum drop in progesterone concentrations to be a causal factor in depressed mood (Harris et al., 1994; Nott, 1976), other studies contradict this (Heidrich et al., 1994; O'Hara et al., 1991). Studies investigating changes in oestradiol, cortisol and prolactin levels relative to mood changes in the perinatal period have similarly failed to establish consistent aetiological roles for these hormones (Harris et al., 1989; O'Hara et al., 1991; Steiner et al., 1986).

Inconsistent findings have also linked androgens, including dehydroepiandrosterone and testosterone (Buckwalter et al., 1999), and the centrally active neurosteroids, including allopregnanolone and pregnanolone (Hill et al., 2000; Pearson Murphy et al., 2001), with changes in mood during pregnancy and the postpartum period.

Despite the lack of evidence for a linear relationship between the level of any particular hormone and symptoms of perinatal depression and/or anxiety, it is clear that hormonal sensitivity is an important risk factor for at least some women. In an elegant study, Bloch et al. (2003) demonstrated that women with a past history of postpartum depression developed mood changes in response to a challenge with exogenous oestrogen and progesterone that had no effect on control subjects without a psychiatric history (Bloch et al., 2003). This suggests that symptoms of perinatal mood disorders may develop as an abnormal response to normal hormonal fluctuations. The factors that determine why some women, and not others, develop symptoms of depression or anxiety in response to these fluctuations, remains to be elucidated (Steiner et al., 2003a).

A relationship between thyroid hormone dysfunction and perinatal mood has also been postulated and thyroid dysfunction has been associated with postpartum depression in thyroid antibody-positive women (Harris, 1999). However, the relationship between the thyroid system and depression seems to be salient only for a sub-group of women and does not explain perinatal mood disorders more generally (Harris, 1999).

Sleep regulation

Finally, the psychobiological pathways involved in sleep may contribute to the development of perinatal mood and anxiety disorders. Women experience dramatic changes to their sleep pattern and sleep quality beginning in late pregnancy and extending well into the postpartum period, including frequent awakenings, fewer hours of total sleep, reduced sleep efficiency, and shorter rapid eye movement (REM) sleep latency (Coble et al., 1994; Karacan et al., 1969). Coble et al. (1994) found that women with a past history of an affective disorder had greater changes in total sleep time and REM sleep latency reduction than did postpartum women with no such history. In another study, the difference in mood experienced by postpartum women in the first week compared to non-postpartum controls was eliminated when the effect of time awake at night was controlled for (Swain et al., 1997). These data are in agreement with a body of evidence that sleep disturbance, insomnia and poor quality of sleep are risk factors for depression in men and women throughout their lifetimes (Ford & Cooper-Patrick, 2001).

Psychosocial factors

In recent years, a sociodemographic profile of women who may be at elevated risk for perinatal mood disorders has begun to emerge. Anxiety disorders have been less well studied in this context, but one assumes a significant overlap in psychosocial causation for anxiety and depression at this time of life.

Marital relationship

Recent studies suggest that women who are not in a stable relationship may be at higher risk for perinatal mood disorders (Beck & Gable, 2001; Bryan et al., 1999). The quality of the marital (or equivalent) relationship is also consistently associated with postpartum depressive symptoms (Beck & Gable, 2001; Johanson et al., 2000; Steinberg & Bellavance, 1999; Wilson et al., 1996).

Education

There are reports that both women with few years of education (Gurel & Gurel, 2000) and highly educated women (Yonkers et al., 2001) are at increased risk of perinatal depression. This may suggest that there is a U-shaped relationship between education level and risk for perinatal depression. Further research is necessary.

Planning of pregnancy

Unplanned or unwanted pregnancy has been associated with increased risk for perinatal depression (Beck & Gable, 2001; Kelly et al., 2001; Kitamura et al., 1998; O'Hara et al., 1984; Verdoux et al., 2002; Warner et al., 1996). Contemplation of termination of the current pregnancy has been associated with prenatal depressive symptoms (Kumar & Robson, 1984), as has previous termination of a pregnancy (Kitamura et al., 1993).

Personality

Neurotic personality style has been linked to depressive symptoms in the postpartum period (Dudley et al., 2001; Matthey et al., 2000), as has high interpersonal sensitivity (Boyce et al., 1991; Matthey et al., 2000) and low self-esteem (Fontaine & Jones, 1997; Hall et al., 1996). Coping styles may mediate vulnerability to perinatal mood disorders (Huizink et al., 2002): an escape-avoidance coping style has been associated with depressive symptoms both during pregnancy (Rudnicki et al., 2001) and the postpartum period (Gotlib et al., 1991).

Social supports, life events, and other factors

Research has consistently found that inadequate social supports, and in particular lack of support from an intimate partner, is associated with depressive symptoms during both pregnancy (Kitamura et al., 1998; Kumar & Robson, 1984) and the postpartum period (Beck & Gable, 2001; Brugha et al., 2000; O'Hara & Swain, 1996). Stressful life events have been associated with depressive symptoms in pregnant women (Rubertsson et al., 2003), and in a number of individual studies and two meta-analyses, in postpartum women (Beck & Gable, 2001; O'Hara & Swain, 1996). Physical pregnancy-related complications have been associated with negative mood throughout pregnancy (Green & Murray, 1994). In multiparous women, negative experience of a previous birth has been associated with depressive symptoms at 15 weeks gestation (Rubertsson et al., 2003). Finally, substance dependency (Pajulo et al., 2001) and particularly cigarette smoking (Kitamura et al., 1998; Marcus et al., 2003) have been associated with prenatal depressive symptoms.

There has been little study of risk factors for perinatal anxiety disorders. However, the available data suggest that many of the risk factors for prenatal depression are also associated with perinatal anxiety. In particular, recent stressful life events and lack of social support have been associated with self-reported anxiety (Norbeck & Anderson, 1989).

Cultural aspects

Most studies on postpartum depression have been conducted in "Western" countries. However, there is increasing interest in the prevalence and presentation of PND in non-Western societies (Chaaya et al., 2002; Chan et al., 2002; Danaci et al., 2002; Hung Chich-Hsiu & Chung Hsin-Hsin, 2001). Until recently, it was believed that, while the prevalence of puerperal psychosis is independent of the culture under study, PND was considered to be more prevalent in Western societies (Cox, 1988). Suggested reasons for the higher prevalence of PND in Western societies have included lower levels of social support, high social expectations without adequate paid leave, and a lack of significant social valuing of the "mother" role (Hayes et al., 2000; Stern & Kruckman, 1983).

More recently, reports have suggested an increase in rates of PND in non-Western societies, with different psychosocial parameters being implicated (Chaaya et al., 2002; Chan et al., 2002; Danaci et al., 2002; Hayes et al., 2001; Hung Chich-Hsiu & Chung Hsin-Hsin, 2001). Levels of PND only slightly lower than those in Western countries have now been cited in Hong Kong, for example (Chan et al., 2002; Hung Chich-Hsiu & Chung Hsin-Hsin, 2001). Many cross-cultural studies have relied upon EPDS scores, despite the fact the instrument is a screening, rather than a diagnostic tool. In some cultures there have been reports of unexpectedly high (14–26%) rates of scoring above the recommended threshold of 12 on the EPDS. Chronic health problems were cited as a reason for this high rate of depression in Beirut (Chaaya et al., 2002), whilst sub-optimal social support, and in particular lack of support from in-laws, was seen as an important determinant in Turkey (Danaci et al., 2002). Economic deprivation and gender of the infant were associated with depression in Indian mothers

(Patel et al., 2002). These data suggest that PND exists in all cultures, though the contributing issues may vary from culture to culture. These issues will require consideration in the management of PND: women immigrating from one culture to another may have factors specifically related to one, or both, of these cultures.

Biopsychosocial models of perinatal mood and anxiety disorders

Although the majority of research studies have evaluated either biological or psychosocial variables in relation to perinatal mood and anxiety disorders, most researchers and clinicians agree that a complex, interactive aetiological pathway is most likely responsible. A multifactorial causal model, incorporating biological (specifically, genetic, which may be linked to evolutionary influences), psychosocial and developmental variables has recently been proposed to describe risk for depression in adult women (Kendler et al., 2002).

There is some empirical evidence that a biopsychosocial model may best account for symptoms of depression and anxiety in perinatal populations as well (Steiner et al., 2003a). The first such model was proposed by O'Hara et al. (1984). Their vulnerability-life stress model demonstrated that personal vulnerability to depression (conferred by cognitive vulnerability and personal and family psychiatric history) interacts with recent life stresses (and particularly childcare-related stressful events) to determine the likelihood of developing postpartum depression (O'Hara et al., 1984).

More recently, Ross et al. (2004) used structural equation modelling techniques to model relationships between biological (including hormonal) and psychosocial variables in the development of pre- and postnatal symptoms of depression and anxiety. In the model of prenatal mood, the biological variables had no direct relationship with symptoms of depression. Rather, they acted indirectly through their effects on psychosocial variables and symptoms of anxiety (Ross et al., 2004). These results were interpreted to suggest that biological vulnerability factors, including hormonal changes, determine the threshold at which psychosocial triggers, including lack of social support, will provoke symptoms of depression and anxiety. As these same relationships could not account for postpartum symptoms of depression and anxiety, the findings await replication (Ross et al., 2004). Future research with biopsychosocial models will likely provide a more complete understanding of both aetiology and treatment of perinatal mood and anxiety disorders.

Detection: A role for screening?

There are currently a number of tools used to screen for perinatal depression. Of these, the EPDS (Cox et al., 1987), is the most widely accepted. It has been used in a number of countries, and has been translated into approximately 30 languages (Cox & Holden, 2003). The EPDS is brief (10 questions), inexpensive to use, and has a high sensitivity and validity for detection of current depression. Although there is controversy about the implementation of routine screening for PND, one report has indicated that up to half of depressed women are not recognized without such a routine measure (Hickie et al., 1991).

Use of the EPDS in research and clinical practice has been criticized by some. During pregnancy in particular, there is debate about the degree to which elevated scores on the EPDS are reflective of clinically significant psychopathology. The optimal cut-off score for the EPDS is 14/15 during pregnancy, two points higher than the threshold recommended for use during the postnatal period (Murray & Cox, 1990). It is notable that the three items of the EPDS that assess components of anxiety, together account for nearly 50% of the total EPDS score in the last weeks of pregnancy. This may suggest that high prenatal EPDS scores are driven by situational anxiety (e.g., normal worries about labour, delivery, and/or the health of the foetus) (Ross et al., 2003).

There is debate about the acceptability of the EPDS to perinatal women (Shakespeare et al., 2003), though this seems to relate primarily to the circumstances in which screening occurs. Concerns have also been raised regarding the economic burden that routine screening could place on already strained healthcare systems. However, most women in Australia (over 90%) see health professionals (general practitioners or/and community nurses) during the postpartum period, and as such, routine screening would be expected to change the context of the interview, rather than to increase the length or number of visits (Mandl et al., 1999).

A number of countries have begun wide-spread screening for perinatal mood disorders: in Canada, emotional health is investigated as part of routine antenatal care; Israel has wide-spread PND screening; and Australia is currently implementing a programme of antenatal and postnatal screening in six states, with subsequent evaluation (Buist et al., 2002).

Prevention

Prevention is considered to be the first line of treatment for postpartum depression (Steiner & Yonkers, 2003b). Having experienced one episode of PND, women will be at a greater risk of relapse or recurrence. Risk estimates vary between 25% and 60%, with a greater risk for puerperal psychosis recurring after future children (Wisner & Wheeler, 1994).

Attempts to prevent PND have been hampered by difficulties in predicting which mothers are at risk. Despite findings that prenatal scores on the EPDS and other symptom scales are strongly and consistently associated with postnatal scores (Da Costa et al., 2000; Josefsson et al., 2002), and that approximately one-third of PNDs have their onset during pregnancy (Murray & Cox, 1990), current methods are unable consistently to identify pregnant women who will go on to develop PND. In a longitudinal study of 1272 women, Green & Murray (1994) found that only 38% of women who scored above the threshold for probable depression at 35 weeks gestation also scored above the threshold at six weeks postpartum. In other words, over 60% of women with postpartum depressive symptoms would not have been predicted on the basis of their prenatal scores. Other variables must therefore be included in an assessment of risk for postpartum depression.

Studies on prevention have generally tested group interventions. Results have been unconvincing, and their validity limited by low sample size, high attrition rates, and lack of ability accurately to predict those at risk (Lumley & Austin, 2001). Debriefing after childbirth has been unhelpful in reducing PND (Priest et al., 2003). Those studies examining prophylactic use of medication have also been disappointing despite optimistic results from an early non-randomized study (Wisner & Wheeler, 1994).

Best practice for the prevention of PND is thus largely based on common sense rather than strong research evidence. This includes minimizing stress and promoting supports, together with close monitoring and aggressive treatment if early signs of depression are detected. Decisions about prophylactic use of pharmacotherapy for women with previous episodes must be made on a case-by-case basis. Severity of illness is a key factor to consider, as are the preferences of the woman and her partner, if she has one. A risk:benefit analysis is required, incorporating risks associated with pharmacotherapy during pregnancy and lactation (see Chapter 9).

Treatment issues

The mother

Psychosocial

A majority of women have significant psychological issues associated with their transition to motherhood. Studies suggest that *supportive counselling* can be adequate to help them deal with their issues of unmet expectations and feelings of failure. Three types of brief psychotherapies were compared to routine primary care, and all were shown to be equally effective in mood improvement (Murray et al., 2003). However, these improvements are only short term.

Evidence suggests that anxiety management and self-feedback components of *cognitive behavioural therapy* (CBT) can help manage anxiety, obsessive thoughts and panic symptoms in the postpartum period. CBT is effective alone or in combination with serotonergic antidepressants (Appleby et al., 1997). Group therapy can potentially provide aspects of both support and CBT as well as providing added social and normalizing benefits (Meager & Milgrom, 1996).

Interpersonal psychotherapy (IPT) has also shown promise in the treatment of depression, both during pregnancy and in the postnatal period. Two controlled trials have found IPT to be more effective than a waiting list or psycho-educational control condition in the treatment of depression in antepartum women (Spinelli & Endicott, 2003; Stuart et al., 1998). Two further controlled trials have shown similar results in postpartum women (O'Hara et al., 2000; Zlotnick et al., 2001). IPT has been used successfully in both predominantly Caucasian, middle-class mothers (O'Hara et al., 2000, Stuart et al., 1998), as well as in immigrant and socioeconomically disadvantaged populations (Spinelli & Endicott, 2003; Zlotnick et al., 2001).

As outlined above, poor *social support* is a key risk factor for PND; it is also a potential key factor in recovery. Specifically, the involvement of the partner in treatment for postpartum depression results in improved outcomes (Misri et al., 2000). With decreasing birth rates and more women joining the work force, traditional social supports such as a network of friends and an extended family are often absent. Thus, maternal child health nurses and PND support groups play a valuable potential role in helping mothers to recover.

Biological

Pharmacological/hormonal interventions

The guidelines which inform *pharmacological treatments* for perinatal psychiatric disorders are generally the same as those used for treatment of the disorders in women at other times in their lives (Altshuler et al., 2001; Steiner & Yonkers, 2003b). However, safety of the therapy for the foetus or breastfed infant is an important consideration in clinical decision-making; this is covered in Chapter 9.

A number of studies have looked at *hormonal treatment* and prevention of perinatal psychiatric disorders. These studies have yielded limited evidence that hormone-based therapies may have some potential for the treatment of postpartum depression in particular. Progesterone therapy was first recommended by Dalton et al. (1983) for treatment of postpartum depression, but without data from well-designed studies to support the recommendation. More recent randomized controlled trials (RCTs) suggest that synthetic progestogens could potentially *cause* depression in at risk women (Granger & Underwood, 2001).

There is more promising evidence for oestrogen therapy of postpartum disorders. Ahokas and colleagues reported on a total on 14 women with severe postpartum depression or postpartum psychosis who responded rapidly to sublingual oestrogen treatment (Ahokas et al., 1999; 2000); and in an open label study of 23 patients receiving sublingual 17-beta-estradiol, 19 achieved clinical recovery within two weeks (Ahokas et al., 2001). However, these findings require replication, and in particular since all patients in these trials were hypoestrogenic at the time therapy was initiated.

A hypoestrogenic state has not been consistently reported across patients with post-partum depression.

High-dose oral oestrogen was used as a prophylactic strategy in seven women with a history of severe postpartum affective disorder (including both postpartum depression and postpartum affective psychosis); six of the seven subjects remained well throughout the first postpartum year (Sichel et al., 1995). However, the high dose (25 mg intravenously 8 hourly, decreasing subsequently) administered in this study is unlikely to be given routinely, as a result of potential safety concerns.

The only published placebo-controlled trial of oestrogen in postpartum depression involved the administration of 200 μg/day of transdermal 17-beta-oestradiol or placebo to 61 women with severe postpartum depression (Gregoire et al., 1996). While the oestrogen-treated participants appeared to improve more rapidly and to a greater extent than controls, differences between the groups were small in magnitude, and potentially confounded by differential use of traditional antidepressant medication. Further research is required to determine whether low-dose oestrogen therapy has a role in the treatment of severe postpartum depression and/or postpartum psychosis.

Electroconvulsive therapy

Electroconvulsive therapy (ECT) has been long considered to have a role in the more severe PNDs and postpartum psychosis. Recent evidence confirms its effectiveness in postnatal mood disorders (Appleby, 1991). Due to issues of stigma, and a high rate of relapse, ECT tends to be reserved for severe cases where there is poor nutritional intake, a strong risk of suicide, or a high level of tormenting thoughts.

Sleep deprivation

Chronic sleep deprivation experienced by women in the late stages of pregnancy and the postpartum period could lead to dysregulation of the circadian rhythm (Review: Ross et al., 2005). Sleep deprivation therapy (Parry et al., 2003) and bright light therapy addressed the issue of disordered mood due to sleep deprivation (Oren et al., 2002). While both have shown promise in preliminary studies, the results need to be replicated. Preliminary evidence suggests that reduction in sleep deprivation in the immediate postpartum period can reduce the prevalence of postpartum depression in high-risk women (Causey et al., 2001). A controlled study is needed to confirm or refute these findings.

Inpatient units

Admitting women without their babies has negative consequences for the mother as it often enhances her guilt for abandoning her child. This separation may have consequences for the child in addition to any consequences of the maternal mental illness itself. As issues of mother–infant attachment are often central to the woman's depression, mother–baby admission allows for issues of parenting and attachment to be addressed as part of the treatment plan (Milgrom et al., 1998).

In response to these needs, mother–baby units originated in the UK with Main's admission of mothers to the paediatric unit in order to prevent separation. Today, dedicated mother–baby units are provided in a number of countries. Reports of the efficacy and effectiveness of these units have been limited to reviews of admitted patients; a randomized control trial would be ethically and practically difficult to implement. A report on a large cohort of women admitted to mother–baby units in the UK over six years found that in a majority of the 848 cases (78%), outcomes were positive with respect to clinical improvement and capacity to care for the child (Salmon et al., 2003).

A smaller review of the admissions to four inpatient units in Melbourne, Australia, in 2002 found similar results. Predictors of poor outcomes (separation from the child, involvement of protective services) included low socioeconomic class, poor relationship to partner, and a diagnosis of schizophrenia (Buist et al., 2004).

Partners and couples

PND in men

In recent years there has been increasing interest in the experience of fathers postpartum. Studies show a higher level of distress in the partners of women with PND and psychosis (Lovestone & Kumar, 1993). This may be due to a number of factors: these men may be subjected to the same stresses as their wives (e.g., financial, moving house); they may have a predisposition to depression or other mental illnesses; and they often take over the child care responsibilities during their wives' illness. Men also have potential psychological issues in dealing with their transition to fatherhood. Recent studies suggest that men in Western societies are grappling with changes in societal expectations, which result in conflicts between the traditional breadwinner role and that of equal sharing of child care responsibilities (Morse et al., 2000), and find pregnancy particularly stressful (Condon et al., 2004).

Couples

Differing expectations of parenthood frequently cause increased stress on relationships. Marital difficulties predating the birth are often accentuated, and these further deplete the support base available to both parties. Relationship counselling is an important part of stress management in this context. Failure to address these factors between couples can result in ongoing marital difficulties and can contribute to parenting difficulties and later marital breakups.

PND in lesbian mothers

Most research on perinatal depression has included samples of predominantly or exclusively heterosexual women. However, increasing numbers of lesbian and bisexual women are choosing to become parents (Patterson & Friel, 2000). In lesbian families, just as in heterosexual families, child adjustment is significantly related to maternal mental health (Fulcher et al., 2002; Golombok et al., 1997; Patterson, 1999), yet little is known about the mental health status of lesbians during the perinatal period. Several studies that have been conducted on the mental health of lesbian mothers of toddlers and school-age children, and found equivalent levels of depressive symptoms relative to either published normal scores (Patterson, 1999) or to heterosexual control groups (Chan et al., 1998a, b; Fulcher et al., 2002; Golombok et al., 1997, 2003). One longitudinal study of 156 lesbian mothers found that 59% of the sample "sought counselling to help them cope with the stresses of new motherhood" (Gartrell et al., 1999).

While many of the fundamental aspects of the transition to parenthood are likely experienced similarly in lesbian and heterosexual mothers, lesbian mothers may differ from heterosexual parents on a number of variables that have been previously associated with parental mental health. For example, the potential lack of family and societal support for lesbian mothers, together with stress associated with homophobia and heterosexism, could make the transition to parenthood difficult for these women, and in particular, for non-biological lesbian parents. However, some characteristics of lesbian families may also protect against perinatal mental illness; for example, their preparedness for pregnancy and their relatively equal division of child care labour (Ross, 2005). Further research is required to clarify the prevalence of and risk factors for perinatal depression in biological and non-biological lesbian mothers. This has the potential to enhance our understanding of the relative importance of social variables in PND in all women.

The child

Obstetric outcomes

Symptoms of depression during pregnancy are consistently associated with a higher risk for pre-term delivery (Dayan et al., 2002; Orr et al., 2002). Studies have demonstrated a similar link between pregnancy-related anxiety or psychosocial stress and pre-term birth (Dole et al., 2003; Newton et al., 1979). Depression in late pregnancy is associated with an increased risk for operative deliveries and admission to a neonatal intensive care unit (Chung et al., 2001). The mechanism for these associations is uncertain, but dysregulation of the maternal-placental-foetal axis as a result of neuroendocrine changes related to depression could be a factor (Wadhwa et al., 2001). However, the importance of potential confounding variables such as maternal smoking, drug/alcohol use, poor nutrition, and a low socioeconomic status should also be considered.

Development

A number of studies have examined cognitive and emotional outcomes of infants of depressed mothers. Both cognitive and developmental delays have been observed, with boys particularly affected. These infants tend to be withdrawn, have behavioural difficulties, and have a higher rate of insecure or avoidant attachments (reviewed by Murray & Cooper, 1997a).

Early childhood studies support the findings recorded in infancy. Delays in children's cognitive, emotional, and social development have been reported by a number of researchers (reviewed by Luoma et al., 2001; Murray & Cooper, 1997b; Weinberg & Tronick, 1998). However, the degree to which a single, treated depressive episode contributes to these problems remains controversial. Further studies controlling for the potential confounder of chronic, untreated maternal depression are needed.

Studies have also linked prenatal symptoms of anxiety with behavioural problems in early childhood (O'Connor et al., 2002), and suggested that physiological changes related to anxiety could affect foetal brain development. In fact, foetal changes, including increased activity and growth delays, as well as low neurotransmitter concentrations and changes in EEG activity in the newborns, have been noted in children of women with high levels of anxiety, depression and anger in the second trimester of pregnancy (Field et al., 2003). There has also been a report of increased risk for criminality in the offspring of women who reported symptoms of depression during pregnancy (Maki et al., 2003). As for the research on developmental effects of postpartum depression, potential confounders such as parenting practices, low socioeconomic status, or childhood abuse (Buist, 1998; Oates, 2002) require further investigation. It appears that adverse outcomes in children are associated with recurrent and untreated depression, and that the likelihood of a negative outcome is low if a single episode of depression is promptly treated (Campbell & Cohn, 1995).

Conclusions

Perinatal psychiatric disorders present a particular challenge to clinicians. Poorly defined and with uncertain aetiology, they are common yet readily missed because of overlap with pregnancy and postnatal symptoms, and social pressures to attain the Western ideal of motherhood. More than at any other time, these disorders confer risks to the whole family, and present an ideal opportunity for early identification and prevention. Research and clinical awareness are imperative in providing a path toward improved treatment outcomes and a clearer understanding of these disorders.

REFERENCES

Abramowitz, J.S., Schwartz, S.A., & Moore, K.M. (2003). Obsessional thoughts in postpartum females and their partners. Content, severity and relationship with depression. *Journal of Clinical Psychology in Medical Settings, 10,* 157–164.

American Psychiatric Association. Diagnostic and statistical manual of mental disorders. DSM IV. 1994; 4th edition, Washington DC.

Ahokas, A., Kaukoranta, J., & Aito, M. (1999). Effect of oestradiol on postpartum depression. *Psychopharmacology Berlin*, *146*, 108–110.

Ahokas, A., Aito, M., & Rimon, R. (2000). Positive treatment effect of estgradiol in postpartum psychosis: A pilot study. *Journal of Clinical Psychiatry*, *61*, 166–169.

Ahokas, A., Kaukoranta, J., Wahlbeck, K., & Aito, M. (2001). Estrogen deficiency in severe post-partum depression: Successful treatment with sublingual physiologic 17-beta-estradiol: A preliminary study. *Journal of Clinical Psychology*, *62*, 332–336.

Altshuler, L.L., Cohen, L.S., Moline, M.L., Kahn, D.A., Carpenter, D., & Docherty, J.P. (2001). The expert consensus guideline series. Treatment of depression in women. *Postgraduate Medicine*, 1–88, 2001 March, 1–107.

Appleby, L. (1991). Suicide during pregnancy and in the first postnatal year. *British Medical Journal*, *302*, 137–140.

Appleby, L., Warner, R., Whitton, A., & Faragher, B. (1997). A controlled study of fluoxetine and cognitive–behavioural counselling in the treatment of postnatal depression. *British Medical Journal*, *314*, 932–936.

Appleby, L., Mortensen, P.B., & Faragher, E.B. (1998). Suicide and other causes of mortality after post-partum psychiatric admission. *British Journal of Psychiatry*, *173*, 209–211.

Arnold, L.M. (1999). A case series of women with postpartum-onset obsessive–compulsive disorder. Primary Care Companion. *Journal of Clinical Psychiatry*, *1*, 103–108.

Beck, C.T. (1998). The effects of postpartum depression on child development: A meta-analysis. *Archives of Psychiatric Nursing*, *1*, 12–20.

Beck, C.T. (2002). Postpartum depression: A metasynthesis. *Qualitative Health Research*, *12*(4), 453–472.

Beck, C.T., & Gable, R.K. (2001). Comparative analysis of the performance of the Postpartum Depression Screening Scale with two other depression instruments. *Nursing Research*, *50*(4), 242–250.

Bergant, A.M., Heim, K., Ulmer, H., & Illmensee, K. (1999). Early postnatal depressive mood: Associations with obstetric and psychosocial factors. *Journal of Psychosomatic Research*, *46*(4), 391–394.

Bloch, M., Daly, R.C., & Rubinow, D.R. (2003). Endocrine factors in the etiology of postpartum depression. *Comprehensive Psychiatry*, *44*(3), 234–246.

Boyce, P., Hickie, I., & Parker, G. (1991). Parents, partners or personality? Risk factors for postnatal depression. *Journal of Affective Disorders*, *21*, 245–255.

Brockington, I.F., Cernik, K.F., Schofield, Em., Downing, A.R., Francis, A.F., & Keelan, C. (1981). Puerperal psychosis, phenomena and diagnosis. *Archives of General Psychiatry*, *38*, 829–833.

Brugha, T.S., Wheatley, S., Taub, N.A., Culverwell, A., Friedman, T., Kirwan, P.H., Jones, D.R., & Shapiro, D.A. (2000). Pragmatic randomised controlled trial of antenatal intervention to prevent postnatal depression by reducing psychosocial risk factors. *Psychological Medicine*, *30*, 1273–1281.

Bryan, T.L., Georgiopoulos, A.M., Harms, R.W., Huxsahl, J.E., Larson, D.R., & Yawn, B.P. (1999). Incidence of postpartum depression in Olmsted Country, Minnesota. A population based retrospective study. *Journal of Reproductive Medicine*, *44*, 351–358.

Buckwalter, J.G., Stanczyk, F.Z., McCleary, C.A., et al. (1999). Pregnancy, the postpartum and steroid hormones: Effects on cognition and mood. 1998 Curt P Richter Award. *Psychoneuroendocrinology*, *24*, 69–81.

Buist, A. (1998). Childhood abuse, postpartum depression and parenting difficulties: A literature review of associations. *Australian New Zealand Journal of Psychiatry*, *32*, 370–378.

Buist, A., Barnett, B., Milgrom, J., Pope, S., Condon, J., Ellwood, D., Boyce, P.M., Austin, M.-P., & Hayes, B. (2002). To screen or not to screen – that is the question in perinatal depression. *Medical Journal of Australia*, (7/10/02 Issue), S101–S105.

Buist, A., Minto, B., Szego, K., Samhuel, M., Shawyer, L., & O'Connor, L. (2004). Mother–Baby Psychiatric Units in Australia – The Victorian Experience. *Archives of Women's Health*, *7*(1), 81–87.

Campbell, S.B., & Cohn, J.F. (1995). Depression in first time mothers: Mother–infant interaction and depression chronicity. *Developmental Psychology*, *31*, 349–357.

Causey, S., Fairman, M., Nicholson, D., & Steiner, M. (2001). Can postpartum depression be prevented? *Archives of Women's Mental Health*, *3*(4), 12–13.

Chaaya, M., Campbell, O.M.R., Kak, F.E., Shaar, D., Harb, H., & Kaddour, A. (2002) Postpartum depression: Prevalence and determinants in Lebanon. *Archives of Women's Health*, *5*, 65–72.

Chan, R.W., Brooks, R.C., Raboy, B., & Patterson, C.J. (1998a). Division of labor among lesbian and heterosexual parents: Associations with children's adjustment. *Journal of Family Health Care*, *12*, 402–419.

Chan, R.W., Raboy, B., & Patterson, C.J. (1998b). Psychological adjustment among children conceived via donor insemination by lesbian and heterosexual mothers. *Child Development*, *69*, 443–457.

Chan, S.W.-C., Levy, V., Chung, T.K.H., & Lee, D. (2002). A qualitative study of the experiences of a group of Hong Kong Chinese women diagnosed with postnatal depression. *Journal of Advanced Nursing*, *39*(6), 571–579.

Chung, T.K., Lau, T.K., Yip, A.S., Chiu, H.F., & Lee, D.T. (2001). Antepartum depressive symptomatology is associated with adverse obstetric and neonatal outcomes. *Psychosomatic Medicine*, *63*, 830–834.

Coble, P.A., Reynolds III, C.F., Kupfer, D.J., Houck, P.R., Day, N.L., & Giles, D.E. (1994). Childbearing in women with and without a history of affective disorder. II. Electroencephalographic sleep. *Comprehensive Psychiatry*, *35*, 215–224.

Cohen, L.S., Sichel, D.A., Dimmock, J.A., & Rosenbaum, J.F. (1994). Impact of pregnancy on panic disorder: A case series. *Journal of Clinical Psychiatry*, *55*, 284–288.

Condon, J.T., Boyce, P., Corkindale, C.J. (2004). The first-time fathers study: a prospective study of the mental health and well being of men during the transition to parenthood. *Australian and New Zealand Journal of Psychiatry*, 38, 56–64.

Coverdale, J.H., McCullough, L.B., Chervenak, F.A., & Bayer, T. (1996). Clinical implications and management strategies when depression occurs during pregnancy. *Australian and New Zealand Journal of Obstetrics and Gynaecology*, *36*, 424–429.

Cox, J. (1988). Childbirth as a life event: Sociocultural aspects of postnatal depression. *Acta Psychiatrica Scandinavica*, *344*(Suppl), 75–83.

Cox, J., & Holden, J. (2003). *Perinatal Mental Health: A guide to the Edinburgh Postnatal Depression Scale (EPDS)*. Glasgow: Gaskell.

Cox, J.L., Holden, J.M., & Sagovsky, R. (1987). Detection of postnatal depression: Development of the 10-item Edinburg postnatal depression scale. *British Journal of Psychiatry*, *150*, 782–786.

Da Costa, D., Larouch, J., Dritsa, M., & Brender, W. (2000). Psychosocial correlates of prepartum and postpartum depressed mood. *Journal of Affective Disorders*, *59*, 31–40.

Dalton, K. (1983). Prophylactic progesterone treatment for postnatal depression. *Marce Society Annual*. London: Marce Society.

Danaci, A.E., Dinc, G., Deveci, A., Firdevs, S.S., & Ilkin, I. (2002). Postnatal depression in Turkey: Epidemiological and cultural aspects. *Social Psychiatry and Psychiatric Epidemiology*, *37*, 125–129.

Dayan, J., Creveuil, C., Herlicoviez, M., et al. (2002). Role of anxiety and depression in the onset of spontaneous preterm labour. *American Journal of Epidemiology*, *155*(4), 292–301.

Dieter, JNI., Field, T., Hernandez-Reif, M., Jones, N.A., Lecanuet, J.-P., Salman, F.A., & Mercedes Redzepi, J. (2001). Maternal depression and increased fetal activity. *Journal of Obstetrics and Gynaecology*, *21*, 468–473.

Dole, N., Savitz, D.A., Hertz-Picciotto, I., Siega-Riz, A.M., McMahon, M.J., & Buekens, P. (2003). Maternal stress and preterm birth. *American Journal of Epidemiology*, *157*, 14–24.

Dudley, M., Roy, K., Kelk, N., & Bernard, D. (2001). Psychological correlates of depression in fathers and mothers in the first postnatal year. *Journal of Reproductive and Infant Psychology*, *19*(3), 187–202.

Elliott, S.A., Rugg, A.J., Watson, J.P., & Brough, D.I. (1983). Mood changes during pregnancy and after the birth of a child. *British Journal of Clinical Psychology*, *22*(Pt 4), 295–308.

Evans, J., Heron, J., Francomb, H., Oke, S., & Golding, J. (2001). Cohort study of depressed mood during pregnancy and after childbirth. *British Medical Journal*, *323*, 257–260.

Field, T., Deigo, M., Hernandex-Reif, M., et al. (2003). Pregnancy anxiety and comorbid depression and anger: Effects on the fetus and neonate. *Depression and Anxiety*, *17*, 140–151.

Fontaine, K.R., & Jones, L.C. (1997). Self esteem, optimism and postpartum depression. *Journal of Clinical Psychology*, *53*, 59–63.

Ford, D.E., & Cooper-Patrick, L. (2001). Sleep disturbances and mood disorders: An epidemiologic perspective. *Depression and Anxiety*, *14*, 3–6.

Fulcher, M., Sutfin, E.L., Chan, R.W., Schieb, J.E., & Patterson, C.J. (2002). In: A. Omoto, & H. Kurtzman (Eds.), *Recent research on sexual orientation, mental health and substance use*. Washington DC. American Psychological Association.

Galler, J.R., Harrison, R.H., Ramsey, F., Forde, V., & Butler, S.C. (2000). Maternal depressive symptoms affect infant cognitive development in Barbados. *Journal of Child Psychology and Psychiatry and Allied Disciplines*, *41*, 747–757.

Gartrell, N., Banks, A., Hamilton, J., Reed, N., Bishop, H., & Rodas, C. (1999). The National Lesbian Family Study: 2. Interviews with mothers of toddlers. *American Journal of Orthopsychiatry*, *69*, 362–369.

Gitau, R., Fisk, N.M., Teixeira, J.M., Cameron, A., & Glover, V. (2001). Fetal hypothalamic-pituitary-adrenal stress responses to invasive procedures are independent of maternal responses. *Journal of Clinical Endocrinology and Metabolism*, *86*(1), 104–109.

Golombok, S., Tasker, F., & Murray, C. (1997). Children raised in fatherless families from infancy: Family relationships and the socioemotional development of children of lesbian and single heterosexual mothers. *Journal of Child Psychology and Psychiatry and Allied Discipline*, *38*, 783–791.

Golombok, S., Perry, B., Burston, A., et al. (2003). Children with lesbian parents: A community study. *Developmental Psychology, 39,* 20–33.

Gotlib, I.H., Whiffen, V.E., Mount, J.H., Milne, K., & Cordy, N.I. (1989). Prevalence rates and demographic characteristics associated with depression in pregnancy and the postpartum. *Journal of Consulting and Clinical Psychology, 57,* 269–274.

Gotlib, I.H., Whiffen, V.E., Wallace, P.M., & Mount, J.H. (1991). Prospective investigation of postpartum depression: Factors involved in onset and recovery. *Journal of Abnormal Psychology, 100,* 122–132.

Grace, S.L., Evindar, A., & Stewart, D.E. (2003). The effect of postpartum depression on child cognitive development and behaviour: A review and critical analysis of the literature. *Archives of Women's Mental Health, 6,* 263–274.

Granger, A.C.P., & Underwood, M.R. (2001). Review of the role of progesterone in the management of postnatal mood disorders. *Journal of Psychosomatic Obstetrics and Gynecology, 22,* 49–55.

Green, J.M., & Murray, D. (1994). In: J. Cox, & J. Holden (Eds.), *Perinatal Psych: Use and Misuse of the Edinburgh Postnatal Depression Scale* (pp. 180–198). London: The Royal College of Psychiatrists.

Gregoire, A.J., Kumar, R., Everitt, B., Henderson, A.F., & Studd, J.W. (1996). Transdermal oestrogen for treatment of severe postnatal depression. *Lancet, 347,* 930–933.

Gurel, S.A., & Gurel, H.G. (2000). The evaluation of determinants of early postpartum low mood: The importance of parity and inter-pregnancy interval. *European Journal of Obstetrics and Gynecology, 91,* 21–24.

Hall, L.A., Kotch, J.B., Browne, D., & Rayens, M.K. (1996). Self-esteem as a mediator of the effects of stressors and social resources on depressive symptoms in postpartum mothers. *Nursing Research, 45,* 231–238.

Harris, B. (1999). Postpartum depression and thyroid antibody status. *Thyroid, 9,* 699–703.

Harris, B., Hucke, P., Thomas, R., Johns, S., & Fung, H. (1989). The use of rating scales to identify postnatal depression. *British Journal of Psychiatry, 154,* 813–817.

Harris, B., Lovett, L., Newcombe, R.G., Read, G.F., Walker, R., & Riad-Fahmy, D. (1994). Maternity blues and major endocrine changes: Cardiff puerperal mood and hormone study II. *British Medical Journal, 308,* 949–953.

Hayes, B., Roberts, S., & Davare, A. (2000). Transactional conflict between psychobiology and culture in the etiology of postpartum depression. *Medical Hypotheses, 54*(1), 7–17.

Hayes, B.A., Muller, R., & Bradley, B.S. (2001). Perinatal depression: A randomized controlled trial of an antenatal education intervention for primiparas. *Birth, 28,* 28–35.

Hedegaard, M., Henriksen, T., Sabroe, S., & Secher, N.J. (1996). The relationship between psychological distress during pregnancy and birth weight for gestational age. *Acta Obstetricia Et Gynecologica Scandinavica, 75,* 32–39.

Heidrich, A., Schleyer, M., Springler, H., et al. (1994). Postpartum blues: Relationship between not-protein bound steroid hormones in plasma and postpartum mood changes. *Journal of Affective Disorders, 30,* 93–101.

Hertzberg, T., & Wahlbeck, K. (1999). The impact of pregnancy and puerperium on panic disorder: A review. *Journal of Psychosomatic Obstetrics and Gynecology, 20*(2), 59–64.

Hickie, I., Parker, G., Wilhelm, K., & Tennant, C. (1991). Perceived interpersonal risk factors of non endogenous depression. *Psychological Medicine*, *21*, 399–412.

Hill, M., Parizek, A., Bicikova, M., et al. (2000). Neuroactive steroids, their precursors and polar conjugates during parturition and postpartum in maternal and umbilical blood: 1. Identification and simultaneous determination of pregnanolone isomers. *Journal of Steroid Biochemistry and Molecular Biology*, *75*, 237–244.

Huizink, A.C., de Robles, M.P.G., Mulder, J.H., Gerard, H.A., & Buitelaar, J.K. (2002). Coping in normal pregnancy. *Annals of Behavioral Medicine*, *24*(2), 132–140.

Hung Chich-Hsiu, & Chung Hsin-Hsin. (2001). The effects of postpartum stress and social support on postpartum women's health status. *Journal of Advanced Nursing*, *36*(5), 676–684.

Johanson, R., Chapman, G., Murray, D., Johnson, I., & Cox, J. (2000). The Northern Staffordshire Maternity Hospital prospective study of pregnancy-associated depression. *Journal of Psychosomatic Obstetrics and Gynecology*, *21*, 93–97.

Johnstone, S.J., Boyce, P.M., Hickey, A.R., Morris-Yates, A.D., & Harris, M.G. (2001). Obstetric risk factors for postnatal depression in urban and rural community samples. *Australian and New Zealand Journal of Psychiatry*, *35*, 69–74.

Jones, N.A., Field, T., Fox, N.A., Davalos, M., Lundy, B., & Hart, S. (1998). Newborns of mothers with depressive symptoms are physiologically less developed. *Infant Behavior and Development*, *21*, 537–541.

Josefsson, A., Angelsioo, L., Berg, G., Ekstrom, C.M., Gunnervik, C., Nordin, C., & Sydsjo, G. (2002). Obstetric, somatic and demographic risk factors for postpartum depressive symptoms. *Obstetrics and Gynecology*, *99*(2), 223–228.

Karacan, I., Williams, R.L., Hursch, C.J., McCaulley, M., & Heine, M.W. (1969). Some implications of the sleep patterns of pregnancy for postpartum emotional disturbances. *British Journal of Psychiatry*, *115*, 929–935.

Kelly, R., Zatzick, D., & Anders, T. (2001). The detection and treatment of psychiatric disorders and substance use among pregnant women cared for in obstetrics. *American Journal of Psychiatry*, *158*, 213–219.

Kendall, R.E., Chalmers, J.C., & Platz, C. (1987). Epidemiology of puerperal psychosis. *British Journal of Psychiatry*, *150*, 662–673.

Kendler, K.S., Gardner, C.O., & Prescott, C.A. (2002). Toward a comprehensive developmental model for major depression in women. *American Journal of Psychiatry*, *159*, 1133–1145.

Kitamura, T., Shima, S., Sugaware, M., & Toda, M.A. (1993). Psychological and social correlates of the onset of affective disorders among pregnant women. *Psychological Medicine*, Nov (23), 967–975.

Kitamura, T., Toda, M.A., Shima, S., Sugawara, K., & Sugawara, M. (1998). Social support and pregnancy: II. Its relationship with depressive symptoms among Japanese women. *Psychiatry and Clinical Neurosciences*, *51*, 37–45.

Kowalcek, I., Mühlhof, A., Bachman, S., & Gemboch, U. (2002). Depressive reactions and stress related to prenatal procedures. *Ultrasound in Obstetrics and Gynecology*, *19*(1), 18.

Kumar, R., & Robson, K. (1984). A prospective study of emotional disorder in childbearing women. *British Journal of Psychiatry*, *144*, 35–47.

Lindgren, K. (2001). Relationships among maternal – fetal attachment, prenatal depression, and health practices in pregnancy. *Research in Nursing Health*, *24*(3), 203–217.

Llewellyn, A., Stowe, Z.N., & Strader, Jr., J.R. (1998). The use of Lithium and management of women with Bipolar Disorder during pregnancy and lactation. *Journal of Clinical Psychiatry*, *59*(Suppl 6), 57–64.

Lockwood, C.H. (1999). Stress-associated preterm delivery: The role of corticotropin-releasing hormone. *American Journal of Obstetrics and Gynecology*, *180*, S264–S266.

Lou, H.C., Hansen, D., Nordentoft, M., Pryds, O., Jensen, F., & Nim, J., et al. (1994). Prenatal stressors of human life affect fetal brain development. *Developmental Medicine and Child Neurology*, *36*, 826–832.

Lovestone, S., & Kumar, R. (1993). Postnatal psychiatric illness: The impact on partners. *British Medical Journal*, *163*, 210–216.

Lumley, J., & Austin, M.P. (2001). What interventions may reduce postpartum depression? *Current Opinion in Obstetrics and Gynecology*, *13*(6), 605–611.

Lundy, B., & Field, T. (1996). Newborns of mothers with depressive symptoms are less expressive. *Infant Behavior and Development*, *19*, 419–424.

Lundy, B., Jones, N.A., Field, T., et al. (1999). Prenatal depression effects on nenonates. *Infant Behavior and Development*, *22*, 119–129.

Luoma, I., Tamminen, T., Kaukonen, P., Laippala, P., Puura, K., Salmelin, R., & Almqvist, F. (2001). Longitudinal study of maternal depressive symptoms and child well-being. *Journal of the American Academy Child and Adolescent Psychiatry*, *40*(12), 1367–1374.

Maki, P., Hakko, H., Joukamaa, M., Laara, E., Isohanni, M., & Veijola, J. (2003). Parental separation at birth and criminal behaviour in adulthood – a long-term follow-up of the Finnish Christmas Seal Home children. *Social Psychiatry and Psychiatric Epidemiology*, *38*(7), 354–359.

Mandl, K., Tronick, E., Brennan, T., Alpert, H., & Homer, C. (1999). Infant health care use and maternal depression. *Archives of Pediatrics and Adolescent Medicine*, (153), 808–813.

Marcus, S.M., Flynn, H.A., Blow, F.C., & Barry, K.L. (2003). Depressive symptoms among pregnant women screened in obstetrics settings. *Journal of Women's Health*, *12*, 373–380.

Martins, C., & Gasffan, E.A. (2000). Effects of early maternal depression on patterns of infant–mother attachment: A meta-analytic investigation. *Journal of Child Psychology and Psychiatry*, *41*, 737–746.

Matthey, S., Barnett, B., Ungerer, J., & Waters, B. (2000). Paternal and maternal depressed mood during the transition to parenthood. *Journal of Affective Disorders*, *60*, 75–85.

Matthey, S., Barnett, B., Howie, B., & Kavanagh, S. (2003). Diagnosing postpartum depression in mothers and fathers: Whatever happened to anxiety? *Journal of Affective Disorders*, *74*, 139–147.

Meager, I., & Milgrom, J. (1996). Group treatment for post-partum depression: A pilot study. *Australian and New Zealand Journal of Psychiatry*, *30*(6), 750–758.

Meltzer, E.S., & Kumar, R. (1985). Puerperal mental illness, clinical feature & classification. A study of 142 mother and baby admissions. *British Journal of Psychiatry*, *147*, 647–654.

Metz, A., Cowen, P.J., Gelder, M.G., Sturp, K., Elliot, J.M., & Graham-Smith, D.G. (1983). Changes in platelet adrenoreceptor binding post partum possible relationship to maternity blues. *Lancet*, March 5, 495–493.

Milgrom Jeannette, Snellen Martien, Stamboulakis Wynne, & Kerryn, B. (1998). Psychiatric illness in women: A review of the function of a specialist mother–baby unit. *Australian and New Zealand Journal of Psychiatry*, *32*, 680–686.

Misri, S., Kostaras, X., Fox, D., & Kostaras, D. (2000). The impact of partner support in the treatment of postpartum depression. *Canadian Journal of Psychiatry*, *45*, 554–558.

Morse, C., Buist, A., & Durkin, S. (2000). First time parenthood: Influences on pre and postnatal adjustment in fathers and mothers. *Journal of Psychosomatic and Gynecology*, *21*, 109–120.

Murray, D., & Cox, J.L. (1990). Screening for depression during pregnancy with the Edinburgh Depression Scale (EPDS). *Journal of Reproductive and Infant Psychology*, (8), 99–107.

Murray, L., & Cooper, P. (1997a). Postpartum depression and child development. *Psychological Medicine*, *27*, 253–260.

Murray, L., & Cooper, P.J. (1997b). Effects of postnatal depression on infant development. *Archives of Disease in Childhood*, *77*(2), 99–101.

Murray Lynne, Woolgar, M., Murray Joseph, & Cooper Peter. (2003). Self-exclusion from health care in women at high risk for postpartum depression. *Journal of Public Health Medicine*, *25*(2), 131–137.

Nappi, R.E., Petraglia, F., Luisi, S., Polatti, F., Farina, C., & Genazzani, A.R. (2001). Serum allopregnanolone in women with postpartum "blues". *Obstetrics and Gynecology*, *97*, 77–80.

Newport, D.J., Stowe, Z.N., & Nemeroff, C.B. (2002). Parental depression: Animal models of an adverse life event. *American Journal of Psychiatry*, *159*(8), 1265–1283.

Newton, R.W., Webster, P.A., Binu, P.S., Maskrey, N., & Phillips, A.B. (1979). Psychological stress in pregnancy and its relation to the onset of premature labour. *British Medical Journal*, *2*, 411–413.

Nonacs, R., & Cohen, L.S. (2003). Assessment and treatment of depression during pregnancy: An update. *Psychiatric Clinics of North America*, *26*, 547–562.

Norbeck, J.S., & Anderson, N.J. (1989). Life stress, social support and anxiety in mid- and late-pregnancy among low income women. *Research in Nursing and Health*, *121*, 281–287.

Northcott, C.J., & Stein, M.B. (1994). Panic disorder in pregnancy. *Journal of Clinical Psychology*, *55*(12), 539–542.

Nott, P.N., Franklin, M., Armitage, C., & Gelder, M.G. (1976). Hormonal changes and mood in the puerperium. *British Journal of Psychiatry*, *128*, 379–383.

Oates, M.R. (2002). Adverse effects of maternal antenatal anxiety on children: Causal effect or developmental continuum? *British Journal of Psychiatry*, *180*, 478–479.

Oates, M. (2003). Postnatal depression and screening: Too broad a sweep? Editorial. *British Journal of General Practice*, *53*, 596–597.

O'Connor, T.G., Heron, J., Golding, J., Beveridge, M., Glover, V., & the ALSPAC Study Team (2002). Antenatal anxiety predicts child behavioural/emotional problems independently of postnatal depression. *Journal of the American Academy Child and Adolescent Psychiatry*, *41*(12), 1470–1477.

O'Hara, M.W., & Swain, A.M. (1996). Rates and risk of postpartum depression – A meta-analysis. *International Review of Psychiatry*, *8*, 37–54.

O'Hara, M.W., Neunaber, D.J., & Zekoski, E.M. (1984). Prospective study of postpartum depression: Prevalence, course and predictive factors. *Journal of Abnormal Psychology*, *93*(2), 158–171.

O'Hara, M.W., Schlechte, J.A., Lewis, D.A., & Varner, M.W. (1991). Controlled prospective study of postpartum mood disorders: Psychological, environmental and hormonal variables. *Journal of Abnormal Psychology, 100*(1), 63–73.

O'Hara, M.W., Stuart, S., Gorman, L.L., & Wenzel, A. (2000). Efficacy of interpersonal psychotherapy for postpartum depression. *Archives of General Psychiatry*, 57, 1039–1045.

Oren, D.A., Wisner, K.L., Spinelli, M., et al. (2002). An open trial of morning light therapy for treatment of antepartum depression. *American Journal of Psychiatry, 159*, 666–669.

Orr, S.T., & Miller, C.A. (1995). Maternal depressive symptoms and the risk of poor pregnancy outcome. Review of the literature and preliminary findings. *Epidemiologic Reviews, 17*(1), 165–171.

Orr, S.T., James, S.A., & Prince, C.B. (2002). Maternal prenatal depressive symptoms & spontaneous preterm births among African-American women in Baltimore, Maryland. *American Journal of Epidemiology, 159*(9), 797–802.

Pajulo, M., Savonlahti, E., Sourander, A., Helenius, H., & Piha, J. (2001). Antenatal depression, substance dependency and social support. *Journal of Affective Disorders*, 65, 9–17.

Parry, B.L., Sorenson, D.L., Meliska, C.J., et al. (2003). Hormonal basis of mood and postpartum disorder. *Current Women's Health Report, 3*(3), 230–235.

Patel, P., Wheatcroft, R., Park, R.J., & Stein, A. (2002). The children of mothers with eating disorders. *Clinical Child and Family Psychological Review, 5*(1), 1–18.

Patterson, C.J. (2001). Families of the lesbian baby boom: Maternal mental health and child adjustment. *Journal of Gay and Lesbian Psychotherapy*, 4, 91–107.

Patterson, C.J., & Friel, L.V. (2000). In: G. Bentley, & N. Mascie-Taylor (Eds.), *Infertility in the modern world: Biosocial perspectives.* Cambridge: Cambridge University Press.

Pearson Murphy, B.E., Steinberg, S.I., Hu, F.Y., & Allison, C.M. (2001). Neuroactive ring A-reduced metabolites of progesterone in human plasma during pregnancy: Elevated levels of 5 alphadihydroprogesterone in depressed patients during the latter half of pregnancy. *Journal of Clinical Endocrinology and Metabolism*, 86, 5981–5987.

Prothoroe, C. (1969). Puerperal psychosis: A long term study 1927–1961. *British Journal of Psychiatry, 11*(518), 9–30.

Radloff, L.S. (1977). The CES-D scale: A self-report depression scale for research in the general population. *Journal of Applied Psychological Measures, 1*, 385–401.

Ross, L.E., Evans, G., Sellers, E.M., & Romach, M.K. (2003). Measurement issues in postpartum depression part 1: Anxiety as a feature of postpartum depression. *Archives of Women's Health*, 6, 51–57.

Ross, L.E., Murray, B.J., Steiner, M. (2005). Sleep and perinatal mood disorders: A critical review. *Journal of Psychiatry and Neuroscience, 30*(4), 247–256.

Ross, L.E. (2005). Perinatal Mental Health in Lesbian mothers: A review of potential risk and protective factors. *Women and Health, 41*(3), 113–128.

Ross, L.E., Sellers, E.M., Gilbert Evans, S.E., & Romach, M.K. (2004). Mood changes during pregnancy and the postpartum period: Development of a biopsychosocial model. *Acta Psychiatrica Scandinavica, 109*, 457–466.

Rubertsson, C., Waldenstrom, U., & Wickberg, B. (2003). Depressive mood in early pregnancy: Prevalence and women at risk in a national Swedish sample. *Journal of Reproductive and Infant Psychology, 21*, 113–123.

Rudnicki, S.R., Graham, J.L., Habbouske, D.F., & Ross, R.D. (2001). Social support and avoidant coping: correlates of depressed mood during pregnancy in minority women. *Women's Health*, *34*, 19–34.

Russell, J.A., Douglas, A.J., & Ingram, C.D. (2001). Brain preparations for maternity – adaptive changes in behavioural and neuroendocrine systems during pregnancy and lactation: An overview. *Brain Research*, *133*, 1–38.

Salmon, M., Abel, K., Cordingley, L., Friedman, T., & Appleby, L. (2003). Clinical and parenting skills. Outcomes following joint mother–baby psychiatric admission. *Australian and New Zealand Journal of Psychiatry*, *37*(5), 556–562.

Sandman, C.A., Wadhwa, P.D., Chicz-DeMet, A., Dunkel-Schetter, C., & Porto, M. (1997). Maternal stress, HPA activity and fetal/infant outcome. *Annals of the New York Academy Sciences*, *814*, 266–275.

Shakespeare, J., Blake, F., & Garcia, J. (2003). A qualitative study of the acceptability of routine screening of postnatal women using the Edinburgh Postnatal Depression Scale. *British Journal of General Practice*, *53*(493), 614–619.

Sichel, D.A., Cohen, L.S., Robertson, L.M., Ruttenberg, A., & Rosenbaum, J.F. (1995). Prophylactic estrogen in recurrent postpartum affective disorder. *Biological Psychiatry*, *38*, 814–818.

Spinelli, M.G., & Endicott, J. (2003). Controlled clinical trial of interpersonal psychotherapy versus parenting education program for depressed pregnant women. *American Journal of Psychiatry*, *160*, 555–562.

Steer, R.A., Scholl, T.O., Hediger, M.L., & Fischer, R.L. (1992). Self-reported depression and negative pregnancy outcomes. *Journal of Clinical Epidemiology*, *45*, 1093–1099.

Steinberg, S.I., & Bellavance, F. (1999). Characteristics and treatment of women with antenatal and postpartum depression. *International Journal of Psychiatry in Medicine*, *29*, 209–233.

Steiner, M., & Born, L. (2002). Anxiety and panic disorders. In: J.P. Pregler, & A.H. DeCherney (Eds.), *Women's health: Principles and clinical practice* (pp. 661–674). Toronto: B.C. Decker.

Steiner, M., Fleming, A.S., Anderson, V.N., Monkhouse, E., & Boulter, G.E. (1986). A psychoneuroendocrine profile for postpartum blues? In: L. Dennerstein, I. Fraser (Eds.) Excerpta Medica: Amsterdam. *Hormones and Behavior*, 327–335.

Steiner, M., & Tam, W.Y.K. (1999). In: L.J. Miller et al. (Eds.), *Postpartum mood disorders*. Washington: American Psychiatric Press.

Steiner, M., Dunn, E., & Born, L. (2003a). Hormones and mood: From menarche to menopause and beyond. *Journal of Affective Disorders*, *74*, 67–83.

Steiner, M., & Yonkers, K.A. (2003b). Evidence-based treatment of mood disorders in women. *Mental Fitness*, *2*, 34–67.

Stern, G., & Kruckman, L. (1983). Multi-disciplinary perspectives on postpartum depression: An anthropological critique. *Social Science and Medicine*, *17*, 1027–1041.

Stuart, S., Couser, G., Schilder, K., O'Hara, M.W., & Gorman, L.L. (1998). Postpartum anxiety and depression: Onset and comorbidity in a community sample. *Journal of Nervous and Mental Disease*, *186*, 420–424.

Swain, A.M., O'Hara, M.W., Starr, K.R., & Gorman, L.L. (1997). A prospective study of sleep, mood and cognitive function in postpartum and non-postpartum women. *Obstetrics and Gynecology*, *90*, 381–386.

Verdoux, H., Sutter, A.L., Glatigny-Dallay, E., & Minisini, A. (2002). Obstetrical complications and the development of postpartum depressive symptoms: A prospective survey of the MATQUID cohort. *Acta Psychiatrica Scandinavica, 106,* 212–219.

Villeponteaux, V.A., Lydiard, R.B., Laraia, M.T., Stuart, G.W., & Ballenger, J.C. (1992). The effects of pregnancy on pre-existing panic disorder. *Journal of Clinical Psychiatry, 53,* 201–203.

Wadhwa, P.D., Sandman, C.A., & Garite, T.J. (2001). The neurobiology of stress in human pregnancy: Implications for prematurity and development of the fetal central nervous system. *Progress in Brain Research, 133,* 131–142.

Warner, R., Appleby, L., Whitton, A., & Faragher, B. (1996). Demographic and obstetric risk factors for postnatal psychiatric morbidity. *British Journal of Psychiatry, 168,* 607–611.

Weinberg, M.K., & Tronick, E.Z. (1998). The impact of maternal psychiatric illness on infant development. *Journal of Clinical Psychiatry, 59*(Suppl 2), 53–61.

Weinstock, M. (1997). Does prenatal stress impair coping and regulation of hypothalamic-pituitary-adrenal axis? *Neuroscience and Biobehavioral Reviews, 21,* 1–10.

Wichers, M.C., Purcell, S., Danckaerts, M., Derom, C., Derom, R., Vlietinck, R., et al. (2002). Prenatal life and post-natal psychopathology: Evidence for negative gene-birth weight interaction. *Psychological Medicine, 32*(7), 1165–1174.

Williams, K.E., & Koran, L.M. (1997). Obsessive–compulsive disorder in pregnancy, the puerperium and the premenstruum. *Journal of Clinical Psychiatry, 58,* 330–334.

Wilson, L.M., Reid, A.J., Midmer, D.K., Biringer, A., Carroll, J.C., & Stewart, D.E. (1996). Antenatal psychosocial risk factors associated with adverse postpartum family outcomes. *Canadian Medical Association Journal, 154,* 785–799.

Wisner, K.L., & Wheeler, S.B. (1994). Prevention of recurrent postpartum major depression: Clinical trial. *Hospital and Community Psychiatry, 45*(12), 1191–1196.

Wisner, K.L., Peindl, K.S., & Hanusa, B.H. (1996). Effects of childbearing on the natural history of panic disorder with comorbid mood disorder. *Journal of Affective Disorders, 41,* 173–180.

Wisner, K.L., Peindl, K.S., Gigliotti, T., & Hanusa, B.H. (1999). Obsessions and compulsions in women with postpartum depression. *Journal of Clinical Psychiatry, 60,* 176–180.

Wisner, K.L., Parry, B.L., & Piontek, C.M. (2002). Clinical practice. Postpartum depression. *New England Journal of Medicine, 347*(3), 194–199.

Yonkers, K.A., Ramin, S.M., Rush, A.J., et al. (2001). Onset and persistence of postpartum depression in an inner city maternal health clinic system. *American Journal of Psychiatry, 158,* 1856–1863.

Zlotnick, C., Johnson, S.L., Miller, I.W., Pearlstein, T., & Howard, M. (2001). Postpartum depression in women receiving public assistance: Pilot study of an interpersonal-therapy-oriented group intervention. *American Journal of Psychiatry, 158,* 638–640.

Zuckerman, B., Amaro, H., Bauchner, H., & Cabral, H. (1989). Depressive symptoms during pregnancy: Relationship to poor health behaviours. *American Journal of Obstetrics and Gynecology, 160*(5), 1107–1111.

Pharmacological treatment of anxiety and depression in pregnancy and lactation

Seetal Dodd[1], Jane Opie[1] and Michael Berk[1,2]

[1]Department of Clinical and Biomedical Sciences, Barwon Health, The University of Melbourne, Geelong, Victoria, Australia
[2]Orygen Youth Health, Parkville, Victoria, Australia

As detailed in Chapter 8 of this volume, pregnancy and the postpartum period may be a stressful and turbulent stage of a woman's life, and is a period of risk for mood and anxiety disorders. Such disorders might require pharmacotherapy. However, the efficacy and safety of pharmacological treatments during pregnancy and lactation require special consideration. Many psychotropic medications have been associated with some adverse effects. These vary in terms of clinical significance. Pregnancy and lactation are times of increased vulnerability to risks associated with pharmacological treatment.

Medications of various classes are routinely administered to pregnant and lactating women. In a study of prescription forms in France, 74.2% of pregnant women had at least one prescription during pregnancy (Haramburu et al., 2000). In a Norwegian study a retrospective questionnaire given to 885 mothers investigated drug utilisation in breastfeeding women and found that 69% of mothers had taken at least one pharmaceutical agent in the 4-month period postpartum. Agents from a wide range of therapeutic classes were taken with the most commonly used agents being analgesics/antipyretics (32%), dermatologicals (19%) and oral contraceptives (13%). Psychotropic agents were taken by only 1.1% of mothers (Matheson et al., 1990).

The decision to use pharmacotherapy, as well as the structure of any treatment schedule during pregnancy and lactation must be made by balancing the risks and benefits of treatment specific to the needs of the individual. If a woman is taking psychotropic medication and desires or achieves pregnancy, treatment decisions must be made with consideration of the possibility of changed dose response properties and safety of medications. Biological changes of pregnancy, including an increase in renal blood flow and changes in plasma volume and plasma proteins can in certain circumstances lead to changes in medication pharmacokinetics resulting in compromised efficacy. Lithium, for example, is eliminated through renal clearance so plasma concentrations of lithium may drop during pregnancy. Most psychotropic agents are eliminated predominantly by hepatic clearance, which remains comparatively unchanged through pregnancy.

Prophylaxis may also be compromised by a clinical decision to reduce the dose of a medication during pregnancy and/or breastfeeding in response to safety concerns. In animal studies high doses of some agents have caused a high incidence of teratogenicity and low doses have not caused teratogenicity. Some evidence is available to suggest a dose response for teratogenicity in humans (Little et al., 1993). However, this does not suggest that if a patient is receiving a therapeutic dose of an agent associated with teratogenic risk, reduction of dose will reduce the risk proportionately. Also the adjusted dose is associated with a risk of being sub-therapeutic. Additionally, prophylaxis may be complicated by individual alteration in susceptibility to anxiety and depression during pregnancy and postpartum. Prevention of breakthrough episodes in these periods of vulnerability may also influence treatment decisions.

Risks associated with pharmacotherapy

Pharmacological treatment during pregnancy and breastfeeding requires serious consideration of safety concerns. Moreover, treatment needs to be tailored to suit the needs of the individual. Medications used for the treatment of mood and anxiety disorders have been associated with toxicity in infants and neonates and teratogenicity in the foetus. Adverse effects of these medications to the mother do not change during pregnancy and lactation; however, some effects, in particular nausea, lethargy, postural hypotension and constipation may compound the so-called "minor symptoms of pregnancy". Weight gain may also be of heightened concern.

Teratogenicity caused by medications is the major concern. Both morphological and neurodevelopmental teratogenicity are considered. If morphological teratogenic events are detected, typically by ultrasound, women are usually counselled regarding options including termination of pregnancy. As teratogenicity occurs in early pregnancy, classically in the first trimester, treatment decisions regarding the use of known or suspected teratogens should be made as early as possible, ideally prior to conception. A management plan for an individual woman's mental illness, discussed and agreed to by the treating clinician and the woman considering pregnancy, should be established prior to pregnancy. All women should have the availability of such information before conception. However, the rate of unplanned pregnancy remains high – one recent study reports rates as high as 48% (Werler et al., 2003).

Physicians will inevitably face the dilemma of unplanned pregnancy in women who are prescribed psychotropic medication. The approach taken will depend on the nature of the prescribed medication; the resultant risk to the pregnancy assessed according to gestational age at exposure; and the woman's preference. Confirmation of gestational age via ultrasound may be prudent. It is important to offer the woman counselling to enable her to make a decision regarding the pregnancy. In some situations this may involve specialist risk counselling, for example, via a genetics unit. Other women may feel strongly that they are unable to continue with a pregnancy given inadvertent exposure. Once again counselling would be advised allowing adequate time for informed decision-making to occur. These women should be offered first trimester ultrasound and maternal serum screening in addition to detailed second trimester ultrasound – however, a normal result cannot guarantee normal development. In those women who elect to continue with the pregnancy, therapeutic decisions should be made by considering the risks and benefits of the various treatment options for the remainder of the pregnancy. This event provides an opportunity to discuss medication management prior to future pregnancies.

Toxicity due to pharmacological treatment can manifest in different phases. These include:

- Antenatally, with intrauterine growth retardation and foetal death-in-utero.
- At parturition (via toxicity or withdrawal) with low birth weight, rash, delirium and "floppy-baby syndrome".
- Postpartum, due to delayed toxicity or withdrawal or from breastfeeding.

The association of a medication with risk of teratogenicity or toxicity does not preclude its use during pregnancy and breastfeeding, provided the benefits are perceived to outweigh the risks and the same benefits cannot be provided by a safer alternative. Similarly, risks associated with many medications vary depending on the stage of pregnancy. The first trimester of pregnancy is when the foetus is vulnerable to medications that may cause developmental abnormalities. Risks associated with the use of these medications are considerably reduced when they are used outside the first trimester.

Risks associated with untreated mental illness

Relapse of mental illness in the mother has also been associated with poor outcomes for the infant. A British population study of all births in the geographical area of Avon investigated the impact of maternal anxiety in 7448 children at 4 years of age. They found maternal anxiety, particularly antenatal anxiety, significantly correlated with behavioural and emotional problems in the children and suggested that maternal anxiety may affect behavioural development in the child. However, the effect size was small (O'Connor et al., 2002). There are reports of potential maternal and foetal consequences with a decision not to treat significant anxiety in pregnancy. A prospective study of 623 nulliparous women in Finland identified significant anxiety in 16% of women in early pregnancy. This group had an increased risk of pre-eclampsia, the interpretation being a link via altered excretion of vasoactive hormones or other neuroendocrine transmitters (Kurki et al., 2000). A French cohort study of 634 pregnant women found an association with anxiety and pre-term labour in women who had a previous history of pre-term labour (Dayan et al., 2002). Quality-of-life issues for the affected woman are also clearly important.

Therapeutic strategies

Some individuals may use herbal or "natural" medications, which lack safety informa-tion on use in pregnancy (Haramburu et al., 2000). Non-pharmacological therapies including cognitive behavioural therapy, relaxation strategies, supportive psychotherapy and lifestyle recommendations relating in particular to sleep hygiene, caffeine, nicotine and alcohol use, and exercise, remain important including for those prescribed phar-macotherapy. Prescribed medication is usually of greater benefit than alternative ther-apies and should, in general, be used at the lowest effective dose for the shortest time necessary, with intermittent use where possible (e.g. with benzodiazepines). Stage of pregnancy should be carefully considered. Predicting time of delivery may be problem-atic – 12.1% of births occurred prior to 37 completed weeks gestation in the USA in 2002 (Martin et al., 2003) – and infants born prematurely will be more susceptible to toxicity. Other "at-risk" neonates include those with hepatic or renal impairment, and those with physiological jaundice. The uncompromised neonate will not achieve hepatic maturation until roughly three months of age (Iqbal, 1999).

The role of lactation is an important consideration. Human milk is nutritionally valuable, has anti-infective properties and breastfeeding aids bonding (Uauy & De Andraca, 1995). Occasionally the risks associated with drug exposure through breast-feeding will outweigh any benefit of breastfeeding. The decision to breastfeed is not risk free and the choice of agent should be carefully considered. Antidepressants, for example, have in general a good safety record with breastfeeding, but risks can be lowered further by choosing a shorter half-life, non-sedating agent with a low milk to plasma ratio. Where possible polypharmacy should be avoided. With agents dosed once daily, the dose should be taken immediately before the infant's feed prior to the infant's longest sleep period in those infants with an established routine.

Balancing risks with benefits

Risk–benefit assessment is a difficult and imprecise challenge that faces the treat-ing clinician. While risks of teratogenic and toxic adverse events may be well docu-mented and can with some degree of accuracy be expressed as a probability, risks of relapse associated with change or dose reduction of medication will be influ-enced by the unique circumstances of each individual. Clinical decisions for treat-ing more severely ill patients during pregnancy and lactation may be easier to make than for less severely ill patients with a history of stability, where a decision to

---

BOX 9.1 Categories of risk related to drug use in pregnancy

Category A: Drugs which have been taken by a large number of pregnant women and women of childbearing age without any proven increase in the frequency of malformations or other direct or indirect harmful effects on the foetus having been observed.

Category B1: Drugs which have been taken by only a limited number of pregnant women and women of childbearing age, without an increase in the frequency of malformation or other direct or indirect harmful effects on the human foetus having been observed. Studies in animals have not shown evidence of an increased occurrence of foetal damage.

Category B2: Studies in animals are inadequate or may be lacking, but available data show no evidence of an increased occurrence of foetal damage.

Category B3: Studies in animals have shown evidence of an increased occurrence of foetal damage, the significance of which is considered uncertain in humans.

Category C: Drugs which owing to their pharmacological effects, have caused or may be suspected of causing, harmful effects on the human foetus or neonate without causing malformations. These effects may be reversible. Accompanying texts should be consulted for further details.

Category D: Drugs which have caused, are suspected to cause or may be expected to cause, an increased incidence of human foetal malformations or irreversible damage. These drugs may also have adverse pharmacological effects. Accompanying texts should be consulted for further details.

Category X: Drugs which have such a high risk of causing permanent damage to the foetus that they should not be used in pregnancy or when there is a possibility of pregnancy.

---

reduce the dose and/or alter medications may appear well founded. Sometimes "correct" decisions can only be made with hindsight.

However, the perception of risk from medication versus illness may be disproportionate. In general, risks are more worrying and less acceptable if they arise from a man-made or unfamiliar source, cause hidden and irreversible damage, threaten a dreaded form of injury, are poorly understood by science, are subject to contradictory opinions and are perceived as involuntary (Bennett, 1997). Conversely "natural" risks are better tolerated. It follows that a discussion about teratogenicity from medication, even if the risk is viewed as small in comparison to risks from untreated mental illness, will invoke fear in most expectant mothers. Pharmacological agents are graded according to potential risk in pregnancy, as shown in Box 9.1.

The clinician's task is challenging – non-pharmacological options should be fully utilised. However, once pharmacotherapy is viewed as necessary, safety and efficacy data need to be presented in an unambiguous and meaningfully interpreted way that offers the woman choice without increasing uncertainty. The ability of the clinician to enable the patient to make a wise decision rather than simply an "informed" decision will require the clinician to consider the needs and capacities of each individual

Table 9.1. Safety in pregnancy and breastfeeding of anxiolytic agents

Anxiolytic	Category in pregnancy*	Compatibility with breastfeeding
Diazepam	C	Compatible in single dose – caution with chronic use
Lorazepam	C	Compatible in single dose – caution with chronic use
Alprazolam	C	Compatible in single dose – caution with chronic use
Oxazepam	C	Compatible in single dose – caution with chronic use
Clonazepam	C	Compatible in single dose – caution with chronic use
Nitrazepam	C	Compatible in single dose – caution with chronic use
Buspirone	Bl	Insufficient data
Propranolol	C	Compatible

Adapted from Dowden J. (2003)

*for definition of categories see Box 9.1 (pg. 167)

regarding the method of presentation of information. This is particularly pertinent with maternal mental illness. The anxious patient, for example, may place excessive emphasis on remote medication risks (Nisselle, 2000). Guilt is common in women during pregnancy if the foetus is felt to be at risk due to the presence or treatment of a maternal medical condition. Such guilt should be addressed openly, and this approach may aid compliance and acceptance.

In this chapter evidence is given for the safety of agents used in the treatment of mood and anxiety disorders during pregnancy and lactation. Where appropriate, treatment guidelines are given. Non-pharmaceutical treatments including herbal and nutritional therapies are also considered.

Benzodiazepines

Benzodiazepines may be prescribed intermittently for breakthrough symptoms, particularly in panic disorder; for regular prophylaxis; to cover the early initiation of serotonin selective reuptake inhibitors (SSRIs); and postnatally, commonly for the short-term management of sleep disturbance.

Benzodiazepine use during pregnancy has been associated with teratogenic outcomes; the risks are tabulated in Table 9.1. Interference with palatal closure with lorazepam has been shown in animal studies (Jurand & Martin, 1994). Human placental transfer of diazepam has been demonstrated to occur from week six of gestation with a preferential transfer to the amniotic cavity and the potential for foetal accumulation (Jauniaux et al., 1996). Human studies have reported an association with benzodiazepines and birth defects (Laegreid, 1990) in particular facial cleft abnormalities (Safra & Oakley, 1975; Saxen, 1975). Some of the early studies have been criticised due to incomplete exposure and dose data, and often limited information on potential confounders. This is relevant when investigating benzodiazepines in anxiety states, as these conditions (particularly social phobia, generalised anxiety disorder, panic disorder and posttraumatic stress disorder) have been associated with higher rates of alcohol and substance use (Vogel & Muskin, 1999). Heavy alcohol intake is associated with craniofacial abnormalities (Dowden, 2003). Tobacco use has been associated with low birth weight, intrauterine growth retardation, miscarriage, infant mortality and adverse health and developmental outcomes for the child (Martin et al., 2003).

A number of prospective studies have looked at benzodiazepines including diazepam, alprazolam, oxazepam, lorazepam, clonazepam and nitrazepam and the results overall do not support an association between benzodiazepines and teratogenicity (Eros et al., 2002; Ornoy et al., 1998; Shiono & Mills, 1984; St Clair & Schirmer, 1992; Weinstock et al., 2001). A meta-analysis of 23 studies determined the pooled cohort studies did not show an association between benzodiazepines and major malformations or oral cleft; however, the pooled case control studies did (Dolovich et al., 1998). Some authors have opined that the cohort evidence is the higher quality evidence so inferences should be based on the outcome of the pooled cohort data (Khan et al., 1999).

Neurodevelopmental teratogenicity also requires consideration. A Swedish study looked at 17 infants born to mothers with continuous benzodiazepine use through pregnancy. The study used the Griffiths' developmental scale and reported a lower mean general development quotient and development quotients for all five sub-scales at 5, 10 and 18 months compared to a control group of 29 infants, concluding a general delay in mental development (Viggedal et al., 1993). A review of 41 studies of psychoactive medications in 1998, including two prospective controlled studies of benzodiazepines, reported no evidence for long-term neurobehavioural sequelae, but acknowledged the limited number of studies (Austin & Mitchell, 1998). A review examined studies on 550 children followed for up to 4 years after exposure to benzodiazepines in pregnancy, and concluded that there was no significant increase in malformation rate or impairment of neurobehavioural development. Note was made of transient developmental delay for a few infants in the first year of life with subsequent catch-up growth by most. There were occasional persistent developmental deficits where other drug therapy or poor environmental and social factors coexisted (McElhatton, 1994). Overall, one cannot be completely reassured about neurodevelopmental or morphological teratogenicity from benzodiazepines, but any risk is likely to be low.

Use of benzodiazepines perinatally has been associated with the floppy infant syndrome with a characteristic clinical pattern of sedation, hypotonia, hypothermia and low Apgar scores (McElhatton, 1994). A syndrome of neonatal withdrawal including hypertonia, hyperreflexia, irritability, seizures, bradycardia and cyanosis is also reported. Signs may take up to 3 weeks to appear and last from hours to months

(Ward et al., 2000). Withdrawal symptoms from shorter acting benzodiazepines may be more severe initially but are less protracted than the longer acting agents such as diazepam and clonazepam (Ward et al., 2000). Regarding *lactation*, particular care is required in infants with prematurity, hepatic or renal insufficiency and physiological jaundice. Diazepam should be used with caution due to its long half-life and association with lethargy, sedation and infant weight loss (Iqbal et al., 2002). A study of 26 infants exposed through breastfeeding to psychoactive medications including benzodiazepines showed infant serum medication levels below the laboratory limit of detection (Birnbaum et al., 1999). In the same study, prenatal exposure resulted in detectable infant serum medication levels.

Benzodiazepine treatment of anxiety during pregnancy should be secondary to other therapies such as SSRIs and psychological approaches. It is prudent to use benzodiazepines at a low dose and intermittently where feasible, with preference given to shorter acting agents such as alprazolam, lorazepam and oxazepam. Women who elect to cease benzodiazepines should taper the dose gradually to avoid maternal discontinuation syndrome (Einarson et al., 2001). Avoidance of all benzodiazepines is wise around the time of delivery. Diazepam in particular should be avoided close to delivery and during lactation. For women requiring regular therapy, high peak concentrations can be avoided by dividing the daily dose (Iqbal et al., 2002). Combinations of benzodiazepines should be avoided. Careful follow-up of infants exposed to benzodiazepines around the time of delivery and during lactation is prudent.

Other anxiolytics

Buspirone is used for its modest anxiolytic effect and low potential for dependence. Full onset of effect may take up to three weeks, which limits intermittent use. Little is known about its use during pregnancy. Animals given high-dose buspirone during pregnancy show reduced maternal weight gain, increased stillbirth rate and lowered vitality of newborns, but no impairment of long-term learning or motor activity (Kai et al., 1990). There are no published reports of human foetal damage attributed to buspirone, but studies are lacking. Its safety during lactation is also not established (Dowden, 2003).

Propranolol may be used to ameliorate the sympathetic arousal associated with anxiety disorders such as performance anxiety in social phobia. Information on its use during pregnancy has been acquired predominantly from women treated for hypertension. Safety concerns are reported. One study, which looked at pregnancy outcome in women treated with propranolol compared with other antihypertensives, reported increased foetal or neonatal deaths in the propranolol group (Lieberman et al., 1978). Growth retardation was higher in propranolol-treated mothers after accounting for the effects of maternal illness (Pruyn et al., 1979). Neonatal bradycardia and hypoglycaemia are also reported (Livingstone et al., 1983). There are no reports of foetal malformations from propranolol. Its use is compatible with breastfeeding – studies have shown that the infant dose is less than 0.1% of the maternal dose (Smith et al., 1983).

Hypnotics

Hypnotics may be required for short-term use in during pregnancy, or postnatally. In addition to benzodiazepines, agents used may include zopiclone, zolpidem and more historically chloral hydrate. The Motherisk Program prospectively followed 40 women who received zopiclone during the first trimester and found no increase in major malformations (Diav-Citrin et al., 1999). There is little information on the use of zolpidem during pregnancy. A small study of nursing infants whose mothers were prescribed zolpidem found no adverse effects (Pons et al., 1989). However, the evidence is too limited to recommend the general use of zopiclone and zolpidem during pregnancy and breastfeeding. Chloral hydrate has been used during pregnancy but has fallen out of favour with many prescribers due to its toxicity in overdose.

Antidepressants

Many antidepressants have well-documented records of safety and have a history of use during pregnancy and breastfeeding. However, a few reports of teratogenicity and toxicity, particularly in neonates, have appeared for some agents. There is a paucity of safety data for some antidepressants, particularly the newer drugs, as these agents have not yet been used by significant numbers of women during pregnancy and breastfeeding. Overall pregnancy risks are summarised in Table 9.2.

Although all antidepressants can be considered for use during pregnancy and breastfeeding, preference should be given to those agents that have been used by a large number of women without serious adverse events. Agents with shorter half-lives are preferred in the perinatal period, as this helps limit neonatal toxicity. Agents associated with discontinuation syndromes may produce such syndromes in neonates exposed antenatally. Toxicity, like many other adverse events, is dose dependant and is considerably less likely when low doses are administered. Consideration should be given towards reducing the dose if possible, especially perinatally.

A European study investigated the outcomes of pregnancies where women were exposed to tricyclic antidepressants ($n = 283$), non-tricyclic antidepressants ($n = 355$) or both tricyclic and non-tricyclic antidepressants ($n = 51$) (McElhatton et al., 1996). Although adverse outcomes were reported in 3% of pregnancies they were not attributed to antidepressant exposure. Antidepressant exposure, analysed by group and for each individual agent, did not affect infant birth weights or rates of spontaneous

Table 9.2. Safety in pregnancy and breastfeeding of antidepressant agents

Antidepressant	Category in pregnancy*	Compatibility with breastfeeding
Sertraline	C	Probably compatible
Fluoxetine	C	Avoid if possible
Paroxetine	C	Probably compatible
Citalopram	C	Probably compatible
Fluvoxamine	C	Probably compatible
Venlafaxine	B2	Probably compatible
Mirtazapine	B3	Insufficient data
Nefazadone	B3	Insufficient data
Bupropion	B2	May be acceptable, very small amounts in breast milk
Mianserin	B2	Insufficient data
Moclobemide	B3	Compatible
Phenylzine	B3	Insufficient data
Tranylcypromine	B2	Insufficient data
Imipramine	C	Compatible
Amitriptyline	C	Compatible
Clomipramine	C	Compatible
Dothiepin	C	Compatible
Doxepin	C	Caution (respiratory depression in a breastfed baby)

Adapted from Dowden J. (2003)

*for definition of categories, see Box 9.1 (pg. 167)

abortion, both of which were within the normal range. Interestingly, the majority of women were receiving drug combination therapies, including benzodiazepines (50%), neuroleptics (20%) and other drugs (40%). Exposures to monoamine oxidase inhibitors were not reported.

Neurodevelopment was investigated in a study of 80 mother–infant pairs with in-utero exposure to tricyclic antidepressants, 55 mother–infant pairs with in-utero exposure to fluoxetine and 84 mother–infant pairs with no in-utero antidepressant exposure (Nulman et al., 1997). Children were assessed between 16 and 86 months of age. The study concluded that neither tricyclic antidepressants nor fluoxetine affected global IQ, language development or behavioural development in the antidepressant-exposed children.

All antidepressants are expressed in breast milk and breastfed infants will be exposed to maternal medications. However, maternal milk to plasma ratios, and consequently the level of exposure to the infant, varies considerably between agents. The exposure of an infant to antidepressant medications can be reduced by choosing a medication with a low milk to plasma ratio and maintaining the mother on the lowest effective dose. The greater vulnerability of women to depression postpartum suggests caution regarding reduction of antidepressant dose. If the dose of an antidepressant was lowered for pregnancy it may be wise to return the dose to pre-pregnancy levels in the postpartum period due to the increased risks of mood disorders in this period. Choosing not to breastfeed can eliminate antidepressant exposure to an infant, but the decision should be made after careful consideration of the individual circumstances. The benefits of breastfeeding will usually outweigh the risks associated with passage of antidepressant medications through breast milk.

SSRIs

SSRIs are often the first choice of antidepressant agent administered to patients presenting with a major depressive episode. A study of 38 pregnancies measured SSRIs in maternal and umbilical cord blood sample collected immediately postpartum. Umbilical cord to maternal serum mean drug concentration ratios were 0.29 for sertraline ($n = 10$), 0.51 for paroxetine ($n = 8$), 0.64 for fluoxetine ($n = 15$) and 0.89 for citalopram ($n = 4$) (Hendrick et al., 2003b). This study suggests a safety advantage for the use of sertraline during pregnancy; larger studies are needed.

A report has suggested that foetal exposure to fluoxetine may be associated with low birth weight (Hendrick et al., 2003a), though this finding was not apparent in the previously cited European study (McElhatton et al., 1996). Suspected cases of postnatal dependence and withdrawal symptoms have been reported in infants exposed to sertraline (Kent & Laidlaw, 1995), paroxetine (Dahl et al., 1997) and fluoxetine (Spencer, 1993). Paroxetine is thought to be associated with a higher rate of neonatal withdrawal syndrome than alternative agents (Nordeng et al., 2001) and is best avoided perinatally. SSRIs may cause serotonergic symptoms such as myoclonus, restlessness, tremor, shivering, hyperreflexia, incoordination and rigidity in infants exposed in-utero (Laine et al., 2003). These findings reinforce the case for dose reduction prior to the expected date of delivery. Caution is advised in not discontinuing SSRIs abruptly during breastfeeding in early infancy.

There is a case report of an association between first trimester exposure to fluoxetine and neural tube malformation (Vendittelli et al., 1995). This association has not been supported by large prospective studies, which have found that rates of abnormalities in neonates are not increased by exposure to fluoxetine (Goldstein et al., 1997). With the large number of in-utero exposures to SSRIs, it is expected that some exposed neonates will be born with abnormalities, but for the SSRIs to be considered causal the abnormalities much either occur at a prevalence greater than that seen in the general community, or must have some common features. Evidence from high-dose animal studies suggests that SSRIs do not cause an increase in the number of foetal malformations. Nevertheless the use of SSRIs during first trimester should be considered carefully, especially if co-administered with other agents.

SSRIs are generally considered to be compatible with breastfeeding, although there have been some concerns about the compatibility of fluoxetine with breast-feeding. The long elimination half-life from plasma is longer for fluoxetine than for other SSRIs, making this drug less suitable for breastfeeding mothers compared with other SSRIs. However, studies of developmental outcomes of infants breast-fed by mothers treated with fluoxetine have not associated fluoxetine with adverse outcomes (Yoshida et al., 1998). SSRIs are expressed in breast milk with maternal milk to plasma ratios of 0.29 to 1.51 for fluoxetine, 1.2 to 3.5 for sertraline, 1.1 to 4.3 for citalopram, 0.09 to 0.9 for paroxetine and 0.29 for fluvoxamine (Dodd et al., 2000a; Berle et al., 2004). At this stage there are no published studies of the safety of escitalopram during pregnancy and breastfeeding, but it is likely to have a safety profile similar to that of citalopram.

Tricyclic antidepressants

In a large prospective follow-up study, in-utero exposure to 10 tricyclic antidepressant agents was not associated with adverse outcomes in pregnancy (McElhatton et al., 1996). The percentage of spontaneous abortions, congenital malformations, premature deliveries and birth weights were within the normal range.

Tricyclic antidepressants are expressed in breast milk with maternal milk to plasma ratios of 0.2–1.9 for amitriptyline, 0.4–3.0 for clomipramine, 1.22 for desipramine, 0.33–4.5 to dothiepin, 1.08 for doxepin and 0.7–1.9 for imipramine (Dodd et al., 2000a), suggesting considerable variability in consequent potential exposure to the infant. Generally, tricyclic antidepressants are considered to be safe during breast-feeding, although a single case of toxicity in an infant attributed to doxepin has been reported (Matheson et al., 1985). The long half-life demethyl metabolite of doxepin was shown to have accumulated in the breastfed infant reaching toxic levels and resulting in respiratory depression.

Other antidepressants

The newer antidepressants, mirtazapine, venlafaxine and nefazadone, have been used during pregnancy and breastfeeding. However, there is less pregnancy data than for SSRIs or TCAs. Consequently, better-studied agents may be the more prudent initial choice of treatment until more information is available on the safety of these agents.

Mirtazapine use in pregnancy has been reported without adverse effects (Kesim et al., 2002). Withdrawal has been reported in a neonate after exposure to venlafaxine (de Moor et al., 2003). Expression of venlafaxine into breast milk is high, with a milk to plasma ratio of 2.5 and 2.7 for the metabolite O-desmethylvenlafaxine (Ilett et al., 2002). This suggests that breastfed infants are exposed to higher percentages of the maternal dose of venlafaxine compared to most other antidepressants. The unusual pharmacokinetics of nefazadone may cause large individual differences in levels of exposure to the foetus and infants of nefazadone treated mothers. Nefazadone milk to plasma ratios of 3.17 and 0.14 were reported for paired specimens collected from two breastfeeding mothers (Dodd et al., 2000b).

There is a paucity of data during pregnancy for bupropion, trazodone, mianserin and moclobemide, and manufacturers discourage use of these agents during pregnancy due to lack of clinical data. In lactation, milk to plasma ratios have been reported as 2.51–8.58 for bupropion, 0.142 for trazodone, 0.8–3.6 for mianserin and 0.39–1.21 for moclobemide (Dodd et al., 2000a). Some data suggest that monoamine oxidase inhibitors, phenelzine and tranylcypromine, may be associated with a low risk when used in pregnancy (Gracious & Wisner, 1997); however, few exposures have been reported.

Mood stabilisers

Treating bipolar disorder during pregnancy and lactation represents a significant challenge (see also Chapter 10). The most commonly used mood stabilising agents for the treatment of bipolar disorder are associated with significant risks of foetal malformations and toxicity. Treatment decisions for sufferers of bipolar disorder need to be made on an individual basis, however for many sufferers reducing or ceasing mood stabilising medication is not a simple option. For a more detailed discussion of the treatment of bipolar disorder during pregnancy and postpartum see Chapter 10.

If a mood stabiliser is required during the first trimester, then counselling, ideally well prior to conception, should be offered. Women should be aware of the benefits of pharmacotherapy as well as the risks associated with drug exposure to the foetus and be advised to undergo ultrasonography. Counselling regarding termination of pregnancy should be provided when serious teratogenic drug effects are detected. Risks associated with exposure of the foetus to the mood stabilisers are summarised in Table 9.3.

Table 9.3. Safety in pregnancy and breastfeeding of mood stabilisers

Mood stabiliser	Category in pregnancy*	Compatibility with breastfeeding
Lithium	D	Avoid
Valproate	D	Compatible
Carbamazepine	D	Compatible, monitor infant for adverse effects
Lamotrigine	B3	Caution, monitor infant plasma concentration

Adapted from Dowden J. (2003)

*for definition of categories, see Box 9.1 (pg. 167)

Lithium

First trimester exposure to lithium during pregnancy has been associated with cardiac malformation of Ebstein type (Jacobson et al., 1992; Schou et al., 1973). Current opinion, however, suggests that the teratogenic risk of exposure to lithium during pregnancy is lower than previously believed (Cohen et al., 1994). Toxicity in neonates due to lithium exposure in pregnancy has been documented, with reports of atrial flutter (Wilson et al., 1983), thyroid toxicity (Karlsson et al., 1975) and goitre (Frassetto et al., 2002), nephrogenic diabetes insipidus (Mizrahi et al., 1979; Pinelli et al., 2002), gross functional lesions of the cardiovascular, renal and neuromuscular systems (Morrell et al., 1983) and floppy baby syndrome (Llewellyn et al., 1998). An association between lithium exposure in-utero and premature birth, macrosomia and perinatal mortality has been suggested (Yoder et al., 1984). The risk of congenital abnormalities with lithium use is estimated as 1 in 1000, while the risk of a recurrent episode of bipolar illness during pregnancy if lithium is discontinued is estimated as one in two (Licht et al., 2003). Lithium exposure carries risks to the foetus; however, its use during pregnancy and breastfeeding is justified in individual cases.

Management is complicated by altered pharmacokinetics during pregnancy. Plasma concentrations of lithium may drop during pregnancy due to increased renal perfusion. Glomerular filtration rate increases by 50%, and remains at this level throughout the pregnancy (Gabbe et al., 1996). To maintain the pre-pregnancy plasma concentration of lithium, the dose needs to be increased by 50%. Caution is urged if the dose of lithium is lowered during pregnancy as the concentration of lithium in plasma may reduce considerably. Similar caution is required in the postpartum period as the glomerular filtration rate quickly returns to pre-pregnancy levels. If the dose is not adjusted, the concentration of lithium in plasma will quickly rise.

Decisions need to be tailored to suit the individual, based on knowledge of the patient's medical history. Most physicians may understandably be reluctant to alter the treatment of patients who have responded well to their current medication. Alterations of a current treatment, which may significantly increase the risk of relapse, should be contextualised to the individual situation. In addition, decisions to reduce or discontinue lithium prior to conception may require extra consideration in older women or others with potentially lower fertility (e.g. women with known polycystic ovarian syndrome), who may take longer to conceive.

An option is to lower the lithium dose prior to conception (see Chapter 10). If clinically indicated, lithium may be slowly tapered off, beginning four weeks prior to parturition and returned to pre-pregnancy levels postpartum. As well as reducing the risk of neonatal toxicity, an argument for lithium discontinuation for parturition is also supported due to slow lithium clearance in the neonate (Arnon et al., 1981). Different options are to discontinue lithium from preconception to the end of the first trimester and again perinatally (Williams & Oke, 2000). Perinatal discontinuation of lithium has, however, been criticised due to its association with a disproportionately high number of induced labours (Kramer et al., 2003). Breastfeeding is not ruled out as an option. During the reproductive period the frequency of visits with the physician treating the woman's bipolar disorder should increase, particularly during times of dose adjustment and during the perinatal period.

Anticonvulsants (see also chapter 10)

Exposure to valproate in-utero has been associated with hydrocephalus and meningomyelocele (Robert & Guibaud, 1982; Weinbaum et al., 1986) and spina bifida (Lindhout & Meinardi, 1984). Other reported severe malformations include skeletal abnormalities and microcephaly (Koch et al., 1983), septo-optic dysplasia (McMahon & Braddock, 1998) and congenital heart defects (Thisted & Ebbesen, 1993). A consistent facial phenotype, termed "foetal valproate syndrome", has been described and consists of recognisable minor abnormalities include epicanthic folds, a small nose with a flat nasal bridge and anteverted nostrils, a long thin upper lip and thickened lower lip, and low-set posteriorly angulated ears (Ardinger et al., 1988; DiLiberti et al., 1984; Winter et al., 1987). Congenital limb defects have also been reported (Rodriguez-Pinilla et al., 2000). Valproate exposure during pregnancy has been associated with intrauterine haemorrhage (Bason et al., 1998), afibrinogenaemia in a neonate (Majer & Green, 1987), hypoglycaemia in a neonate (Thisted & Ebbesen, 1993) and fatal liver atrophy and cholestasis in two infant siblings (Legius et al., 1987). Valproate has a good history of safety in use during breastfeeding. Haematological adverse events with exposure through breast milk may occur but are very rare.

Exposure to carbamazepine in-utero has been associated with spina bifida (Rosa, 1991), and less severely, developmental delays, minor craniofacial defects and fingernail hypoplasia (Jones et al., 1989). Possible carcinogenesis has been suggested from a single report of congenital neuroblastoma (Baptista et al., 1998). Carbamazepine exposure has additionally been associated with transient hepatic toxicity. There is some evidence to suggest that carbamazepine exposure through breastfeeding may result in transient cholestatic hepatitis (Frey et al., 1990) and hepatic dysfunction (Merlob et al., 1992). Both cases were resolved by ceasing carbamazepine exposure.

Valproate and carbamazepine are believed to deplete selenium and folate. Nutritional supplementation has been demonstrated to be useful for women not exposed to anticonvulsants and is recommended for all women considering pregnancy. There is some evidence to suggest that the benefits of nutritional supplementation with folate prior to conception and in early pregnancy may be lessened by anticonvulsant administration (Yerby, 2003). The effects of carbamazepine on vitamin levels are detailed in Chapter 10.

There is a paucity of data concerning the safety of newer anticonvulsants, such as lamotrigine and oxcarbazepine, during pregnancy and breastfeeding, although adverse events have been reported in animal studies. Lamotrigine clearance from plasma steadily increases during pregnancy, peaking at an average of >350% of clearance pre-pregnancy at 32 weeks gestational age, then trending downwards and rapidly returning to pre-pregnancy values postpartum (Pennell, 2003). Newer anticonvulsants should be considered potentially harmful to the foetus and breastfed infant. As clinical experience with these agents in the reproductive period increases, a clearer picture of the associated risks will emerge. For more explicit guidelines about the use of anticonvulsants during pregnancy and post-partum, see Chapter 10.

Herbal remedies and supplements

Alternative agents, herbal remedies and nutritional supplements are commonly taken for symptoms of depression and anxiety. Some agents are taken as primary treatment, such as St John's wort (*Hypericum perforatum*) for depressive disorders and kava kava (*Piper methysticum*) for generalised anxiety disorder. Other agents are taken for the treatment of specific symptoms, such as valerian root (*Valerian officinalis*) for insomnia and damiana (*Turnera diffusa*) to treat sexual dysfunction associated with antidepressant therapy. Nutritional supplements, such as B complex vitamins, mineral supplements and omega-3-fatty acid, are also used. Alternative agents have considerable appeal but their efficacy and safety has often been poorly researched. There is a mistaken belief that herbal products are necessarily safe. There is also significant variability in contents of the various preparations.

Few data are available on the use of alternative agents during pregnancy and lactation. A cohort study of 33 breastfeeding women receiving St John's wort reported minor adverse events in infants included two cases of colic, two of drowsiness and one of lethargy (Lee et al., 2003). Hyperforin, an active constituent of St John's wort, has been measured in milk samples from a breastfeeding mother (Klier et al., 2002), demonstrating that breastfed infants may be exposed to at least one component of this herbal preparation. St John's wort is an inducer of hepatic CYP450 enzymes and this requires consideration with respect to concomitant medications.

Ginseng should not be used during pregnancy because of hormonal effects, including neonatal androgenisation (Koren et al., 1990), and valerian should be avoided in pregnancy as in-vitro studies have demonstrated cytotoxic and mutagenic activity (Tesch, 2003). At present there is insufficient evidence on safety and efficacy to recommend the use of alternative agents during pregnancy and lactation.

Conclusions

Pharmacological treatment during pregnancy and lactation is commonly required, and needs to be considered on a basis of balancing risks with clinical need.

Key points are:

- The risk associated with exposure during pregnancy and lactation to individual agents varies considerably. Preference should be given to better-studied agents with a good history of safety during reproductive events.
- Minimal effective medication doses for the shortest time necessary should be employed, with intermittent prescribing where feasible.
- In most cases the benefits of breastfeeding outweigh the risks associated with infant exposure via breast milk and, with a few exceptions, the continuation of breastfeeding is usually advised.
- During lactation, preference should be given to agents with shorter half-lives, that are less sedating, with low milk to plasma ratios. Dividing the daily dose where appropriate may reduce peak levels.

Risks associated with medications used during pregnancy and lactation need to be considered on the basis of available evidence. The relative safety of many conventional agents in pregnancy and breastfeeding has been established through clinical use. Clinical decisions can be made by carefully balancing the risks and benefits associated with treatment and by tailoring treatments to suit the individual.

REFERENCES

Ardinger, H.H., Atkin, J.F., Blackston, R.D., Elsas, L.J., Clarren, S.K., Livingstone, S., Flannery, D.B., Pellock, J.M., Harrod, M.J., Lammer, E.J., et al. (1988). Verification of the fetal valproate syndrome phenotype. *American Journal of Medical Genetics, 29*, 171–185.

Arnon, R.G., Marin-Garcia, J., & Peeden, J.N. (1981). Tricuspid valve regurgitation and lithium carbonate toxicity in a newborn infant. *American Journal of Diseases of Children, 135*, 941–943.

Austin, M.P., & Mitchell, P.B. (1998). Psychotropic medications in pregnant women: Treatment dilemmas. *Medical Journal of Australia, 169*, 428–431.

Baptista, T., Araujo, H., Rada, P., & Hernandez, L. (1998). Congenital neuroblastoma in a boy born to a woman with bipolar disorder treated with carbamazepine during pregnancy. *Progress in Neuro-psychopharmacology & Biological Psychiatry, 22*, 445–454.

Bason, L., Ming, J.E., & Zackal, E.H. (1998). Intrauterine hemorrhage associated with prenatal valproate exposure. *American Journal of Human Genetics, 63*, A159.

Bennett, P. (1997). *Communicating about risks to public health: Pointers to good practice.* London: Department of Health, EOR division.

Birnbaum, C.S., Cohen, L.S., Bailey, J.W., Grush, L.R., Robertson, L.M., & Stowe, Z.N. (1999). Serum concentrations of antidepressants and benzodiazepines in nursing infants: A case series. *Pediatrics, 104*, e11.

Cohen, L.S., Friedman, J.M., Jefferson, J.W., Johnson, E.M., & Weiner, M.L. (1994). A reevaluation of risk of in utero exposure to lithium. *Journal of the American Medical Association, 271*, 146–150.

Dahl, M.L., Olhager, E., & Ahlner, J. (1997). Paroxetine withdrawal syndrome in a neonate. *British Journal of Psychiatry, 171*, 391–392.

Dayan, J., Creveuil, C., Herlicoviez, M., Herbel, C., Baranger, E., Savoye, C., & Thouin, A. (2002). Role of anxiety and depression in the onset of spontaneous preterm labor. *American Journal of Epidemiology, 155*, 293–301.

de Moor, R.A., Mourad, L., ter Haar, J., & Egberts, A.C. (2003). Withdrawal symptoms in a neonate following exposure to venlafaxine during pregnancy. *Nederlands Tijdschrift Voor Geneeskunde, 147*, 1370–1372.

Diav-Citrin, O., Okotore, B., Lucarelli, K., & Koren, G. (1999). Pregnancy outcome following first-trimester exposure to zopiclone: A prospective controlled cohort study. *American Journal of Perinatology, 16*, 157–160.

DiLiberti, J.H., Farndon, P.A., Dennis, N.R., & Curry, C.J. (1984). The fetal valproate syndrome. *American Journal of Medical Genetics, 19*, 473–481.

Dodd, S., Buist, A., & Norman, T.R. (2000a). Antidepressants and breast-feeding: A review of the literature. *Paediatric Drugs, 2*, 183–192.

Dodd, S., Maguire, K.P., Burrows, G.D., & Norman, T.R. (2000b). Nefazodone in the breast milk of nursing mothers: A report of two patients. *Journal of Clinical Psychopharmacology, 20*, 717–718.

Dolovich, L.R., Addis, A., Vaillancourt, J.M., Power, J.D., Koren, G., & Einarson, T.R. (1998). Benzodiazepine use in pregnancy and major malformations or oral cleft: Meta-analysis of cohort and case-control studies. *British Medical Journal, 317*, 839–843.

Dowden, J. (2003). *Therapeutic guidelines. Psychotropic version 5.* North Melbourne, Australia: Therapeutic Guidelines Limited.

Einarson, A., Selby, P., & Koren, G. (2001). Discontinuing antidepressants and benzodiazepines upon becoming pregnant. Beware of the risks of abrupt discontinuation. *Canadian Family Physician, 47*, 489–490.

Eros, E., Czeizel, A.E., Rockenbauer, M., Sorensen, H.T., & Olsen, J. (2002). A population-based case-control teratologic study of nitrazepam, medazepam, tofisopam, alprazolum and clonazepam treatment during pregnancy. *European Journal of Obstetrics Gynecology and Reproductive Biology, 101*, 147–154.

Frassetto, F., Tourneur Martel, F., Barjhoux, C.E., Villier, C., Bot, B.L., & Vincent, F. (2002). Goiter in a newborn exposed to lithium in utero. *Annals of Pharmacotherapy, 36*, 1745–1748.

Frey, B., Schubiger, G., & Musy, J.P. (1990). Transient cholestatic hepatitis in a neonate associated with carbamazepine exposure during pregnancy and breast-feeding. *European Journal of Pediatrics, 150*, 136–138.

Gabbe, S.G., Niebyl, J.R., & Simpson, J.L. (1996). *Obstetrics: Normal and problem pregnancies.* New York: Churchill Livingstone Inc.

Goldstein, D.J., Corbin, L.A., & Sundell, K.L. (1997). Effects of first-trimester fluoxetine exposure on the newborn. *Obstetrics and Gynecology, 89*, 713–718.

Gracious, B.L., & Wisner, K.L. (1997). Phenelzine use throughout pregnancy and the puerperium: Case report, review of the literature, and management recommendations. *Depression and Anxiety, 6*, 124–128.

Haramburu, F., Miremont-Salame, G., & Moore, N. (2000). Good and bad drug prescription in pregnancy. *Lancet, 356*, 1704.

Hendrick, V., Smith, L.M., Suri, R., Hwang, S., Haynes, D., & Altshuler, L. (2003a). Birth outcomes after prenatal exposure to antidepressant medication. *American Journal of Obstetrics and Gynecology, 188*, 812–815.

Hendrick, V., Stowe, Z.N., Altshuler, L.L., Hwang, S., Lee, E., & Haynes, D. (2003b). Placental passage of antidepressant medications. *American Journal of Psychiatry, 160*, 993–996.

Ilett, K.F., Kristensen, J.H., Hackett, L.P., Paech, M., Kohan, R., & Rampono, J. (2002). Distribution of venlafaxine and its O-desmethyl metabolite in human milk and their effects in breastfed infants. *British Journal of Clinical Pharmacology, 53*, 17–22.

Iqbal, M.M. (1999). Effects of antidepressants during pregnancy and lactation. *Annals of Clinical Psychiatry, 11*, 237–256.

Iqbal, M.M., Sobhan, T., & Ryals, T. (2002). Effects of commonly used benzodiazepines on the fetus, the neonate, and the nursing infant. *Psychiatric Services, 53*, 39–49.

Jacobson, S.J., Jones, K., Johnson, K., Ceolin, L., Kaur, P., Sahn, D., Donnenfeld, A.E., Rieder, M., Santelli, R., Smythe, J., et al. (1992). Prospective multicentre study of pregnancy outcome after lithium exposure during first trimester. *Lancet, 339*, 530–533.

Jauniaux, E., Jurkovic, D., Lees, C., Campbell, S., & Gulbis, B. (1996). In-vivo study of diazepam transfer across the first trimester human placenta. *Human Reproduction, 11*, 889–892.

Jones, K.L., Lacro, R.V., Johnson, K.A., & Adams, J. (1989). Pattern of malformations in the children of women treated with carbamazepine during pregnancy. *New England Journal of Medicine, 320*, 1661–1666.

Jurand, A., & Martin, L.V. (1994). Cleft palate and open eyelids inducing activity of lorazepam and the effect of flumazenil, the benzodiazepine antagonist. *Pharmacology and Toxicology, 74*, 228–235.

Kai, S., Kohmura, H., Ishikawa, K., Ohta, S., Kuroyanagi, K., Kawano, S., Kadota, T., Chikazawa, H., Kondo, H., & Takahashi, N. (1990). Reproductive and developmental toxicity studies of buspirone hydrochloride (II) – Oral administration to rats during perinatal and lactation periods. *Journal of Toxicology and Science, 15*(Suppl 1), 61–84.

Karlsson, K., Lindstedt, G., Lundberg, P.A., & Selstam, U. (1975). Letter: Transplacental lithium poisoning: Reversible inhibition of fetal thyroid. *Lancet, 1*, 1295.

Kent, L.S., & Laidlaw, J.D. (1995). Suspected congenital sertraline dependence. *British Journal of Psychiatry, 167*, 412–413.

Kesim, M., Yaris, F., Kadioglu, M., Yaris, E., Kalyoncu, N.I., & Ulku, C. (2002). Mirtazapine use in two pregnant women: is it safe? *Teratology, 66*, 204.

Khan, K.S., Wykes, C., & Gee, H. (1999). Benzodiazepine use in pregnancy and major malformations or oral clefts. Quality of primary studies must influence inferences made from meta-analyses. *British Medical Journal, 319*, 919.

Klier, C.M., Schafer, M.R., Schmid-Siegel, B., Lenz, G., & Mannel, M. (2002). St John's wort (Hypericum perforatum) – is it safe during breastfeeding? *Pharmacopsychiatry, 35*, 29–30.

Koch, S., Jager-Roman, E., Rating, D., & Helge, H. (1983). Possible teratogenic effect of valproate during pregnancy. *Journal of Pediatrics, 103*, 1007–1008.

Koren, G., Randor, S., Martin, S., & Danneman, D. (1990). Maternal ginseng use associated with neonatal androgenization. *Journal of the American Medical Association, 264*, 2866.

Kramer, A., Knoppert-Van der Klein, E.A.M., Van Kamp, I.L., Walter, F.J., Van Vliet, I.M., & Zitman, F.G. (2003). Bipolar and pregnant? No problem! A clinical evaluation of lithium use during pregnancy. *European Neuropsychopharmacology, 13*, S246.

Kurki, T., Hiilesmaa, V., Raitasalo, R., Mattila, H., & Ylikorkala, O. (2000). Depression and anxiety in early pregnancy and risk for preeclampsia. *Obstetrics and Gynecology, 95*, 487–490.

Laegreid, L. (1990). Clinical observations in children after prenatal benzodiazepine exposure. *Developmental Pharmacology and Therapeutics, 15*, 186–188.

Laine, K., Heikkinen, T., Ekblad, U., & Kero, P. (2003). Effects of exposure to selective serotonin reuptake inhibitors during pregnancy on serotonergic symptoms in newborns and cord blood monoamine and prolactin concentrations. *Archives of General Psychiatry, 60*, 720–726.

Lee, A., Minhas, R., Matsuda, N., Lam, M., & Ito, S. (2003). The safety of St John's wort (Hypericum perforatum) during breastfeeding. *Journal of Clinical Psychiatry, 64*, 966–968.

Legius, E., Jaeken, J., & Eggermont, E. (1987). Sodium valproate, pregnancy, and infantile fatal liver failure. *Lancet, 2*, 1518–1519.

Licht, R.W., Vestergaard, P., Kessing, L.V., Larsen, J.K., & Thomsen, P.H. (2003). Psychopharmacological treatment with lithium and antiepileptic drugs: Suggested guidelines from the Danish Psychiatric Association and the Child and Adolescent Psychiatric Association in Denmark. *Acta Psychiatrica Scandinavica Supplement*, 1–22.

Lieberman, B.A., Stirrat, G.M., Cohen, S.L., Beard, R.W., Pinker, G.D., & Belsey, E. (1978). The possible adverse effect of propranolol on the fetus in pregnancies complicated by severe hypertension. *British Journal of Obstetrics and Gynaecology*, 85, 678–683.

Lindhout, D., & Meinardi, H. (1984). Spina bifida and in-utero exposure to valproate. *Lancet, 2*, 396.

Little, B.B., Santos-Ramos, R., Newell, J.F., & Maberry, M.C. (1993). Megadose carbamazepine during the period of neural tube closure. *Obstetrics and Gynecology, 82*, 705–708.

Livingstone, I., Craswell, P.W., Bevan, E.B., Smith, M.T., & Eadie, M.J. (1983). Propranolol in pregnancy three year prospective study. *Clinical and Experimental Hypertension B, 2*, 341–350.

Llewellyn, A., Stowe, Z.N., & Strader Jr, J.R. (1998). The use of lithium and management of women with bipolar disorder during pregnancy and lactation. *Journal of Clinical Psychiatry, 59*(Suppl 6), 57–64, discussion 65.

Majer, R.V., & Green, P.J. (1987). Neonatal afibrinogenaemia due to sodium valproate. *Lancet, 2*, 740–741.

Martin, J.A., Hamilton, B.E., Sutton, P.D., Ventura, S.J., Menacker, F., & Munson, M.L. (2003). Births: Final data for 2002. *National Vital Statistical Report, 52*, 1–113.

Matheson, I., Pande, H., & Alertsen, A.R. (1985). Respiratory depression caused by N-desmethyldoxepin in breast milk. *Lancet, 2*, 1124.

Matheson, I., Kristensen, K., & Lunde, P.K. (1990). Drug utilization in breast-feeding women. A survey in Oslo. *European Journal of Clinical Pharmacology, 38*, 453–459.

McElhatton, P.R. (1994). The effects of benzodiazepine use during pregnancy and lactation. *Reproductive Toxicology, 8*, 461–475.

McElhatton, P.R., Garbis, H.M., Elefant, E., Vial, T., Bellemin, B., Mastroiacovo, P., Arnon, J., Rodriguez-Pinilla, E., Schaefer, C., Pexieder, T., Merlob, P., & Dal Verme, S. (1996). The outcome of pregnancy in 689 women exposed to therapeutic doses of antidepressants. A collaborative study of the European Network of Teratology Information Services (ENTIS). *Reproductive Toxicology, 10*, 285–294.

McMahon, C.L., & Braddock, S.R. (1998). Septo-optic dysplasia in a child exposed to valproic acid in utero. *Teratology, 57*, 284.

Merlob, P., Mor, N., & Litwin, A. (1992). Transient hepatic dysfunction in an infant of an epileptic mother treated with carbamazepine during pregnancy and breastfeeding. *Annals of Pharmacotherapy, 26*, 1563–1565.

Mizrahi, E.M., Hobbs, J.F., & Goldsmith, D.I. (1979). Nephrogenic diabetes insipidus in transplacental lithium intoxication. *Journal of Pediatrics, 94*, 493–495.

Morrell, P., Sutherland, G.R., Buamah, P.K., Oo, M., & Bain, H.H. (1983). Lithium toxicity in a neonate. *Archives of Disease in Childhood, 58*, 539–541.

Nisselle, P. (2000). Informed consent. In: F. Bochner (Ed.), *Therapeutic guidelines, psychotropic version 4* (p. 39). North Melbourne, Australia: Therapeutic Guidelines Limited.

Nordeng, H., Lindemann, R., Perminov, K.V., & Reikvam, A. (2001). Neonatal withdrawal syndrome after in utero exposure to selective serotonin reuptake inhibitors. *Acta Paediatrica, 90*, 288–291.

Nulman, I., Rovet, J., Stewart, D.E., Wolpin, J., Gardner, H.A., Theis, J.G., Kulin, N., & Koren, G. (1997). Neurodevelopment of children exposed in utero to antidepressant drugs. *New England Journal of Medicine, 336*, 258–262.

O'Connor, T.G., Heron, J., Golding, J., Beveridge, M., & Glover, V. (2002). Maternal antenatal anxiety and children's behavioural/emotional problems at 4 years. Report from the Avon Longitudinal Study of Parents and Children. *British Journal of Psychiatry, 180*, 502–508.

Ornoy, A., Arnon, J., Shechtman, S., Moerman, L., & Lukashova, I. (1998). Is benzodiazepine use during pregnancy really teratogenic? *Reproductive Toxicology, 12*, 511–515.

Pennell, P.B. (2003). Antiepileptic drug pharmacokinetics during pregnancy and lactation. *Neurology, 61*, S35–S42.

Pinelli, J.M., Symington, A.J., Cunningham, K.A., & Paes, B.A. (2002). Case report and review of the perinatal implications of maternal lithium use. *American Journal of Obstetrics and Gynecology, 187*, 245–249.

Pons, G., Francoual, C., Guillet, P., Moran, C., Hermann, P., Bianchetti, G., Thiercelin, J.F., Thenot, J.P., & Olive, G. (1989). Zolpidem excretion in breast milk. *European Journal of Clinical Pharmacology, 37*, 245–248.

Pruyn, S.C., Phelan, J.P., & Buchanan, G.C. (1979). Long-term propranolol therapy in pregnancy: Maternal and fetal outcome. *American Journal of Obstetrics and Gynecology, 135*, 485–489.

Robert, E., & Guibaud, P. (1982). Maternal valproic acid and congenital neural tube defects. *Lancet, 2*, 937.

Rodriguez-Pinilla, E., Arroyo, I., Fondevilla, J., Garcia, M.J., & Martinez-Frias, M.L. (2000). Prenatal exposure to valproic acid during pregnancy and limb deficiencies: A case-control study. *American Journal of Medical Genetics, 90*, 376–381.

Rosa, F.W. (1991). Spina bifida in infants of women treated with carbamazepine during pregnancy. *New England Journal of Medicine, 324*, 674–677.

Safra, M.J., & Oakley Jr, G.P. (1975). Association between cleft lip with or without cleft palate and prenatal exposure to diazepam. *Lancet, 2*, 478–480.

Saxen, I. (1975). Associations between oral clefts and drugs taken during pregnancy. *International Journal of Epidemiology, 4*, 37–44.

Schou, M., Goldfield, M.D., Weinstein, M.R., & Villeneuve, A. (1973). Lithium and pregnancy. I. Report from the Register of Lithium Babies. *British Medical Journal, 2*, 135–136.

Shiono, P.H., & Mills, J.L. (1984). Oral clefts and diazepam use during pregnancy. *New England Journal of Medicine, 311*, 919–920.

Smith, M.T., Livingstone, I., Hooper, W.D., Eadie, M.J., & Triggs, E.J. (1983). Propranolol, propranolol glucuronide, and naphthoxylactic acid in breast milk and plasma. *Therapeutic Drug Monitoring, 5*, 87–93.

Spencer, M.J. (1993). Fluoxetine hydrochloride (Prozac) toxicity in a neonate. *Pediatrics*, *92*, 721–722.

St Clair, S.M., & Schirmer, R.G. (1992). First-trimester exposure to alprazolam. *Obstetrics and Gynecology*, *80*, 843–846.

Tesch, B.J. (2003). Herbs commonly used by women: An evidence-based review. *American Journal of Obstetrics and Gynecology*, *188*, S44–S55.

Thisted, E., & Ebbesen, F. (1993). Malformations, withdrawal manifestations, and hypoglycaemia after exposure to valproate in utero. *Archives of Disease in Childhood*, *69*, 288–291.

Uauy, R., & De Andraca, I. (1995). Human milk and breast feeding for optimal mental development. *Journal of Nutrition*, *125*, 2278S–2280S.

Vendittelli, F., Alain, J., Nouaille, Y., Brosset, A., & Tabaste, J.L. (1995). A case of lipomeningocele reported with fluoxetine (and alprazolam, vitamins B1 and B6, heptaminol) prescribed during pregnancy. *European Journal of Obstetrics Gynecology and Reproductive Biology*, *58*, 85–86.

Viggedal, G., Hagberg, B.S., Laegreid, L., & Aronsson, M. (1993). Mental development in late infancy after prenatal exposure to benzodiazepines – a prospective study. *Journal of Child Psychology and Psychiatry and Allied Disciplines*, *34*, 295–305.

Vogel, L., & Muskin, P. (1999). Anxiety disorders. In: J. Cutler, & P. Marcus (Eds.), *Psychiatry* USA: W.B. Saunders Company.

Ward, R.M., Bates, B.A., McCarver, D.G., Notterman, D.A., & Walson, P.D. (2000). Use of psychoactive medication during pregnancy and possible effects on the fetus and newborn. Committee on drugs. American Academy of Pediatrics. *Pediatrics*, *105*, 880–887.

Weinbaum, P.J., Cassidy, S.B., Vintzileos, A.M., Campbell, W.A., Ciarleglio, L., & Nochimson, D.J. (1986). Prenatal detection of a neural tube defect after fetal exposure to valproic acid. *Obstetrics and Gynecology*, *67*, 31S–33S.

Weinstock, L., Cohen, L.S., Bailey, J.W., Blatman, R., & Rosenbaum, J.F. (2001). Obstetrical and neonatal outcome following clonazepam use during pregnancy: A case series. *Psychotherapy and Psychosomatics*, *70*, 158–162.

Werler, M.M., Bower, C., Payne, J., & Serna, P. (2003). Findings on potential teratogens from a case-control study in Western Australia. *Australian and New Zealand Journal of Obstetrics and Gynecology*, *43*, 443–447.

Williams, K., & Oke, S. (2000). Lithium and pregnancy. *Psychiatric Bulletin*, *24*, 229–231.

Wilson, N., Forfar, J.D., & Godman, M.J. (1983). Atrial flutter in the newborn resulting from maternal lithium ingestion. *Archives of Disease in Childhood*, *58*, 538–539.

Winter, R.M., Donnai, D., Burn, J., & Tucker, S.M. (1987). Fetal valproate syndrome: Is there a recognisable phenotype? *Journal of Medical Genetics*, *24*, 692–695.

Yerby, M.S. (2003). Clinical care of pregnant women with epilepsy: Neural tube defects and folic acid supplementation. *Epilepsia*, *44*(Suppl 3), 33–40.

Yoder, M.C., Belik, J., Lannon, R.A., & Pereira, G.R. (1984). Infants of mothers treated with lithium during pregnancy have an increased incidence of prematurity, macrosomia and perinatal mortality. *Pediatric Research*, *18*, 163A.

Yoshida, K., Smith, B., Craggs, M., & Kumar, R.C. (1998). Fluoxetine in breast-milk and developmental outcome of breast-fed infants. *British Journal of Psychiatry*, *172*, 175–178.

10

Bipolar affective disorder: Special issues for women

Shaila Misri[1,2], Diana Carter[2] and Ruth M. Little[2]

[1]Department of Psychiatry and OB/GYN, University of British Columbia, Columbia, SC, USA
[2]Reproductive Mental Health Program, St. Paul's Hospital and BC Women's Hospital, Vancouver BC, Canada

"Oddly enough, it had never occurred to me not to have children simply because I had manic-depressive illness … Of course, I had had serious concerns: How could one not? Would I, for example, be able to take care of my children properly? What would happen to them if I got severely depressed? Much more frightening still, what would happen to them if I got manic, if my judgment became impaired, if I became violent or uncontrollable? How would it be to watch my own children struggle with depression, hopelessness, despair, or insanity if they themselves became ill? Would I watch them too hawkishly for symptoms or mistake their normal reactions to life as signs of illness?"

Kay Redfield Jamison, *An Unquiet Mind* (1995, p. 191–192)

This poignant quote depicts the difficult and painful struggle that women with bipolar disorder (BD) face when contemplating motherhood. Generally a life-long condition beginning in late adolescence and early adulthood, most women with BD will experience this illness during their child-bearing years (Viguera et al., 2002a). For treating physicians, the event of pregnancy in a woman with BD creates a challenging clinical dilemma. Essential to successful treatment is an understanding of the two ways this condition is manifested during childbearing. Firstly, women with a *known* history of BD are particularly vulnerable during pregnancy and the postpartum. The second manifestation of this condition is that of *new onset* BD in the postpartum; the adverse effects of puerperal psychosis are well documented. Faced with these considerations, the management of women with BD throughout pregnancy and/or in the postpartum requires the delicate and dynamic balancing of the risks and benefits of different treatment options.

This chapter describes the gender differences relevant to BD; general reproductive health issues for women with BD; risk factors for relapse or new onset BD during childbearing; the impact of untreated BD in pregnancy and the postpartum; and the management issues and strategies during preconception and the prenatal, perinatal and post-natal periods. Relevant other chapters in this volume include Chapters 8 and 9.

Gender differences in BD

The prevalence of BD in the USA is 0.5–1.5% (Yonkers et al., 2004). Whilst men and women are equally affected by BD, the expression of this condition and course of illness differs between the sexes in various ways (Arnold, 2003; Leibenluft, 1997). An understanding of the interplay between gender and BD is vital so that this information can be incorporated into clinical decision-making, to optimize patient management.

The onset of BD

The mean age of onset of BD has been reported as later in women than men in most studies (Hendrick et al., 2000; Robb et al., 1998). Viguera et al. (2001) studied a cohort of patients with BD (I or II) and found that the onset of BD was a mean 3.2 years later in women than men. By age 25 years, more men (71%) than women (52.8%) had BD, and more women (33.6%) had onset after 30 years than men (22.1%). Notably, women may be more likely than men to develop late onset (45–49 years) BD (Leibenluft, 1996).

The later onset of BD for women appears to be a blessing of epidemiology which grants women several extra disease-free years. However, this phenomenon may actually be due, in part, to delayed diagnosis or misdiagnosis with depression. Women are more likely to have a depressive index episode and have bipolar II (which typically follows a depressive trajectory) (Viguera et al., 2001). Women are also misdiagnosed with unipolar depression for longer than men; a study reporting that females were thought to have unipolar depression for 3.9 years before bipolar was diagnosed, versus 2.0 years for males (Viguera et al., 2001). This is not surprising considering that unipolar depression is more common in women (Blazer et al., 1994). However, the impact of delayed or misdiagnosis is significant, and can include adverse experiences accumulated in the interim as well as potential complications of treatment such as rapid cycling secondary to antidepressant administration (Robb et al., 1998).

Symptoms, course of illness and treatment

There are differences in the expression of BD in males and females, with women more commonly experiencing rapid cycling, depressive episodes and possibly mixed mania (Leibenluft, 1996; Robb et al., 1998). The relationship between rapid cycling and gender is well established. According to Diagnostic and Statistical Manual of Mental Disorders, Edition IV, Text Revision (DSM-IV-TR), about 10–20% of patients with BD experience rapid cycling; and 70–90% of the patients with BD who suffer from rapid cycling are female (American Psychiatric Association, 2000). Rapid cycling is also more common in patients with bipolar II, which women are 1.6 times more likely to develop (Tondo et al., 1998; Viguera et al., 2001).

These differences in symptomatology affect the age of onset, course of illness and treatment options for women. Viguera et al. (2001) found that the period between the onset of BD and beginning treatment was 24.4 months longer for females, likely due to initial misdiagnosis with unipolar depression and a time lag between diagnosis and starting treatment. Women were as likely as men to stop lithium treatment and to stop it abruptly/quickly, but were in treatment for 10.7 months longer and had their first recurrence during lithium maintenance, on average 6 months later (Viguera et al., 2001). Lithium-related side effects can also differ between the sexes, one study reporting weight gain and clinical hypothyroidism to be more likely to be experienced by women; however, tremor was more common amongst men (Henry, 2002). Seasonal variations in mood, depressive episodes and hospital admissions also vary between the sexes (D'Mello et al., 1995; Faedda et al., 1993).

Co-morbidity and gender

BD is not a lonely diagnosis: common co-morbidities include anxiety disorders, alcohol and substance abuse, hypothyroidism, migraines and obesity (Arnold, 2003). The prevalence of most co-morbid conditions differs between the sexes. McElroy et al. (2001) examined the relationship between BD and anxiety disorders, substance abuse and eating disorders for 288 outpatients with BD. The majority (65%) had a lifetime axis I co-morbid disorder. A reported 42% had a substance use disorder, and 5% had an eating disorder. Lifetime anxiety disorders were found in 42% of cases, the most common subtypes being panic disorder/agoraphobia (20%) and social phobia (16%). Anxiety disorders are more common in women than men in general (see Chapter 4), and there are data suggesting that panic disorder disproportionately affects women with BD (Arnold, 2003; Kessler et al., 1994; MacKinnon et al., 2002). A study exploring the clinical significance of this co-morbidity, found that patients with bipolar I and lifetime panic symptoms had more depression, suicidal ideation and a six month longer time lag between acute treatment and achieving remission (Frank et al., 2002).

Alcohol and substance abuse in individuals with BD is reported as more common amongst men than women in most research, a pattern that mimics the gender distribution of these conditions in the general population (Cassidy et al., 2001; Frye et al., 2003; Kessler et al., 1994; and see Chapter 3). Nonetheless, alcohol and substance abuse remain an important co-morbidity for women with BD, who have higher lifetime rates than the general community for alcohol abuse (37.8% versus 14.6%) and drug abuse (33.8% versus 9.4%). Notably, lifetime drug abuse rates were greatest for marijuana followed by cocaine (Cassidy et al., 2001).

It is not only psychiatric disorders but general medical conditions that can occur in bipolar patients, and women again tend to be disproportionately affected. Migraine, obesity and thyroid disease are more frequently experienced by individuals with BD, with women affected more than men (Arnold, 2003; Elmslie et al., 2000; Johnston & Eagles, 1999).

The high prevalence of one or more co-morbidity amongst patients with BD increases the complexity of the clinical treatment of women with BD.

BD and reproduction

Reproductive health

The relationship between mood and the menstrual cycle in BD is debatable. Some researchers have found that there are mood disturbances related to the menstrual cycle in patients with BD, but no clear pattern has been found for cohorts at large (Blehar et al., 1998; Leibenluft et al., 1999; Rasgon et al., 2003).

It is not known whether a direct relationship exists between BD and polycystic ovaries (PCO) or whether PCO is an effect of treatment or of medication-induced obesity. Burt & Rasgon, 2004; Isojarvi et al., 1993, 1996; Rasgon et al., 2000).

Preconception

"The fact that manic-depressive illness is a genetic disease brings with it, not surprisingly, very complicated and often difficult emotions. At one extreme is the shame and guilt one can be made to feel. Many years ago, when I was living in Los Angeles, I went to a physician recommended to me by a colleague. After examining me, and finding out that I had been on lithium for many years, he asked me an extended series of questions about my psychiatric history. He also asked me whether or not I planned to have children … I asked him if his concerns about my having children stemmed from the fact that, because of my illness, he thought I would be an inadequate mother or simply that he thought it was best to avoid bringing another manic-depressive into the world. Ignoring or missing my sarcasm, he replied 'Both'."

Kay Redfield Jamison, *An Unquiet Mind* (1995, p. 190–191)

The decision whether or not to have children can be difficult and conflicting for women with BD. Preconception counselling provides an ideal opportunity to assist women with this decision-making process, and inform them about the risks and benefits of their therapeutic options during pregnancy. Preconception counselling allows a pregnancy to be planned and occur when a women is as stable and in the most supportive environment feasible. Planning may also permit a trial free of medications, and discussions about fertility – a potential issue for some patients due to BD and its treatments.

Genetic counselling is also essential, to address patient fears and to educate them about disease inheritance. Whilst the genetics of BD are not yet fully determined, it is clear that the offspring of individuals with this condition have an increased risk of psychiatric illness. A population-based study reported a 14-fold greater risk of BD in individuals with a first-degree relative with BD. A maternal history of BD conferred a relative risk of 12, a paternal history 15 and both parents a 113-fold greater risk than individuals without such a family history (Mortensen et al., 2003). A meta-analysis comparing children of individuals with BD with offspring of those without a mental illness, found that the former group had a 4-fold greater likelihood of an affective disorder and a 2.7-fold greater risk of any mental disorder (Lapalme et al., 1997). Such risk must, however, be discussed within the context of the relationship between genetic and environmental factors. Monozygotic twin studies show concordance rates greater than those of dizygotic twins, but less than 100%; illustrating that whilst genetic factors are strong, environmental factors do influence the expression of this condition (Smoller & Finn, 2003).

Viguera et al. (2002b) examined the choices made by women with BD who received a preconception psychiatric consultation to inform them about the risks/benefits of medication during pregnancy. A reported 45% of women had been previously advised by health professionals not to conceive; 69% of these were mental health professionals. Opposition to pregnancy had also been voiced by spouses (21%) and parents/siblings (45%). Following this consultation, 63% of women tried to conceive whilst 37% avoided conceiving. Reasons for avoiding pregnancy were:

- fear of adverse effects of medicines on foetal development (56%);
- risk of relapse with medication cessation (50%);
- fear of their child inheriting BD (22%);
- fears of recurrent illness negatively impacting upon the foetus/existing children (17%);
- reluctance to repeat past pregnancy-related illness (17%).

In reality, up to 40% of pregnancies in the general US population are unplanned, and 50% of individuals with planned pregnancies will not have seen a health care provider prior to conception (American Academy of Neurology, 1998). A substantial proportion of women with BD will thus present already pregnant. The concern is that women will discover their pregnancy in the first trimester, by which time the foetus has already been exposed to psychoactive medications (Yonkers et al., 2004).

Potential effects of untreated BD during childbearing

In the USA, only around a quarter of people with BP are thought to receive treatment (Goodwin & Jamison, 1990). Untreated BD during pregnancy and the postpartum can impact upon both the woman and her unborn child. Acute episodes during pregnancy are of concern due to the risks of substance abuse, neglect of antenatal care, poor judgment, impulsive behaviour, poor nutrition, increased risk of committing or being a victim of violence and the risk of self-harm, including suicide in major depression (Finnerty et al., 1996; Viguera et al., 2000). In the postpartum period, maternal recurrences can affect practical infant care and mother–infant attachment (Brockington, 2004; Brockington et al., 1982). Severe psychiatric illness (usually psychosis) in the postpartum period also carries the risk of neonaticide and infanticide, particularly in the early months (Overpeck et al., 1998; Spinelli, 2001).

BD, childbearing and risk factors for relapse

The debate about whether or not pregnancy is protective against BD recurrence is unresolved. Viguera et al. (2000) reported similar rates of illness recurrence in pregnant (52%) and non-pregnant (58%) women who discontinued lithium maintenance therapy over 1–40 weeks. These rates were higher than the preceding year, when 21% of the then-medicated cohort relapsed. In patients who were euthymic during weeks 1–40, relapse in weeks 41–64 was greater for the pregnant (postpartum) group (70% versus 24% in the non-pregnant group). The authors commented that either pregnancy is not specifically protective or that any protective effects are negated by factors such as medication cessation. In contrast, Grof et al. (2000) reported that women with bipolar I had fewer recurrences and shorter duration of recurrences during pregnancy than in the nine months before conception and the nine months after delivery. Overall, pregnancy may confer some protection for stable women with single episodes, no recurrences for an extended period and a good response to pharmacotherapy; however, this protection may not be enough to permit medication discontinuation in most cases. Pregnancy is unlikely to be protective for women with refractory illness, an early age of illness onset, multiple episodes and who experience a high relapse rate when unmedicated.

There are several known risk factors for postpartum BD episodes. A family history of postpartum psychosis is a key risk factor. Jones and Craddock (2001) reported that 74% of women with BD suffering from puerperal psychosis had a family history of postpartum psychosis (first-degree relatives). Comparatively, only 30% of women with bipolar and no family history developed puerperal psychosis. A personal past history is another major risk factor; postpartum psychotic episodes carry a 30–50% chance of recurrence in each future pregnancy (American Psychiatric Association, 2000). The maternal course of illness during pregnancy may also be predictive of postpartum mental health, one study reporting that a postpartum episode was more likely to occur in women whose depressive symptoms worsened during pregnancy (Freeman et al., 2002). However, postpartum prophylaxis with a mood stabilizer may be protective; Cohen et al. (1995) found that women with known BD who did not receive prophylaxis with a mood stabilizer had an 8.6 times greater relative risk of postpartum relapse in the first 3 months after childbirth than women administered postpartum prophylaxis (mostly lithium).

There is limited information on the influence of socio-economic and obstetric factors on the course of illness of childbearing women with BD. Kendell et al. (1987)

commented that the risk of severe puerperal psychiatric illness included being primi-parae, without a husband at the time of delivery, having a Caesarean section and peri-natal death. The potential link between sleep disturbances and postnatal psychosis is unclear. Sharma and Mazmanian (2003, p. 102) comment that "*sleep loss may be the final common pathway by which various putative risk factors produce psychosis in susceptible women*".

Childbirth is a well documented risk factor for psychiatric morbidity in women, particularly primiparae. The risk of bipolar relapse is highest in the immediate post-partum period, but stays higher than the pre-pregnancy risk for several years there-after. Kendell et al. (1987) reported the relative risk of psychiatric admission 30 days from birth was 6.0, and for primiparae only the risk was 10.9. The relative risk of admission with psychosis within 30 days of delivery was 21.7 (35.0 for primiparae) and the relative risk of admission within two years of parturition was 1.6 (or 3.5 for admission with psychosis within two years). Of the general childbearing population, 1–2 per 1000 will be effected by postpartum psychosis (Kendell et al., 1987). For a detailed discussion of these issues, see Chapter 8.

Management of BD in pregnancy

Principles of management

Experts recommend classifying all pregnant women with BD as "high-risk" preg-nancies (Viguera et al., 2002a). Holistic prenatal care of these "high-risk" cases has several elements, including:

- maintaining the best possible control of BD;
- intensive psychiatric follow-up and a multidisciplinary specialist team approach;
- addressing co-morbid conditions;
- attending to issues relevant to any pregnant woman such as antenatal care, diet and avoidance of smoking (Brockington 2004; Viguera et al., 2002a; Yonkers et al., 2004).

Only the first of these facets are addressed here.

In order to ascertain the treatment options for each individual during pregnancy, key patient information required includes a past history of BD (related and unrelated to pregnancy), a family history of puerperal psychosis and a medication history (response to different agents, time to relapse) (Jones & Craddock, 2001; Yonkers et al., 2004). There are no failsafe rules to follow when treating women with BD during preg-nancy. The management of each patient must be decided on a case-by-case basis after evaluating the risk/benefit ratio for every individual (see also Chapter 9). However, there are some general principles of management. Viguera et al. (2002a) state that patients who have had one manic episode with rapid, total recovery and subsequent stability may be able to taper medication gradually, prior to conception. A recognized drawback of this approach is the risk of relapse while awaiting conception, yet waiting until pregnancy before stopping medication can be problematic, as rapid or abrupt cessation of medication increases the risk of early relapse (Viguera et al., 2000, 2002a; Yonkers et al., 2004). Furthermore, by the time conception is determined the period of greatest risk of foetal exposure may already be passed. Home pregnancy tests can detect conception from 10 days and embryonic exposure is minimal as it takes about 14 days before utero-placental circulation is established (Viguera et al., 2002a). If the patient discontinues medication, it should be reinstituted if they become symptomatic, even during trimester one. In women with brittle BD, with a past history of numerous severe recurrences (and potentially psychosis or suicidality), maintaining medication prior to and throughout the pregnancy is typically recommended (Viguera et al., 2002a; Yonkers et al., 2004).

The US Food and Drug Administration are yet to approve the use of psychotropic agents in pregnant women (Altshuler et al., 1996). The principles of drug administration during pregnancy include using the lowest possible therapeutic dose, monotherapy and using agents with the lowest potential for adverse foetal effects. Medication is more difficult to titrate during childbearing as drug pharmacokinetics are affected by the physiological changes of pregnancy and delivery, particularly shifting fluid loads and altered drug clearance rates (Altshuler et al., 1996; Burt & Rasgon, 2004; Yonkers et al., 2004). Regular monitoring of blood levels is essential, as these physiological changes can mean higher doses are required to achieve therapeutic levels. During parturition and the early postpartum period, the levels of some agents may increase rapidly with abrupt fluid losses; thus, intensive monitoring of maternal hydration status and drug levels is advised (Yonkers et al., 2004).

All psychotrophic agents cross the placenta, and thus can affect foetal organ development and growth in utero, and cause neonatal toxicity or withdrawal at birth (Altshuler et al., 1996; American Academy of Pediatrics (AAP): Committee on Drugs, 2000). Little is known about the impact of these drugs upon long-term behaviour and development. There are specific periods of gestation during which drug exposure increases the risk of particular conditions. For example, exposure on days 21–56 can impact upon cardiac formation, on days 42–63 can affect palate and lip formation and up to day 32 can impact upon neural tube formation and closure. Exposure in trimesters two and three carries the potential risks of low birth weight, preterm delivery, minor malformations and behavioural sequelae (Yonkers et al., 2004). Notably, information on psychoactive drugs in pregnancy generally comes from retrospective cohort studies or case reports; there are few less biased prospective studies or randomized controlled trials due to practical and ethical reasons (AAP: Committee on Drugs, 2000; Shader & Greenblatt, 1995). The reader is also referred to Chapter 9.

Lithium

Foetal and neonatal effects

Lithium is the first line agent for mood stabilization in pregnant women with BD (Viguera et al., 2002a). Lithium is not as dangerous as once perceived (Cohen et al., 1994), with most exposed infants being born normal. The risk of Ebstein's anomaly was perceived as 400-fold greater for the children of women taking lithium (Schou et al., 1973a), but the rate is now recalculated at 1 in 1000 compared with the general population rate of 1 in 20,000 (Altshuler et al., 1996; Cohen et al., 1994). Due to this heightened risk, a high-resolution ultrasound and foetal echocardiograph are recommended at 16–18 weeks gestational age for women taking lithium in trimester one (Cohen et al., 1991).

Lithium exposure during delivery can result in neonatal toxicity: hallmarks of the "floppy baby syndrome" include neonatal cyanosis and hypotonicity (Altshuler et al., 1996). Nephrogenic diabetes insipidus and neonatal hypothyroidism have also been reported (Mizrahi et al., 1979; Nars & Girard, 1977). Foetal thyroid goitre infrequently occurs with exposure to lithium during trimesters two and three (AAP: Committee on Drugs, 2000), and can complicate delivery. The birth weight of neonates with trimester one exposure has been reported as significantly greater than controls by a mean of 92 g (Jacobson et al., 1992). Long-term neurobehavioural and developmental effects from lithium exposure in utero have been researched in follow-up studies, with no consistent negative consequences described (Jacobson et al., 1992; Schou, 1976; Yonkers et al., 2004).

Therapy during pregnancy and delivery

The narrow therapeutic window of lithium makes it a difficult drug to regulate, particularly during pregnancy and delivery when fluid shifts occur, and pharmacokinetics change. Due to the short half-life of lithium (8–10 h), dosing is recommended 3–4 times/day to maintain the best possible steady state levels (Yonkers et al., 2004). Adequate hydration (particularly during concurrent medical illness) is important to avoid lithium toxicity. Maternal polyuria and polydypsia during pregnancy can be aggravated by lithium (Misri & Lusskin, 2004). Lithium levels should be monitored monthly during pregnancy, with increasing frequency as pregnancy progresses and delivery approaches. The required lithium dose typically increases with advancing pregnancy, due to greater drug clearance (Misri & Lusskin, 2004; Schou et al., 1973; Yonkers et al., 2004). To avoid maternal and neonatal toxicity at birth, decreasing the lithium dose 25–30% just prior to parturition is advised (Altshuler et al., 1996). This decision must be balanced against risk of maternal relapse in labour or thereafter. Preserving the patient's hydration status and intensive monitoring of maternal symptoms and lithium levels is recommended, because of the risk of toxicity or relapse during childbirth and the immediate postpartum (Viguera et al., 2000; Yonkers et al., 2004; and see Chapter 9).

Anti-convulsants

One in three patients with BD does not respond to or tolerate lithium (AAP: Committee on Drugs, 2000), and most of these individuals receive anti-convulsant therapy. Our understanding of the effect of anti-convulsant exposure on foetal development is mainly limited to research on pregnant women with epilepsy, who typically receive higher doses of anti-convulsants than patients with BD. Although this group is thought to have increased rates of malformations per se, if epilepsy is removed from the equation the frequency of congenital anomalies still remains increased with anti-convulsant exposure (Altshuler et al., 1996). Due to the risks to the foetus associated with carbamazepine and valproate therapy, these agents are not generally recommended for use in pregnancy, unless other agents are unavailable (Misri & Lusskin, 2004; Yonkers et al., 2004; and see Chapter 9).

Valproate

Foetal and neonatal effects

One of the primary concerns of valproate use in pregnancy is the 1–5% risk of neural tube defects (NTDs), particularly lumbosacral meningomyelocele (Altshuler et al., 1996; Kennedy & Koren, 1998). This risk is considered dose-related and coincides with the impact of drug exposure on days 17–30 (Yonkers et al., 2004). Notably, valproate reduces folate levels (Altshuler et al., 1996). Folic acid before as well as during pregnancy is recommended, as closure of the neural tube occurs on days 26–27 (Wild et al., 1997). Although folate supplementation is effective in lowering the risk of NTD in the general community, it has not been systematically assessed in women taking anticonvulsants (Yonkers et al., 2004). Advice on the amount of folic acid which should be administered to these patients varies. Crawford et al. (1999) recommend 5 mg/day for epileptic women taking anticonvulsants, beginning prior to conception and until the completion of trimester one as a minimum. The AAP refers to women using this drug in pregnancy for its psychoactive properties, and suggests using 4 mg/day before pregnancy and 400 μg when not trying to conceive (AAP: Committee on Drugs, 2000). Measuring vitamin B_{12} levels prior to folate administration is advised to rule out pernicious anaemia (Yonkers et al., 2004). Prenatal testing for NTDs includes maternal serum α-fetoprotein, targeted ultrasound and amniocentesis for α-fetoprotein levels.

DiLiberti et al. (1984) coined the term "foetal valproate syndrome" to describe the pattern of malformation of the "anticonvulsant face"; however, it is unclear whether intrauterine growth retardation and mental retardation form part of this syndrome

(Yonkers et al., 2004). Neonatal toxicity (heart rate decelerations) and symptoms of withdrawal (irritability, jitteriness, abnormal tone and feeding problems) have been described from valproate administration in pregnant women with epilepsy (Jager-Roman, 1986; Thisted & Ebbesen, 1993). Hepatotoxicity, hypoglycaemia and reduced neonatal fibrinogen have also been reported, as has transient neonatal hyperglycinemia (Kennedy & Koren, 1998; Majer & Green, 1987; Thisted & Ebbesen, 1993). Intrauterine growth retardation, hyperbilirubinemia, skeletal dysplasia and foetal/neonatal distress have also been linked to valproic acid (AAP: Committee on Drugs, 2000). Valproate has a Food and Drug Administration (FDA) warning against use in children below the age of two years (Yonkers et al., 2004).

Therapy during pregnancy and delivery

Intensive monitoring of serum levels is required as levels can change over the course of the pregnancy. Experts also warn against drug dosing once per day, as this regime can result in unpredictably high peak concentrations (Yonkers et al., 2004).

Carbamazepine

Foetal and neonatal effects

Carbamazepine, like many other psychotropic agents, crosses the placenta, and foetal serum levels have been reported as 50–80% of maternal levels (Nau et al., 1982). Carbamazepine use in pregnancy carries a risk of NTDs reported as 0.5–1.0% after trimester one exposure, compared to a population rate of 0.03% (Altshuler et al., 1996; Heinonen et al., 1997; Rosa, 1991). Therefore, as with valproate, folate is advised for women taking carbamazepine. A form of facial malformation from exposure to carbamazepine (or valproate) termed the "anticonvulsant face" can also occur, with mid-face hypoplasia, small nose, anteverted nostrils and a long upper lip (Jones et al., 1989; Yonkers et al., 2004). A two-fold greater rate of major congenital anomalies and lower birth weight of about 250 g with trimester one carbamazepine exposure has been reported (Diav-Citrin et al., 2001). A lower mean head circumference has been described (Hiilesmaa et al., 1981), as have craniofacial defects, fingernail hypoplasia and developmental delay (Jones et al., 1989). Carbamazepine exposure also increases the risk of microencephaly (Viguera et al., 2002a). Neurobehavioral effects were not documented in a follow-up study (to 18–36 months) of 36 mother–infant pairs exposed in utero to carbamazepine monotherapy (Scolnick, 1994).

Therapy during pregnancy and delivery

Clinicians treating women on carbamazepine during pregnancy must be aware that this agent can result in foetal vitamin K deficiency. This can affect midface development and lower levels of vitamin K dependent clotting factors (Leibenluft, 1997;

Yonkers et al., 2004), risking neonatal bleeding including intracerebral haemorrhage (AAP: Committee on Drugs, 2000). The AAP advises maternal treatment with 10–20 mg/day oral vitamin K for the final month of pregnancy (AAP: Committee on Drugs, 2000) and neonates should receive 1 mg intramuscular vitamin K (Yonkers et al., 2004). Measuring unbound drug levels is also recommended when monitoring carbamazepine use in pregnancy (Yonkers et al., 2004).

It is also important to note that the contraceptive efficacy of the oral contraceptive pill (OCP) can by effected by medications used to treat BD. Carbamazepine is known to induce cytochrome p450, lowering levels of the OCP (Arnold, 2003; Leibenluft, 1996).

Lamotrigine

Foetal and neonatal effects

Data on newer anticonvulsants is emerging, and lamotrigine is now a first line treatment in epileptic women of reproductive age. The Lamotrigine Pregnancy Register (GlaxoSmithKline) as of September 30, 2003, reported a 2% estimated rate of major malformations from lamotrigine monotherapy, which was comparable to general population rates. Greater malformation rates were described with polytherapy, particular with valproic acid (Yonkers et al., 2004). Information on intrauterine growth with lamotrigine exposure in utero has not been described and in a study of development at 1 year, no abnormalities were reported (Mackay et al., 1997). Experts warn about hepatotoxicity which has occurred in adults receiving lamotrigine, and about skin rashes (Yonkers et al., 2004).

Therapy during pregnancy and delivery

A small study of epileptic women reported lamotrigine clearance increased by over 50% during pregnancy and rapidly decreased in the postpartum to preconception levels (Tran et al., 2002). Ohman et al. (2000) reported that maternal lamotrigine levels increased significantly in the early postpartum period, most likely a consequence of changes to drug clearance after delivery. Changing lamotrigine clearance highlights the importance of monitoring drug levels and dosing over pregnancy and the postpartum, particularly immediately postpartum (see also Chapter 9).

Topiramate

Topiramate may impact upon the contraceptive efficacy of the OCP by reducing OCP ethinyl oestradiol levels, but as a new anticonvulsant such information is very limited (Rosenfeld et al., 1997). Ohman et al. (2002) studied topiramate levels in five mother–infant pairs in women with epilepsy (who all concommittently received either valproic acid or carbamazepine). No malformations were reported, though one woman delivered preterm at 36 weeks. The study also found that top-iramate crosses the placenta in significant amounts.

Anti-psychotics

First-generation anti-psychotics

Foetal and neonatal effects

A study of pregnant women with psychosis compared those administered or not administered chlorpromazine during pregnancy. The rates of foetal malformation were similar between groups but about double that of the general population; thus, non-pharmacological factors may have contributed to the higher rates (Sobel, 1960; Yonkers et al., 2004). A meta-analysis reported that amongst non-psychotic women administered low-potency phenothiazines in the first trimester, offspring had a 0.4% increased risk of congenital anomalies (Altshuler et al., 1996). Neonatal toxicity has been described in the context of both withdrawal and extra-pyramidal symptoms with conventional anti-psychotics, but it is unclear whether this is due to the disease or to anti-cholinergic or anti-histaminergic properties of these agents. Neurobehavioral effects have not been reported (Yonkers et al., 2004).

Therapy during pregnancy and delivery

First generation anti-psychotics have several applications in pregnant women with BD. Firstly, they are used in acute manic episodes. Secondly, some advocate their use instead of lithium or anticonvulsants in pregnancy/trimester one, because they confer a lower foetal risk. Thirdly, they may be chosen for women who are unmedicated during their pregnancy and become symptomatic (Yonkers et al., 2004). High potency anti-psychotics are recommended by the AAP, as they "minimize maternal anti-cholinergic, hypotensive and antihistamineric effects", and as mentioned, low-potency agents have been associated with an increased risk of malformations. Notably, this AAP advice does not apply to loxapine, mesoridazine, chlorprothixene, molindone or pimozide, due to inadequate data. The AAP also advises against the use of long-acting depot preparations of high-potency agents, to minimize the time of potential infant exposure to toxic drug levels (AAP: Committee on Drugs, 2000).

Second-generation or novel anti-psychotics

Foetal and neonatal effects

Olanzapine is approved for use in acute mania, but little data are available on this agent during pregnancy. The manufacturer's registry collected data prospectively ($N = 23$) and retrospectively ($N = 11$) on pregnant women taking olanzapine. The latter group reported two cases of major malformations, which the authors thought were unlikely to be caused by olanzapine (Goldstein et al., 2000). Whether or not olanzapine can cause neonatal toxicity is unknown. *Quetiapine* was recently approved by the US FDA for use in acute mania but data in pregnancy and the postpartum are currently unavailable, except for a case report with no adverse infant effects (Tenyi et al., 2002). *Risperidone* is another novel anti-psychotic which is used for the treatment of BD, but data on its use in pregnancy are limited to two case reports, for which there were no maternal and neonatal complications, and no developmental abnormalities at 9–12 months (Ratnayake & Libretto, 2002). Regarding *clozapine*, there are a few case reports with no major malformations reported, and the manufacturer's registry notes that of 28 babies exposed to clozapine in utero, 25 were healthy and 4 had complications. White cell counts are required in infants of mothers of clozapine, as agranulocytosis can occur in adult patients receiving this medication (Patton et al., 2002).

Therapy during pregnancy and delivery

Experts recommend close monitoring of blood pressure, blood sugar levels and weight increases in pregnant women taking olanzapine, because data have linked olanzapine with weight gain, insulin resistance, gestational diabetes and preeclampsia (Yonkers et al., 2004). It is important to note that the prolactin-sparing qualities of some novel anti-psychotics can mean an increased risk of conception when changing between an older agent and a prolactin-sparing anti-psychotic (Gregoire & Pearson, 2002).

Benzodiazepines

Benzodiazepines (BDPs) are not primary agents for the treatment of BD but are used to help alleviate associated symptoms such as anxiety, agitation and sleeping difficulties (Yonkers et al., 2004). Pregnant women may also be exposed to BDPs when they are required for medical reasons, such as preterm labor.

Foetal and neonatal effects

Whilst teratogenic effects have not been described for lorazepam or clonazepam (which are most often used in BD), it is unclear whether or not BDPs cause cleft lip/palate (Yonkers et al., 2004; and see Chapter 9). Many women become pregnant on BDPs since pregnancies are not always planned. Therefore, it is very important to advise women on BDPs with regard to the safety of these agents. In a review by Dolovich et al. (1998) of over 14,000 studies, it appeared that the analysis of cohort studies reported no increased risk of major malformations or oral cleft with trimester one maternal BDP use. However, case-control studies showed a small increased risk of the development of major malformations or oral cleft of with BDP use. It is now recommended that a level two ultrasound be performed when BDPs are used in the first trimester, to exclude visible oral cleft (Dolovich et al., 1998) which can be corrected at birth.

Cases of neonatal toxicity from BDP exposure in trimester three or at delivery have been reported; features include low-apgar scores, muscular hypotonicity, failure to feed, apnoea and impaired temperature regulation (Altshuler et al., 1996). Withdrawal symptoms (infant irritability, tremor, vomiting and diarrhoea, hypertonicity and vigorous sucking) have also been reported from chronic maternal BDP use; however, another report of maternal clonazepam use for panic disorder did not report neonatal toxicity (Weinstock, 1996; Yonkers et al., 2004). The risk of long-term developmental delay is unclear, as data are limited and existing studies have produced contradictory results (Altshuler et al., 1996; Yonkers et al., 2004).

Therapy during pregnancy and delivery

In pregnant women, high-potency BDPs may be the best option, because of the shorter half-life, decreased chance of sedation and reduced accumulation (Yonkers et al., 2004).

Electroconvulsive therapy

Once contraindicated in pregnancy, electroconvulsive therapy (ECT) now has an important role in the management of symptomatic pregnant women with BD, particularly for urgent therapy (i.e., when a woman is acutely suicidal or has homicidal thoughts and poses a risk to herself or others). In most cases these women are acutely psychotic. ECT is considered a relatively safe and effective treatment (Altshuler et al., 1996), and should be undertaken by a multidisciplinary team of obstetricians, anaesthetists and psychiatrists. In an examination of 300 reported cases of ECT in pregnancy from 1942 to 1991, complications were described in 28 cases (9.3%). These included mild vaginal bleeding, transient benign foetal dysrhythmias, abdominal pain and a few cases of self-limiting uterine contractions (Miller, 1994). Maternal risks which are infrequently experienced can be minimized in the hands of expert obstetricians and anaesthetists. Risks to the mother and foetus can also be minimized by adequate oxygenation, right hip elevation and avoiding both atropine and hyperventilation (Yonkers et al., 2004).

Postpartum, ECT risks are considered minimal, but breastfeeding is not recommended for several hours after the ECT because of co-administered pharmacotherapy (Rabheru, 2001). There are important ethical issues when ECT is used in pregnant patients, as obtaining informed consent for a women and her unborn child can be difficult if a patient's mental state is adversely affected or impacts upon her understanding of the situation. Furthermore, the attending physician is treating two patients and must consider the health of both the mother and the unborn child (Miller, 1994).

Psychosocial therapies

Pharmacotherapy is the mainstay of treatment for BD. However, the chronicity and adverse effect of BD on function mean that psychosocial therapies have an important role to play in improving outcomes for patients with BD and their families. Although not studied extensively, individual and/or group cognitive behavioural therapy may have a role in patients with BD for improving compliance, increasing function and quality of life, improved early detection of symptoms and reduced relapse and depressive symptoms (Patelis-Siotis, 2001). Limited research has been undertaken on the effect of psychosocial therapies on families and partners of individuals with BD. In a study of patients with a major affective disorder or BD married about 17 years, those who had psychoeducational marital intervention had improvements in compliance and overall function (but not symptoms), as compared with individuals receiving medication only (Clarkin et al., 1998).

Management of BD in the postpartum period

The postpartum period is a time of physiological and hormonal change, as well as the stressors of a newborn child such as disrupted sleep and shifting family dynamics. Common psychological conditions associated with this period include the postpartum "blues", puerperal depression (1 in 10) and puerperal psychosis (1–2 per 1000) (Chamberlain & Steer, 1999; Kendell et al., 1987). The reader is also referred to Chapter 8 for an overview of postpartum mood disorders.

Postpartum psychosis

"A 30 year old woman delivered 6 days ago of her 4th infant was suddenly seized by a "délire furieux". The first sign was that she wanted to put her baby (whom she was suckling) in a stove to cook him. The family managed to stop her, but only against her vociferous and violent resistance. When the doctor arrived it required 4 men to restrain her. She didn't recognize anyone and repeated the same words in a violent voice. She was treated with ether and immediately fell asleep for two hours. When she awoke she was in a rational frame of mind, though tired, and remembered nothing of the incident. She resumed her normal life two days later. Some years later (unrelated to childbirth) she had a similar attack."

Louis Marcé, 1858 (Brockington et al., 1982, p. 40–41)

Puerperal psychosis is a medical conundrum that physicians have been trying to solve for centuries. Whilst the mainstay of treatment in developed nations today lies in the realm of pharmacology, the "magic bullet" for the prevention of this condition remains elusive. Postpartum psychosis is considered a clinical emergency, potential sequelae including infanticide and maternal suicide (American Psychiatric Association, 2000; Appleby et al., 1998). Onset occurs within two weeks of delivery in over two-thirds of cases, and patients can manifest symptoms of a manic, depressed or mixed state (Chaudron & Pies, 2003).

There has been significant debate about whether postpartum psychosis is a distinct psychiatric condition or a time- and situation-specific expression of BD, for which the trigger is childbirth (see also Chapter 8). In a review of the relationship between BD and postpartum psychosis, Chaudron and Pies (2003, p. 1286) commented that "*postpartum psychosis is not a discrete nosologic entity, but a postpartum presentation of an underlying mood disorder. In many, if not most cases, this underlying disorder appears to be within the bipolar spectrum*". Comparatively, DSM-IV-TR refers to a postpartum onset specifier for mood disorders (major depressive, manic or mixed episode of major depressive disorder, bipolar I or II disorder, or brief psychotic disorder) which can occur in the presence/absence of psychotic features. DSM-IV-TR also defines postpartum onset as within four weeks of delivery, whilst others extend this time period (American Psychiatric Association, 2000; Kendell et al., 1987; Videbech & Gouliaev, 1995).

There are strong links between BD and puerperal psychosis, therefore clinicians should maintain a high index of suspicion for BD in patients presenting with puerperal depression or mania, especially in cases with psychotic symptoms. Red flags include a family history of BD or puerperal psychosis, a past history of misdiagnosed or missed mood episodes and past mania or hypomania. (Chaudron & Pies, 2003)

Treatment of postpartum psychosis

The acute treatment of postpartum psychosis typically involves hospital admission and anti-psychotic medication. Due to the association between BD and postpartum psychosis, experts recommend administering mood stabilizers with anti-psychotics and the careful use of antidepressants because of the risk rapid of cycling (Chaudron & Pies, 2003). The potential side effects of these medications are outlined below.

The use of ECT in patients with acute postpartum psychosis is recommended in situations as previously discussed. ECT was shown in a preliminary study to be effective in women with puerperal psychosis (Reed et al., 1999). Long-term follow-up of new cases of BD is also required, and information about seeking preconception counselling with future pregnancies should be supplied.

Breastfeeding and medication

For women with BD, the decision whether or not to breastfeed is complex (see also Chapter 9). The health benefits of breastfeeding for both mother and child are well documented and publicly promoted. However, prophylactic or therapeutic mood stabilization may be recommended during this high risk period, and all these agents pass into the breastmilk and infant serum in varying amounts.

Numerous factors may influence a women's decision whether or not to breastfeed. These include previous puerperal episodes, a family history of postpartum psychosis, the mother's desire to breastfeed, risks and benefits to the neonate and maternal risks from breastfeeding (e.g., sleep deprivation may trigger a manic episode) (Chaudron, 2000a; Leibenluft, 2000). Providing patients with information about the risks and benefits of breastfeeding and unknown risks such as long-term sequelae is advised (Chaudron & Jefferson, 2000b). In women who choose to breastfeed and require mood stabilization, the principles governing drug administration are similar to those used in pregnancy such as monotherapy where possible, and using the lowest therapeutic dose. Selecting treating agents based on the patient's current condition and past responses to medication is also recommended (Chaudron & Jefferson, 2000b). Viguera et al. (2002a) suggest beginning postpartum prophylaxis with a mood stabilizer 2–4 weeks before parturition to ensure a degree of pharmalogical protection against the onset of the postpartum disorder, but they recognize that no empirical data supports this strategy. Furthermore, as outlined in Chapter 9, exposure of the foetus to lithium in late pregnancy can result in neonatal toxicity.

Lithium

Postpartum lithium prophylaxis has been reported to decrease the relapse rate in women with BD from about 50% to 10%. (Cohen et al., 1995; Stewart et al., 1991) The AAP states that lithium should be administered to breastfeeding women "with caution", as infant blood concentrations 1/3–1/2 therapeutic levels have been reported (AAP: Committee on Drugs, 2001; Schou & Amdisen, 1973). Studies have found breastmilk lithium concentrations about 40% (range 24–72%) and infant levels 5–200% of maternal levels (Chaudron & Jefferson, 2000b). Yonkers et al. (2004) recommend monitoring lithium concentrations and the Certified Breastfeeding Counselor (CBC) of infants with breastfeeding mothers taking lithium, and also warn of the risk of toxicity from rapid dehydration in febrile neonates. The long-term impact of extended lithium exposure has not been determined (Yonkers et al., 2004).

Anti-convulsants

Both valproic acid and carbamazepine are considered "usually compatible with breastfeeding" by the AAP: Committee on Drugs (2001). Notably, most studies on valproate and carbamazepine are very small and typically case reports of epileptic women administered one or more anticonvulsant (Chaudron & Jefferson, 2000b).

Valproate

Valproate levels in breastmilk have been reported as under 1% and up to 10.5% of maternal serum levels, with infant levels varying from undetectable to 40% of maternal levels (Chaudron & Jefferson, 2000b). No adverse effects were reported in two breastfed infants whose mothers received valproate for BD (Wisner & Perel, 1998) whilst a case of thrombocytopenia purpura, anaemia and reticulocytosis has been described in a breastfed 3-month-old infant whose mother received valproic acid for epilepsy; these symptoms resolved with the cessation of breastfeeding (Stahl et al., 1997). Hepatotoxicity has been reported in children less than 24 months receiving valproate directly (not through breastmilk). Whilst it is unclear whether nursing infants are at a similar risk, some authors recommend avoiding its use (Chaudron & Jefferson, 2000b).

Carbamazepine

Low levels of carbamazepine are found in breastmilk (Yonkers et al., 2004), but reports have ranged from 7% to 95% of maternal serum levels (Chaudron & Jefferson, 2000b). Infant serum levels vary from 6% to 65% of maternal concentrations. Notably, in most cases exposure also has occurred in utero (Chaudron & Jefferson, 2000b). Transient hepatotoxicity has been twice reported, one a newborn exposed to transplacental carbamazepine, and the other an infant whose symptoms resolved with the cessation of breastfeeding (Frey et al., 1990; Merlob et al., 1992). There have also been four reports of poor feeding in infants of mothers taking carbamazepine (Chaudron & Jefferson, 2000b).

Lamotrigine

Like other psychoactive agents, lamotrigine crosses into the breastmilk. Ohman et al. (2000) studied nine women with epilepsy treated with lamotrigine, who breastfed their ten children. At birth the umbilical cord blood/maternal lamotrigine ratio was a median 0.9 (range 0.6–1.3), which gradually decreased with time. At 2–3 weeks after birth the median milk/maternal plasma concentration ratio was 0.61. Infant plasma levels varied from 23% to 50% (median 30%) of maternal plasma levels, and adverse effects were not reported. The AAP classifies lamotrigine as an agent of unknown effect which may be of concern because of potentially therapeutic serum levels in infants (AAP: Committee on Drugs, 2001). Careful monitoring of infants for rashes is advised, as children receiving lamotrigine for epilepsy are at a heightened risk of life-threatening skin reactions (Chaudron & Jefferson, 2000b).

Topiramate

In a study of five mother–infant pairs in women with epilepsy taking topiramate (who all concommittently received either valproic acid or carbamazepine), three of the pairs were breastfed. Topiramate was found to be excreted into the breastmilk in large amounts, the milk/maternal plasma topiramate concentration ratio being high. Infant levels were about 10–20% maternal serum levels, and adverse effects were not reported in the infants (Ohman et al., 2002). However, there are very little data on this agent.

Anti-psychotics

First-generation anti-psychotics

The AAP classifies numerous anti-psychotics (including chlorprozamine, chlor-prothixene, haloperidol, mesoridazine and trifluoperazine) as having an "unknown" effect but which may be of concern in breastfed infants. The AAP also mentions the possible effect of decline in developmental scores with exposure to haloperidol and chlorprozamine through breastfeeding, and the potential for infant lethargy and drowsiness and maternal galactorrhoea with chlorprozamine (AAP: Committee on Drugs, 2001). A few case reports have been published describing exposure to anti-psychotic agents through nursing, with minimal adverse events (Yonkers et al., 2004).

Second-generation or novel anti-psychotics

The side-effect profile of atypical antipsychotics means they are often favoured in clinical practice. Information on these drugs in lactating women is scant, being limited to case reports. According to the AAP, clozapine has an unknown effect but may be of concern in breastfed infants (AAP: Committee on Drugs, 2001). In a study of seven breastfeeding women taking olanzapine, a relative infant dose of about 1% was reported, with undetectable plasma levels in six of the seven infants; no infant adverse effects were found (Gardiner et al., 2003). A few other reported cases also describe no infant adverse effects caused by olanzapine exposure during breastfeeding (Goldstein et al., 2000; Kirchheiner et al., 2000). There is even less information on risperidone. In a study of two breastfed infants whose mothers took risperidone, the maternal milk/plasma concentration ratio was $\leqslant 0.5$, the relative infant dose ranged from 2.3% to 4.7% of the maternal weight-adjusted dose; the drug was undetectable in the infant serum and no adverse effects were described (Ilett et al., 2004). Although these very limited data suggests olanzapine, risperidone and clozapine may be used in nursing women, the nursing infant should be monitored for any adverse effects.

BDPs

The primary role of BDPs in the postpartum period is alleviation of anxiety, agitation, panic and sleeping difficulties. Adverse effects of lorazepam and clonazepam use have not been reported, but diazepam was linked with neonatal sedation in one case report (Yonkers et al., 2004). The AAP classifies diazepam, lorazepam, midazolam, temazepam and several other anxiolytics as having an unknown effect on breastfed infants, but which may be of concern, particularly if administered for extended periods (AAP: Committee on Drugs, 2001).

Conclusions

The reproductive lifecycle of a woman with BD is dynamic. There are mental health concerns that arise with each phase – whether mania or depression. Physicians require a flexible outlook and a keen awareness of the issues pertinent to each stage, so that their therapeutic approach can shift as their patients transition each phase. During the childbearing era, women with BD face specific risks, particularly illness exacerbation. For some individuals, this period may be their first presentation of the disorder.

1 BD affects women during their child-bearing years, therefore has implications for both the mother and baby given the chronic and disruptive nature of the illness.

2 Pregnancy planning, postpartum prophylaxis and intensive monitoring by a team of psychiatrists, obstetricians and paediatricians is recommended in the treatment of patients with BD in pregnancy and the postpartum.

3 Each case must be individually analysed from a risk/benefit perspective and management planned accordingly.

4 Pharmacotherapy is challenging but with proper preconception counselling and ongoing monitoring during pregnancy and the postpartum, the risks to the mother and baby can be minimized.

REFERENCES

Altshuler, L.L., Cohen, L., Szuba, M.P., Burt, V.K., Gitlin, M., & Mintz, J. (1996). Pharmacologic management of psychiatric illness during pregnancy: Dilemmas and guidelines. *American Journal of Psychiatry, 153*, 592–606.

American Academy of Neurology. (1998). Practice parameter: Management issues for women with epilepsy (summary statement). Report of the Quality Standards Subcommittee of the American Academy of Neurology. *Neurology, 51*, 944–948.

American Academy of Pediatrics. Committee on Drugs (2000). Use of psychoactive medication during pregnancy and possible effects on the fetus and newborn. *Pediatrics, 105*, 880–887.

American Psychiatric Association. (2000). *Diagnostic and statistical manual of mental disorders, 4th edn, Text revision*, Washington, DC: American Psychiatric Association.

Appleby, L., Mortensen, P.B., & Faragher, E.B. (1998). Suicide and other causes of mortality after post-partum psychiatric admission. *British Journal of Psychiatry, 173*, 209–211.

Arnold, L.M. (2003). Gender differences in bipolar disorder. *Psychiatric Clinics of North America, 26*, 595–620.

Blazer, D.G., Kessler, R.C., McGonagle, K.A., & Swartz, M.S. (1994). The prevalence and distribution of major depression in a national community sample: The National Comorbidity Survey. *American Journal of Psychiatry, 151*, 979–986.

Blehar, M.C., DePaulo Jr., J.R., Gershon, E.S., Reich, T., Simpson, S.G., & Nurnberger Jr., J.I. (1998). Women with bipolar disorder: Findings from the NIMH genetics initiative sample. *Psychopharmacology Bulletin, 34,* 239–243.

Brockington, I. (2004). Postpartum psychiatric disorders. *Lancet, 363,* 303–310.

Brockington, I., Winokur, G., & Dean, C. (1982). Puerperal psychosis. In: I.F. Brockington, & R. Kumar (Eds.), *Motherhood and mental illness.* New York: Grune and Stratton Inc.

Burt, V.K., & Rasgon, N. (2004). Special considerations in treating bipolar disorder in women. *Bipolar Disorders, 6,* 2–13.

Cassidy, F., Ahearn, E.P., & Carroll, B.J. (2001). Substance abuse in bipolar disorder. *Bipolar Disorders, 3,* 181–188.

Chamberlain, G., & Steer, P. (1999). ABC of labour care: Obstetric emergencies. *British Medical Journal, 318,* 1342–1345.

Chaudron, L.H. (2000a). When and how to use mood stabilizers during breastfeeding. *Primary. Care Update Obstetrics and Gynaecologists, 7,* 113–117.

Chaudron, L.H., & Jefferson, J.W. (2000b). Mood stabilizers during breastfeeding: A review. *Journal of Clinical Psychiatry, 61,* 79–90.

Chaudron, L.H., & Pies, R.W. (2003). The relationship between postpartum psychosis and bipolar disorder: A review. *Journal of Clinical Psychiatry, 64,* 1284–1292.

Clarkin, J.F., Carpenter, D., Hull, J., Wilner, P., & Glick, I. (1998). Effects of psychoeducational intervention for married patients with bipolar disorder and their spouses. *Psychiatric Services, 49,* 531–553.

Cohen, L.S., Rosenbaum, J.F., & Heller, V.L. (1991). Psychotrophic drug use in pregnancy. In: A.J. Gelenberg, E.L. Bassuk, & S.C. Schoonover (Eds.), *The practitioner's guide to psychoactive drugs* (pp. 389–405). New York: Plenum Medical Book Co.

Cohen, L.S., Friedman, J.M., Jefferson, J.W., Johnson, E.M., & Weiner, M.L. (1994). A reevaluation of risk of in utero exposure to lithium. *Journal of the American Medical Association, 271,* 146–150.

Cohen, L.S., Sichel, D.A., Robertson, L.M., Heckscher, E., & Rosenbaum, J.F. (1995). Postpartum prophylaxis for women with bipolar disorder. *American Journal of Psychiatry, 152,* 1641–1645.

Crawford, P., Appleton, R., Betts, T., Duncan, J., Guthrie, E., & Morrow, J. (1999). Best practice guidelines for the management of women with epilepsy. The women with epilepsy guidelines development group. *Seizure, 8,* 201–217.

Diav-Citrin, O., Shechtman, S., Arnon, J., & Ornoy, A. (2001). Is carbamazepine teratogenic? A prospective controlled study of 210 pregnancies. *Neurology, 57,* 321–324.

DiLiberti, J.H., Farndon, P.A., Dennis, N.R., & Curry, C.J. (1984). The fetal valproate syndrome. *American Journal of Medical Genetics, 19,* 473–481.

D'Mello, D.A., McNeil, J.A., & Msibi, B. (1995). Seasons and bipolar disorder. *Annals of Clinical Psychiatry, 7*(1), 11–18.

Dolovich, L.R., Addis, A., Vaillancourt, J.M., Power, J.D., Koren, G., & Einarson, T.R. (1998). Benzodiazepine use in pregnancy and major malformations or oral cleft: Meta-analysis of cohort and case-control studies. *British Medical Journal, 317,* 839–843.

Elmslie, J.L., Silverstone, J.T., Mann, J.I., Williams, S.M., & Romans, S.E. (2000). Prevalence of overweight and obesity in bipolar patients. *Journal of Clinical Psychiatry, 61,* 179–184.

Faedda, G.L., Tondo, L., Teicher, M.H., Baldessarini, R.J., Gelbard, H.A., & Floris, G.F. (1993). Seasonal mood disorders. Patterns of seasonal recurrences in mania and depression. *Archives of General Psychiatry*, *50*(1), 17–23.

Finnerty, M., Levin, Z., & Miller, L.J. (1996). Acute manic episodes in pregnancy. *American Journal of Psychiatry*, *153*, 261–263.

Frank, E., Cyranowski, J.M., Rucci, P., Shear, M.K., Fagiolini, A., Thase, M.E., Cassano, G.B., Grochocinski, V.J., Kostelnik, B., & Kupfer, D.J. (2002). Clinical significance of lifetime panic spectrum symptoms in the treatment of patients with bipolar I disorder. *Archives of General Psychiatry*, *59*, 905–911.

Freeman, M.P., Smith, K.W., Freeman, S.A., McElroy, S.L., Kmetz, G.E., Wright, R., & Keck Jr., P.E. (2002). The impact of reproductive events on the course of bipolar disorder in women. *Journal of Clinical Psychiatry*, *63*, 284–287.

Frey, B., Schubiger, G., & Musy, J.P. (1990). Transient cholestatic hepatitis in a neonate associated with carbamazepine exposure during pregnancy and breast-feeding. *European Journal of Pediatrics*, *150*, 136–138.

Frye, M.A., Altshuler, L.L., McElroy, S.L., Suppes, T., Keck, P.E., Denicoff, K., Nolen, W.A., Kupka, R., Leverich, G.S., Pollio, C., Grunze, H., Walden, J., & Post, R.M. (2003). Gender differences in prevalence, risk, and clinical correlates of alcoholism comorbidity in bipolar disorder. *American Journal of Psychiatry*, *160*, 883–889.

Gardiner, S.J., Kristensen, J.H., Begg, E.J., Hackett, L.P., Wilson, D.A., Ilett, K.F., Kohan, R., & Rampono, J. (2003). Transfer of olanzapine into breast milk, calculation of infant drug dose, and effect on breast-fed infants. *American Journal of Psychiatry*, *160*, 1428–1431.

Goldstein, D.J., Corbin, L.A., & Fung, M.C. (2000). Olanzapine-exposed pregnancies and lactation: Early experience. *Journal of Clinical Psychopharmacology*, *20*, 399–403.

Goodwin, F.D., & Jamison, K.R. (1990). *Manic-depressive illness* (3pp.), New York: Oxford University Press.

Gregoire, A., & Pearson, S. (2002). Risk of pregnancy when changing to atypical antipsychotics. *British Journal of Psychiatry*, *180*, 83–84.

Grof, P., Robbins, W., Alda, M., Berghoefer, A., Vojtechovsky, M., Nilsson, A., & Robertson, C. (2000). Protective effect of pregnancy in women with lithium-responsive bipolar disorder. *Journal of Affective Disorders*, *61*, 31–39.

Heinonen, O.P., Slone, D., & Shapiro, S. (1997). *Birth defects and drugs in pregnancy* (447 pp.), Littleton, MA: Publishing Services Group.

Hendrick, V., Altshuler, L.L., Gitlin, M.J., Delrahim, S., & Hammen, C. (2000). Gender and bipolar illness. *Journal of Clinical Psychiatry*, *61*, 393–396.

Henry, C. (2002). Lithium side-effects and predictors of hypothyroidism in patients with bipolar disorder: Sex differences. *Journal of Psychiatry and Neuroscience*, *27*, 104–107.

Hiilesmaa, V.K., Teramo, K., Granstrom, M.L., & Bardy, A.H. (1981). Fetal head growth retardation associated with maternal antiepileptic drugs. *Lancet*, *2*, 165–167.

Ilett, K.F., Hackett, L.P., Kristensen, J.H., Vaddadi, K.S., Gardiner, S.J., & Begg, E.J. (2004). Transfer of risperidone and 9-hydroxyrisperidone into human milk. *Annals of Pharmacotherapy*, *38*, 273–276.

Isojarvi, J.I., Laatikainen, T.J., Pakarinen, A.J., Juntunen, K.T., & Myllyla, V.V. (1993). Polycystic ovaries and hyperandrogenism in women taking valproate for epilepsy. *New England Journal of Medicine, 329*, 1383–1388.

Isojarvi, J.I., Laatikainen, T.J., Knip, M., Pakarinen, A.J., Juntunen, K.T., & Myllyla, V.V. (1996). Obesity and endocrine disorders in women taking valproate for epilepsy. *Annals of Neurology, 39*(5), 579–584.

Jacobson, S.J., Jones, K., Johnson, K., Ceolin, L., Kaur, P., Sahn, D., Donnenfeld, A.E., Rieder, M., Santelli, R., Smythe, J., et al. (1992). Prospective multicentre study of pregnancy outcome after lithium exposure during first trimester. *Lancet, 339*, 530–533.

Jager-Roman, E. (1986). Fetal growth, major malformations, and minor anomalies in infants born to women receiving valproic acid. *Journal of Pediatrics, 108*, 997–1004.

Johnston, A.M., & Eagles, J.M. (1999). Lithium-associated clinical hypothyroidism. Prevalence and risk factors. *British Journal of Psychiatry, 175*, 336–339.

Jones, I., & Craddock, N. (2001). Familiality of the puerperal trigger in bipolar disorder: Results of a family study. *American Journal of Psychiatry, 158*, 913–917.

Jones, K.L., Lacro, R.V., Johnson, K.A., & Adams, J. (1989). Pattern of malformations in the children of women treated with carbamazepine during pregnancy. *New England Journal of Medicine, 320*, 1661–1666.

Kendell, R.E., Chalmers, J.C., & Platz, C. (1987). Epidemiology of puerperal psychoses. *British Journal of Psychiatry, 150*, 662–673.

Kennedy, D., & Koren, G. (1998). Valproic acid use in psychiatry: Issues in treating women of reproductive age. *Journal of Psychiatry and Neuroscience, 23*, 223–228.

Kessler, R.C., McGonagle, K.A., Zhao, S., Nelson, C.B., Hughes, M., Eshleman, S., Wittchen, H.U., & Kendler, K.S. (1994). Lifetime and 12-month prevalence of DSM-III-R psychiatric disorders in the United States. Results from the National Comorbidity Survey. *Archives of General Psychiatry, 51*, 8–19.

Kirchheiner, J., Berghofer, A., & Bolk-Weischedel, D. (2000). Healthy outcome under olanzapine treatment in a pregnant woman. *Pharmacopsychiatry, 33*, 78–80.

Lapalme, M., Hodgins, S., & LaRoche, C. (1997). Children of parents with bipolar disorder: A metaanalysis of risk for mental disorders. *Canadian Journal of Psychiatry, 42*, 623–631.

Leibenluft, E. (1996). Women with bipolar illness: Clinical and research issues. *American Journal of Psychiatry, 153*, 163–173.

Leibenluft, E. (1997). Issues in the treatment of women with bipolar illness. *Journal of Clinical Psychiatry, 58*(Suppl 15), 5–11.

Leibenluft, E. (2000). Women and bipolar disorder: An update. *Bulletin of the Menninger Clinic, 64*, 5–17.

Leibenluft, E., Ashman, S.B., Feldman-Naim, S., & Yonkers, K.A. (1999). Lack of relationship between menstrual cycle phase and mood in a sample of women with rapid cycling bipolar disorder. *Biological Psychiatry, 46*, 577–580.

Mackay, F.J., Wilton, L.V., Pearce, G.L., Freemantle, S.N., & Mann, R.D. (1997). Safety of long-term lamotrigine in epilepsy. *Epilepsia, 38*, 881–886.

MacKinnon, D.F., Zandi, P.P., Cooper, J., Potash, J.B., Simpson, S.G., Gershon, E., Nurnberger, J., Reich, T., & DePaulo, J.R. (2002). Comorbid bipolar disorder and panic disorder in families with a high prevalence of bipolar disorder. *American Journal of Psychiatry*, *159*, 30–35.

Majer, R., & Green, P. (1987). Neonatal afibrinogenaemia due to sodium valproate. *Lancet, 2*, 740–741.

McElroy, S.L., Altshuler, L.L., Suppes, T., Keck Jr., P.E., Frye, M.A., Denicoff, K.D., Nolen, W.A., Kupka, R.W., Leverich, G.S., Rochussen, J.R., Rush, A.J., & Post, R.M. (2001). Axis I psychiatric comorbidity and its relationship to historical illness variables in 288 patients with bipolar disorder. *American Journal of Psychiatry*, *158*, 420–426.

Merlob, P., Mor, N., & Litwin, A. (1992). Transient hepatic dysfunction in an infant of an epileptic mother treated with carbamazapine during pregnancy and breastfeeding. *Annals of Pharmacotherapy*, *26*, 1563–1565.

Miller, L.J. (1994). Use of electroconvulsive therapy during pregnancy. *Hospital and Community Psychiatry*, *45*, 444–450.

Misri, S., & Lusskin, S.I. (2004). Postpartum mood disorders. In: B.D. Rose (Ed.), *UpToDate. Version 11.3.* MA: Wellesly.

Mizrahi, E.M., Hobbs, J.F., & Goldsmith, D.I. (1979). Nephrogenic diabetes insipidus in transplacental lithium intoxication. *Journal of Pediatrics*, *94*, 493–495.

Mortensen, P.B., Pedersen, C.B., Melbye, M., Mors, O., & Ewald, H. (2003). Individual and familial risk factors for bipolar affective disorders in Denmark. *Archives of General Psychiatry*, *60*, 1209–1215.

Nars, P.W., & Girard, J. (1997). Lithium carbonate intake during pregnancy leading to large goiter in a premature infant. *American Journal of Diseases of Children*, *131*, 924–925.

Nau, H., Kuhnz, W., Egger, H., Rating, D., & Hedge, H. (1982). Anticonvulsants during pregnancy and lactation: Transplacental, maternal and neonatal pharmacokinetics. *Clinical Pharmacokinetics*, *6*, 508–543.

Ohman, I., Vitols, S., & Tomson, T. (2000). Lamotrigine in pregnancy: Pharmacokinetics during delivery, in the neonate, and during lactation. *Epilepsia*, *41*, 709–713.

Ohman, I., Vitols, S., Luef, G., Soderfeldt, B., & Tomson, T. (2002). Topiramate kinetics during delivery, lactation, and in the neonate: Preliminary observations. *Epilepsia*, *43*, 1157–1160.

Overpeck, M.D., Brenner, R.A., Trumble, A.C., Trifiletti, L.B., & Berendes, H.W. (1998). Risk factors for infant homicide in the United States. *New England Journal of Medicine*, *339*, 1211–1216.

Patelis-Siotis, I. (2001). Cognitive-behavioral therapy: Applications for the management of bipolar disorder. *Bipolar Disorders*, *3*, 1–10.

Patton, S.W., Misri, S., Corral, M.R., Perry, K.F., & Kuan, A.J. (2002). Antipsychotic medication during pregnancy and lactation in women with schizophrenia: Evaluating the risk. *Canadian Journal of Psychiatry*, *47*(10), 959–965.

Rabheru, K. (2001). The use of electroconvulsive therapy in special patient populations. *Canadian Journal of Psychiatry*, *46*, 710–719.

Rasgon, N.L., Altshuler, L.L., Gudeman, D., Burt, V.K., Tanavoli, S., Hendrick, V., & Korenman, S. (2000). Medication status and polycystic ovary syndrome in women with bipolar disorder: A preliminary report. *Journal Clinical of Psychiatry*, *61*, 173–178.

Rasgon, N., Bauer, M., Glenn, T., Elman, S., & Whybrow, P.C. (2003). Menstrual cycle related mood changes in women with bipolar disorder. *Bipolar Disorders*, *5*, 48–52.

Ratnayake, T., & Libretto, S.E. (2002). No complications with risperidone treatment before and throughout pregnancy and during the nursing period. *Journal of Clinical Psychiatry*, *63*(1), 76–77.

Redfield Jamison, K. (1995). *An unquiet mind.* New York: Alfred A. Knopf.

Reed, P., Sermin, N., Appleby, L., & Faragher, B. (1999). A comparison of clinical response to electroconvulsive therapy in puerperal and non-puerperal psychoses. *Journal of Affective Disorders*, *54*, 255–260.

Robb, J.C., Young, L.T., Cooke, R.G., & Joffe, R.T. (1998). Gender differences in patients with bipolar disorder influence outcome in the medical outcomes survey (SF-20) subscale scores. *Journal of Affective Disorders*, *49*, 189–193.

Rosa, F. (1991). Spina bifida in infants of women treated with carbamazepine during pregnancy. *New England Journal of Medicine*, *324*, 674–677.

Rosenfeld, W.E., Doose, D.R., Walker, S.A., & Nayak, R.K. (1997). Effect of topiramate on the pharmacokinetics of an oral contraceptive containing norethindrone and ethinyl estradiol in patients with epilepsy. *Epilepsia*, *38*, 317–323.

Schou, M. (1976). What happened later to the lithium babies? A follow-up study on children born without malformations. *Acta Psychiatrica Scandinavica*, *54*, 193–197.

Schou, M., & Amdisen, A. (1973). Lithium and pregnancy, III: Lithium ingestion by children breast-fed by women on lithium treatment. *British Medical Journal*, *2*, 138.

Schou, M., Goldfield, M.D., Weinstein, M.R., & Villeneuve, A. (1973a). Lithium and pregnancy, I: Report from the register of lithium babies. *British Medical Journal*, *2*(5859), 135–136.

Schou, M., Amdisen, A., & Steenstrup, O.R. (1973b). Lithium and pregnancy, II: Hazards to women given lithium during pregnancy and delivery. *British Medical Journal*, *2*, 137–138.

Scolnick, D. (1994). Neurodevelopment of children exposed in utero to phenytoin and carbamazepine monotherapy. *Journal of the American Medical Association*, *271*, 767–770.

Shader, R.I., & Greenblatt, D.J. (1995). More on drugs and pregnancy. *Journal of Clinical Psychopharmacology*, *15*, 1–2.

Sharma, V., & Mazmanian, D. (2003). Sleep loss and postpartum psychosis. *Bipolar Disorders*, *5*, 98–105.

Smoller, J.W., & Finn, C.T. (2003). Family, twin, and adoption studies of bipolar disorder. *American Journal of Medical Genetics*, *123C*, 48–58.

Sobel, D. (1960). Fetal damage due to ECT, insulin coma, chlorpromazine or reserpine. *Archives of General Psychiatry*, *2*, 606–611.

Spinelli, M.G. (2001). A systematic investigation of 16 cases of neonaticide. *American Journal of Psychiatry*, *158*, 811–813.

Stahl, M.M., Neiderud, J., & Vinge, E. (1997). Thrombocytopenic purpura and anemia in a breast-fed infant whose mother was treated with valproic acid. *Journal of Pediatrics*, *130*, 1001–1003.

Stewart, D.E., Klompenhouwer, J.L., & Van Hulst, A.M. (1991). Prophylactic lithium in puerperal psychosis: The experience of three centers. *British Journal of Psychiatry*, *158*, 393–397.

Tenyi, T., Trixler, M., & Keresztes, Z. (2002). Quetiapine and Pregnancy, *American Journal of Psychiatry*, *159*(4), 674.

Thisted, E., & Ebbesen, F. (1993). Malformations, withdrawal manifestations, and hypoglycaemia after exposure to valproate in utero. *Archives of Disease in Childhood*, *69*, 288–291.

Tondo, L., Baldessarini, R.J., Hennen, J., & Floris, G. (1998). Lithium maintenance treatment of depression and mania in bipolar I and bipolar II disorders. *American Journal of Psychiatry, 155,* 638–645.

Tran, T.A., Leppik, I.E., Blesi, K., Sathanandan, S.T., & Remmel, R. (2002). Lamotrigine clearance during pregnancy. *Neurology, 59,* 251–255.

Videbech, P., & Gouliaev, G. (1995). First admission with puerperal psychosis: 7–14 years of follow-up. *Acta Psychiatrica Scandinavica, 91,* 167–173.

Viguera, A.C., Nonacs, R., Cohen, L.S., Tondo, L., Murray, A., & Baldessarini, R.J. (2000). Risk of recurrence of bipolar disorder in pregnant and nonpregnant women after discontinuing lithium maintenance. *American Journal of Psychiatry, 157,* 179–184.

Viguera, A.C., Baldessarini, R.J., & Tondo, L. (2001). Response to lithium maintenance treatment in bipolar disorders: Comparison of women and men. *Bipolar Disorders, 3,* 245–252.

Viguera, A.C., Cohen, L.S., Baldessarini, R.J., & Nonacs, R. (2002a). Managing bipolar disorder during pregnancy: Weighing the risks and benefits. *Canadian Journal of Psychiatry, 47,* 426–436.

Viguera, A.C., Cohen, L.S., Bouffard, S., Whitfield, T.H., & Baldessarini, R.J. (2002b). Reproductive decisions by women with bipolar disorder after prepregnancy psychiatric consultation. *American Journal of Psychiatry, 159,* 2102–2104.

Weinstock, L. (1996). Obstetrical and neonatal outcome following clonazepam use during pregnancy; A case series. *Psychotherapy and Psychosomatics, 70,* 158–162.

Wild, J., Sutcliffe, M., Schorah, C.J., & Levene, M.I. (1997). Prevention of neural-tube defects. *Lancet, 350,* 30–31.

Wisner, K.L., & Perel, J.M. (1998). Serum levels of valproate and carbamazepine in breastfeeding mother–infant pairs. *Journal of Clinical Psychopharmacology, 18,* 167–169.

Yonkers, K.A., Wisner, K.L., Stowe, Z., Leibenluft, E., Cohen, L., Miller, L., Manber, R., Viguera, A., Suppes, T., & Altshuler, L. (2004). Management of bipolar disorder during pregnancy and the postpartum period. *American Journal of Psychiatry, 161,* 608–620.

11

Mood and menopause

Lorraine Dennerstein[1] and Jeanne Leventhal Alexander[2]

[1]Office for Gender and Health, Department of Psychiatry, The University of Melbourne, Parkville, Vic., Australia
[2]Northern California Kaiser Permanente Medical Group Psychiatry Women's Health Program, CA; Department of Psychiatry, Stanford Medical School, Palo Alto, CA; Alexander Foundation for Women's Health, Alexander Foundation, Berkeley, CA, USA

There has been much controversy over the relationship between menopause and depression. Earlier psychiatric terminology had a special term, "involutional melancholia," to refer to depression presenting in women in association with the menopausal years (Burrows & Dennerstein, 1981). These midlife years also coincide with other stressors for women, including their children reaching the developmental stage of independence and leaving home, ill health of elderly parents, health problems for the spouse or for women themselves, confrontation with ageing, the need to re-evaluate life expectations and goals, work stressors, and so on. In addition, it was not clear whether chronologic ageing predisposed women to depression.

Psychological symptoms are frequently reported by mid-aged women (Boulet et al., 1994; Dennerstein et al., 1994b). Mood problems are known to be among the three most common problems reported to specialist menopause clinics (Sarrel & Whitehead, 1985). They are also reported in association with other phases of exogenous and endogenous change in ovarian steroid hormones (see Chapter 7). The greatest sense of well-being has been found to occur during the follicular and ovulatory phases of the menstrual cycle (Dennerstein et al., 1994a). The majority of reproductive-age women report that symptoms of tension and depression increase in the premenstruum (Dennerstein et al., 1988). Some of these women find the symptoms problematic enough to seek medical intervention. A small minority of women (<5%) in the peak reproductive phase experience severe cyclical premenstrual depression and meet criteria for premenstrual dysphoric disorder (American Psychiatric Association, (APA), 1994). Depressive mood changes (and adverse effects on sexual functioning) are reported to be among the most frequent symptoms cited by women for ceasing the oral contraceptive pill (Dennerstein, 1999).

Women presenting for treatment of mood complaints associated with the menstrual cycle are more likely to report adverse mood experience with oral contraceptives

(Dennerstein et al., 1994a). There has also been increasing concern about the high prevalence of minor and major depression in pregnancy and postnatally (Dennerstein et al., 1989). There are associations between premenstrual mood complaints and experience of postnatal depression (Dennerstein et al., 1989) and between premenstrual dysphoric disorder and lifetime experience of depression (APA, 1994). Thus, these findings suggest a strong link between underlying ovarian steroid changes and depression.

This chapter explores how mood problems (depressive symptoms or major depressive disorder) relate to the endocrine changes of the natural menopausal transition (MT). The chapter utilizes soundly conducted epidemiological studies to identify any relationship between depressed mood, menopausal status and hormone levels and to determine the relative importance in the aetiology of mid-aged women's depression of hormonal change, chronologic ageing, health problems and other stressors. The clinical implications are outlined.

Meanings of menopause

Menopause literally means cessation of menstruation. Scientifically, menopause refers to the moment of last menstruation. More recent definitions come from the Stages of Reproductive Ageing Workshop (STRAW; Soules et al., 2001). Natural menopause is recognized to have occurred when there has been 12 consecutive months of amenorrhoea, generally in women over 40 years of age, for which there is no other cause, pathologic or physiologic. The endocrine changes underlying menopause take place over a number of years. This period of time, both before and for the first 12 months after cessation of menses, is often termed the perimenopause or the climacteric. Most women are aware of changes in menstrual flow and frequency for a variable number of years preceding the last menses. The term early MT is used when the mid-aged woman notices changes in her menstrual cycle length. The term late MT is used when there are two or more skipped cycles (corresponding to amenorrhoea lasting between 90 days and 12 months). The term late reproductive phase refers to the phase in which mid-aged women experience regular cycles and have not yet entered the MT; this phase is sometimes referred to as premenopause in the literature. Induced menopause is the cessation of menses that occurs following either surgical removal of both ovaries (with or without hysterectomy) or other iatrogenic ablation of ovarian function (chemotherapy, radiation, etc.). The term postmenopause refers to 12 months or more of amenorrhoea.

The criteria women use to self-define their menopausal status have not been fully elucidated. In a population study of 2000 Australian women between 45 and 55 years of age, a question was asked about where each woman placed herself with regard to menopause (Garamszegi et al., 1998). The responses were the following: lack of any sign; just beginning; in the middle; near the end; or completed. There were discrepancies between women's self-reported menopausal status and menopausal status defined objectively (Garamszegi et al., 1998). Interestingly, self-reported menopausal status (i.e., a woman's own concept of where she is in the MT) was more strongly related to symptom experience scores than was menstrually determined menopausal status (Garamszegi et al., 1998). In a later analysis based on prospectively acquired menstrual diaries in the Melbourne Women's Midlife Health Project, self-rated menopausal status increased the likelihood of the woman reaching final menstrual period in a shorter time interval (Taffe & Dennerstein, 2000). Further research needs to explore the basis women use for determining their menopausal status.

Endocrine changes associated with menopause

The MT is characterized by underlying endocrine changes. Using annually collected hormone measures, the Melbourne Women's Midlife Health Project (MWMHP; Burger et al., 1999) has shown that follicle-stimulating hormone (FSH) levels begin to rise during the early MT. During this phase, oestradiol levels are highly variable and may even increase initially in some women. The rise in FSH seems to be driven by a decrease in the level of inhibin B (Burger et al., 1998) and, to some extent, oestradiol (Burger et al., 1998). Not all cycles will be ovulatory and women report menstrual irregularity. The late MT (characterized by amenorrhoea of 3–11 months' duration in the Melbourne study) coincides with the steepest decline in oestradiol levels and a corresponding steep increase in FSH (Burger et al., 1999). FSH levels stabilize at an elevated level during the early postmenopause, while oestradiol levels stabilize at low levels during the same phase. Women's experience of bothersome hot flashes increases significantly during the late MT (Dennerstein et al., 2000). The MWMHP (Burger et al., 2000) has also shown that total testosterone levels do not significantly change with the MT or over eight years of follow-up. However, the amount of bioavailable testosterone (free testosterone index (FTI)) increased as a result of a corresponding decrease in sex hormone-binding globulin (Burger et al., 2000). Dehydroepiandrosterone sulphate (DHEAS) is not affected by the MT, but shows a steady decline with age (Burger et al., 2000).

While natural menopause appears to have less impact than age on testosterone levels (Burger et al., 2000), bilateral oophorectomy in both the premenopausal and postmenopausal woman leads to an approximately 50% fall in circulating levels of testosterone (Judd et al., 1974). Oestrogen levels also decline significantly with oophorectomy in premenopausal women (Shifren, 2002).

Methodological aspects of studies of depression and menopause

Clinical conclusions regarding the relationship between menopause and mood are based on a small proportion of self-selecting women who may not be representative of most women's experience (Morse et al., 1994). Observational studies of women drawn from general populations provide the opportunity to investigate whether depressed mood symptoms are related directly to the hormonal changes of the MT or to other concurrent factors occurring in midlife. Methodological issues limiting the inferences which can be drawn from published epidemiological studies include those of:

- design (cross-sectional versus longitudinal);
- lack of hormone measures (Bromberger & Matthews, 1996; Greene & Cooke, 1980; Kaufert et al., 1992; McKinley et al., 1987);
- a short length of time of follow-up (Bromberger & Matthews, 1996; Kaufert et al., 1992; Woods & Mitchell, 1997);
- validity of the mood measures used; and
- type of statistical analysis (Lehert & Dennerstein, 2002).

Studies using symptom checklists differ in terms of the method of construction and selection of these lists, number of symptoms, order of symptoms, whether factor analysis or simple categorization is used to obtain sub-scales, cut-point for factor loading, time frame used for recall, and how the study has been presented to the sample (which may lead to expectancy bias). Varying instruments have been used, with the Centre for Epidemiological Studies Depression scale (CES-D) being the most common measure of depressed mood. There are marked differences in age ranges studied, inclusion and exclusion categories (e.g., hormone users are variously identified and included), and whether the sample is clinic or community based.

Most earlier studies did not control for other factors known to affect mood. These include: vasomotor symptoms, sleep disturbance, quality of perceived health, education, financial and other stressors, employment status and perceived social support. Multivariate analysis is needed to take the effect of these factors into account.

Culture/race

Most studies of the effects of the MT have been conducted amongst Caucasian women from Western cultures. The few studies available in non-Western countries are limited, inter alia, by: small sample size; non-standardized measures; and failure to use clear definitions of menopausal status. There is also a problem of use of clinic or other convenience samples which could not be considered representative and limit the generalizability of findings (Boulet et al., 1994; Punyahotra & Dennerstein, 1997a).

One of the few studies conducted outside of Western countries (Boulet et al., 1994) found considerable differences in symptom reporting between Asian countries. Another cross-cultural comparison study reported that rates of nearly every symptom were lower in Japanese than in US and Canadian women of similar ages (Avis et al., 1993). The symptom rate of feeling blue/depressed was highest in the USA. There was a significant interaction between country and menopause status with regard to this symptom. In the Japanese and Canadian women the highest rates of feeling depressed were in the premenopausal women while in the USA, the highest rates were reported in perimenopausal women.

More recent studies such as the USA based Study of Women's Health Across the Nation (SWAN; Avis et al., 2001b) provide an indication of the role of ethnic factors in women's experience of the menopause. Using linear regression and controlling for age, education, health and economic strain, psychosomatic symptoms (tense, depressed, irritable, forgetful, headaches) differed by both race/ethnicity and menopausal status. Caucasian women reported significantly more of these symptoms than did other groups. Chinese and Japanese women reported fewer of the symptoms. Such differences could reflect: differing beliefs and expectations regarding menopause; ageing and the status and roles of women; sensitivity to specific hormones; biological differences (hormone levels, polymorphisms); dietary and lifestyle factors; and health behaviours such as willingness to perceive and/or report symptoms. Across all racial/ethnic groups, the factors of menopausal symptoms (hot flashes and night sweats) and psychological and psychosomatic symptoms nevertheless emerged in symptom checklists (Avis et al., 2001b).

Results of cross-sectional studies

Table 11.1 summarizes the results of cross-sectional studies which have examined for relationship of menopausal status and various measures of mood disturbance. The table includes information on sampling, measure, age group, relationship of mood to menopausal status and hormone levels, and also outlines the major limitations of the studies.

These studies are divided as to whether there is a relationship between menopausal status and depressed mood. Many of the studies report no relationship between mood and menopausal status (Dennerstein et al., 1993, 1994b; Greene & Cooke, 1980; Holte & Mikkelsen, 1982; McKinley et al., 1987; Oldenhave et al., 1993; Pop et al., 1998; Stadberg et al., 2000; Woods & Mitchell, 1997). Some studies do report more psychological or mood symptoms amongst those women in the MT (perimenopausal women) (Avis et al., 2001a; Ballinger, 1975; Bromberger et al., 2001; Hunter et al., 1986; Jaszmann et al., 1969; Punyahotra et al., 1997; Tam et al.,

Table 11.1. Mood and menopausal status. Results of cross-sectional studies

Citation	Size	Admission criteria	Measures	Results	Comments/possible biases
Neugarten and Kraines (1965)	N = 460	Convenience sample. Ages 13–64 years. Excluded: history of major physical illness, disability, or induced menopause.	Blatt Menopausal Index	Decreased psychological and psychosomatic symptoms in women aged >55 years. Self-defined menopausal women did not differ from others aged 45–54 years on psychological symptoms.	Bias due to high educational level; lack of statistical analysis; lack of factor analysis or multivariate analysis. No hormone levels.
Jaszmann et al. (1969)	N = 3000	Survey. Ages 40–60 years.	SCL	More reports of fatigue, headaches, irritability amongst women in MT.	Descriptive analysis only. Insufficient detail. No hormone levels.
Ballinger (1975)	N = 539	Postal survey of 760 women on UK GP practice list. Ages 40–55 years. Response rate = 71%.	GHQ. Cut-off score >11 = case	Significantly more cases in late MT, and women aged 45–49 years.	Simple analysis not controlling for confounding variables. Clinic sample. No hormone levels.
Greene and Cooke (1980)	N = 408	Population sample from electoral role Glasgow. Ages 25–64 years. Response rate = 77%.	SCL	Highest rate of psychological symptoms was in age 35–44 years. Menstrual status did not affect psychological symptom reporting.	Number of women in each age group small. Hierarchical stepwise multiple regression. No hormone levels.
Holte and Mikkelsen (1982)	N = 200	Population sample Norwegian women. Ages 45–55 years.	SCL	Psychological symptoms not explained by menopausal status.	Small sample. No hormone levels.

(*Continued*)

Table 11.1. (*Continued*)

Citation	Size	Admission criteria	Measures	Results	Comments/ possible biases
Hunter et al. (1986)	N = 682	Convenience sample of 850 recruited for ovarian screening. Ages 45–65 years.	Women's Health questionnaire, depressed mood sub-scale	Multiple regression analysis. Menopausal status explained 3% of variance. Depressed mood increased in MT and postmenopausal women.	Convenience sample. No hormone levels.
McKinlay et al. (1987)	N = 2500	Population sample from Massachusetts census lists (N = 8,050). Ages: 45–55 years. Inclusion: menses in prior 3 months; uterus; at least 1 ovary. Followed up for 27 months. But CES-D completed only once.	CES-D	Depression associated with surgical menopause but not the natural MT. Increase (not significantly higher) observed for MT (perimenopausal) but declines again for postmenopausal.	Pooled, cross-sectional analysis. No hormone levels.
Gath et al. (1987)	N = 521	Population sample of 600 women from two Oxford group practices. Response rate = 87%. Ages 35–59 years.	Present State Examination, GHQ	No relationship of psychiatric state to menstrual status.	No multivariate analysis. No hormone levels. Menopausal status defined atypically.
Dennerstein et al. (1993)	N = 2000	Population sample of 2000 Melbourne women by random telephone dialling. Ages 45–55 years. Response rate = 71%.	Dysphoria sub-scale of SCL (2 weeks recall)	ANOVA found dysphoria not affected by menopausal status.	MT not sub-divided. No hormone levels.

Avis et al. (1993)	N = 10,334	Population samples from Manitoba, Massachusetts, Japan. Ages 45–55 years. Response rates = 68–77%.	SCL. Recall 2 weeks	For Japanese and Canadian women, the highest rates of feeling depressed were for premenopausal women. USA women, highest rates were in perimenopausal (MT) women.	No hormone levels. Perimenopause not split into early and late MT.
Oldenhave et al. (1993)	N = 5213	Population sample of Dutch Town. Ages 39–60 years. Response rate = 71% (N = 7256). Excluded: surgical, oral contraceptive users and those not speaking Dutch.	A typical complaints symptom list. Recall = prior month	Menstruating women report more severe "atypical" complaints than non-menstruating women with similarly severe vasomotor symptoms. No clear link to menopausal status.	No multivariate analysis. No hormone levels. No standardized scale.
Boulet et al. (1994)	N = 2992	Convenience samples of mid-aged women in Hong Kong, Korea, Indonesia, Malaysia, Philippines, Singapore, Taiwan.	SCL	Pattern of psychological symptoms with menopausal status varied by country. Indonesian, Korean, Malaysian and Taiwan women had less psychological symptoms in premenopause than in the MT or post. Multivariate analysis related these symptoms to postmenopausal status.	Small samples for each ethnic group. Bias in convenience samples. No hormone levels.
Dennerstein et al. (1994b)	N = 1503	Population sample of 2000 Melbourne women by random telephone dialling. Ages 45–55 years. Response rate = 71%.	Affectometer 2, Recall = 2 weeks	Analysis = ANOVA. No relationship of mood to menopausal status.	No separation of early and late MT. No hormone levels.

(Continued)

Table 11.1. (Continued)

Citation	Size	Admission criteria	Measures	Results	Comments/possible biases
Collins et al. (1995)	N = 1399	Population sample of Stockholm women aged 48 years. Response rate = 70%	SCL	One way ANOVA showed significantly, higher scores for negative moods for postmenopausal women and HT users compared with premenopausal. Multiple regression found negative moods explained by vasomotor symptoms and other factors but not menopausal status.	No hormone levels. One age group. Menopausal status categories not standard. No hormone levels.
Harlow et al. (1995)	N = 688	Population sample of 10,000 Boston women. Ages 45–54 years. Compared 344 who reached menopause before age 40 years with others.	Interview	Medically treated depression associated with early menopause.	Differing age groups. Confounding psychological factors in premature menopause. Case control design.
O'Connor et al. (1995)	N = 381	Population sample of 600 Australian women. Response rate = 83% of those contactable. Ages 45–54 years.	SCL	Postmenopausal women had lowest rate of psychological symptoms, then premenopausal. Higher rates for MT, surgical menopause and HT users.	No hormone levels. Perimenopause not split into early and late MT.
Porter et al. (1996)	N = 6096	Population sample of 8000 Scottish women. Response rate = 78%.	CES-D, SCL recall 6 months	Non-HT users did not differ on psychological symptoms. HT users reported higher levels of	No multivariate analysis. No hormone levels. Perimenopause not split

	N	Sample	Measure	Findings	Comments
		Ages 45–54 years.		psychological symptoms. Surgical menopause and HT users had higher CES-D scores.	into early and late MT.
Cawood and Bancroft (1996)	$N = 141$	Convenience sample of women volunteers. Ages 40–60 years not using HT, must have intact uterus.	SCL. MAACL for prior week. Weekly plasma samples for 4 weeks	No relationship of psychological symptoms to menopausal status. DHEA related to positive affect.	Pooled analysis. Did have four hormone levels.
Punyahotra et al. (1997)	$N = 268$	Convenience sample women accompanying outpatients in Thailand. Ages 40–59 years.	SCL, 2 weeks recall	Depression and tiredness significantly higher prevalence for MT and postmenopausal women. No differences for irritability, nervousness.	No multivariate analysis for depression. No hormone levels.
Woods and Mitchell (1997)	$N = 337$	Population sample, Seattle. Ages 35–55 years. Response rate = 75%. Eligibility: menses in prior year, no HRT, not pregnant, intact uterus and at least 1 ovary.	CES-D, SCL 90	No effect of change in menstrual frequency on depression scores.	Multiethnic sample. Only type of MT analysed was that of change in menstrual frequency.
Kuh et al. (1997)	$N = 1498$	Population sample UK. Response rate = 84% to questionnaire at age 47 years.	SCL for prior 12 months	Logistic regression found that psychological symptoms not significantly related to natural menopausal status. Significantly higher for hysterectomized and HRT users.	No hormone levels. One age only.
Cagnacci et al. (1997)	$N = 1031$	Clinic sample 275 perimenopause (MT) 509 postmenopause	Zung Depression Scale	Depression and anxiety scores lower in MT women than untreated postmenopausal	Bias in sample.

(Continued)

Table 11.1. (*Continued*)

Citation	Size	Admission Criteria	Measures	Results	Comments/possible biases
		247 postmenopause (HT)		women. HT users had lower scores than postmenopausal. Combined E + P lower scores than E.	
Pop et al. (1998)	$N = 583$	Population sample. Ages: 47–57 years living in Eindhoven (78% Response rate to first study).	Edinburgh Depression Scale	No relationship to menopausal status using multiple logistic regression.	No hormone levels.
Tam et al. (1999)	$N = 100$	Convenience clinic sample of 121 Californian women. Ages 45–65 years. Response rate = 21%.	BDI, psychiatric assessment	On ANOVA perimenopausal women had higher BDI scores than pre- or postmenopausal ($p < 0.0001$).	Bias in sample. Early and late MT not separated. Small sample size. No hormone levels.
Zhao et al. (2000)	$N = 806$	Multistage cluster sampling of rural farmers and professional urban women. Ages 41–60 years. Response rate = 95%.	E2, FSH, LH SCL Recall = 1 year	Psychological symptoms (particularly irritability) less frequent in older women (>55) and postmenopausal, and are frequent in perimenopausal women. No relationship between hormone levels and psychological symptoms.	No multivariate analysis of psychological symptoms carried out. Does have hormone levels.
Stadberg et al. (2000)	$N = 5990$	Random sample Goteborg women. Ages 42–62 years. Response rate = 76%.	Visual analogue score well-being	Well-being not associated with menstrual status on stepwise multiple regression.	No hormone levels. No standardized measure of depressed mood analysed.

Study	N	Sample	Measure	Results	Comments
Barentsen et al. (2001)	N = 269	Convenience Dutch sample. Ages 45–65 years.	Green Climacteric Scale	No significant change in depression sub-scale with menopausal status. MT and postmenopausal scored higher than premenopausal on psychological sub-scale.	No hormone levels. Possible bias in sampling. No valid measure of depression.
Bromberger et al. (2001)	N = 16,065	Community sample from seven USA sites. Ages 40–55 years. Over sampling to obtain Caucasian, African-American, Japanese, Chinese and Hispanic samples.	Psychological distress (tense, irritable and depressed in prior 2 weeks)	Higher distress in early MT than pre- or postmenopausal. Caucasian higher odds ratios than other ethnicities.	Multivariate analysis. Did adjust for covariates. No hormones. Distress not a standardized measure. Hormone levels not reported.
Avis et al. (2001b)	N = 14,906	Population samples from Manitoba, Massachusetts, Japan. Ages 45–55 years. Response rates = 68–77%.	SCL and telephone interview	Premenopausal women had significantly less psychosomatic symptoms than MT, surgical menopausal or HRT users. Caucasian women had more psychosomatic symptoms than all other ethnicities.	Validity and clinical meaning of psychosomatic symptoms factor? Hormone levels not reported.
Joffe et al. (2002)	N = 476	Primary care sample, Boston. Ages 40–60 years. Response rate = 55%.	CES-D	Perimenopausal women with vasomotor symptoms more likely to be depressed than postmenopausal or older premenopausal women with vasomotor symptoms.	No hormone levels. Early and late MT not separated.

ANOVA: analysis of variance; BDI: Beck depression inventory; CES-D: Centre for Epidemiological Studies Depression scale; DHEA: Dehydroepiandrosterone; GHQ: general health questionnaire; HT: hormone therapy; HRT: hormone replacement therapy; MAACL: multiple affect adjective checklist; SCL: symptom checklist

1999). Some of these studies did not control for vasomotor symptoms (Ballinger, 1975; Jaszmann et al., 1969). As Avis et al. (2001b) point out, when vasomotor symptoms are included in the model, the relationship with menopausal status attenuates (Avis et al., 1994; Collins & Landgren, 1995).

Study findings are also mixed as to whether any increased risk of depression associated with the MT is related to the early- or late MT. For example, Avis et al. (2001b) found that women who were in the MT, hormone therapy (HT) users and surgical menopause women reported more symptoms than did premenopausal women. The authors did not divide the MT into early and late phases. Interestingly postmenopausal women did not differ from premenopausal women. Jaszmann et al. (1969) associated increased psychological symptoms with change in menstrual pattern (early MT) whereas Ballinger (1975) found more "cases" in those with at least three months amenorrhoea (late MT). Further examples are shown in Table 11.1.

The biological link between menopause and depression is based on the hypothesis that low levels of oestrogen are associated with depressed mood (Bromberger et al., 2001). If this is so then the postmenopause, when oestrogen levels are stable and low, would be expected to be associated with higher levels of depression. Yet with few exceptions, most studies show either no relationship with menopausal status or that perimenopausal women have higher psychological symptom levels. Findings from the SWAN study (Bromberger et al., 2001) suggest that any change in psychological symptoms associated with transiting the menopause may be more likely associated with the phase when gonadal hormones are fluctuating; that is, the early MT. These authors found a 20% higher risk for the presence of psychological symptoms in the two weeks prior to the interview for women in the early MT after adjusting for all other factors. Unfortunately there were no hormone levels published in this paper, although hormone levels have been collected in the SWAN study. The absence of a significant interaction with race/ethnicity in this study indicates that for all women regardless of race, the probability of distress is greater at the start of the MT and is likely to decrease with time. This study was able to identify this effect of the early MT as the study included women aged as young as 40, many of whom were still in the late reproductive phase (premenopause).

Many of the studies listed in Table 11.1 began with women already aged 45, most of whom would have entered the MT. Also, not all studies separated the effect of early and late MT. In an earlier study, Oldenhave et al. (1993) demonstrated that menstruating women had more "atypical" complaints than non-menstruating women whatever the level of vasomotor symptoms. A possible mechanism is suggested by the study of Joffe et al. (2002) who found that perimenopausal (menopausal transition) women with vasomotor symptoms were significantly more likely to be depressed than were older premenopausal or postmenopausal women who suffered from vasomotor symptoms.

Tam et al. (1999), using a small clinical sample, found that perimenopausal women had significantly higher Beck Depression Inventory scores than did pre-menopausal or postmenopausal women. Psychiatric interview found that the most common diagnosis was major depressive disorder, recurrent. Of the 11 perimeno-pausal women diagnosed with major depressive disorder, recurrent, six reported postpartum depressive symptoms lasting longer than two weeks.

A number of studies have found age to be negatively related to psychological symptoms (Avis et al., 2001b; Greene & Cooke, 1980; Neugarten & Kraines, 1965; Zhao et al., 2000).

In those studies which did not exclude surgical menopause, there were reports that women who had undergone surgical menopause had higher levels of depressed mood than premenopausal women (Avis et al., 2001a, b; Kaufert et al., 1992; McKinley et al., 1987). Very few of the cross-sectional studies reported included hormone levels (Zhao et al., 2000). More information on the role of hormonal factors in depressed mood is available from longitudinal studies.

Longitudinal studies

Longitudinal population-based studies that include concomitant measures of mood using validated instruments, menstrual cycle status, psychosocial and life-style factors and hormones are a more powerful and reliable methodology for revealing the proportion of women who will experience depression in relation to underlying endocrine changes and the MT. These rich sources of data can also be used to explore the roles of hormonal change relative to ageing, psychosocial factors, health and lifestyle factors. This in turn can aid clinicians by highlighting risk factors for depression.

Table 11.2 outlines longitudinal studies of psychological parameters in the menopause: again these are divided in finding an association with MT. Thus, some studies (Avis et al., 2001a; Bromberger & Matthews, 1996; Dennerstein et al., 1999, 2000; Hallstrom & Samuelsson, 1985; Matthews et al., 1990; Woods & Mitchell, 1996) reported no association with the MT. For example, using data from the Massachusetts Women's Health Study, Avis et al. (1994) found that onset of natural menopause was not associated with an increased risk of depression. Experiencing a long MT (27 months or more) was, however, associated with an increased risk of depression. This appeared to be explained by increased symptoms rather than menopausal status itself. These authors concluded that any effect of MT on mood appears transitory. The study reported did not include hormone levels. A later study by the same research group in Massachusetts (Avis et al., 2001a) reported a 3-year follow-up involving a smaller sample group who were seen annually and had blood drawn for hormone levels during the follicular phase. Again, depression

Table 11.2. Mood and menopausal status. Results of observational longitudinal studies

Citation	Size	Admission criteria	Measures	Results	Comments/possible biases
Hallstrom and Samuelsson (1985)	$N = 899$	Population sample Gothenberg. Ages 38–54 years, 85% response second interview. 6 years follow-up.	GHQ and interview measure of depressed mood.	Menopause not associated with risk of onset of psychiatric disorder.	One of few studies to use psychiatric interview rather than self-report of symptoms. No hormone levels.
Matthews et al. (1990)	$N = 541$	Population sample Pennsylvania driver's license list. Ages 42–50 years. Inclusion; healthy, menses in prior 3 months. Follow-up 3 years later.	BDI	Scores for pre-post compared with those who stayed pre over 3 years. Found no increase in psychological symptoms with transition to postmenopause.	Short follow-up. Only 13% became postmenopausal. No hormone levels reported.
Hunter (1992)	$N = 36$	Convenience sample. 850 south-east England women at ovarian screening clinic. Inclusion >47 years, premenopausal at outset. Follow-up 3 years. $N = 56$.	Women's Health Questionnaire	Increase in depressed mood (due to greater dysphoria and irritability) with transition from pre to peri/postmenopausal (paired t-test, $p < 0.05$).	Combined MT (irregular menses) and postmenopause. Small sample size, short follow-up, bias in selection (negative attitudes to menopause). No logistic regression including menopausal status with psychosocial variables. No hormone levels.

Study	N	Sample	Measure	Results	Comments
Kaufert et al. (1992)	$N = 469$	Population sample from Manitoba. Ages 45–55 years baseline. Followed for 2½ years. Response rate = 68%. Inclusion: menses in prior 3 months or hysterectomies. Response rate = 87%.	CES-D	No relationship between depression and menopausal status but increased risk of depression for hysterectomized.	Pooled analysis, no hormone levels. No separation of early and late MT. Short follow-up.
Avis et al. (1994)	$N = 2565$	Population sample Massachusetts census. Ages 45–55 years. Inclusion: Menses in prior 3 months, uterus, at least 1 ovary. Response rate at baseline = 77%. Response rate at 3 years = 92%. Analysis based on 27 months follow-up.	CES-D by telephone	Controlling for baseline CES-D, HRT use. Significant effect ($p = 0.03$). OR = 2.05 ($p < 0.05$) for remained in MT for 27 months. Effect of MT not significant if menopausal symptoms included.	Logistic regression. CES-D only given twice. Short follow-up, (27 months). No hormone levels.
Khan et al. (1994)	$N = 46$	Convenience sample recruited from a clinic list. Eligibility: 39–51 years, in good health, not using HT, not postmenopausal or hysterectomized. 560	SCL	Four mood symptoms and breast discomfort improved after menses ceased.	Paired t-test. Scale not validated, small sample size, did not control for confounders, short follow-up and only 46 had reached late MT. No hormone levels.

(Continued)

Table 11.2. (*Continued*)

Citation	Size	Admission criteria	Measures	Results	Comments/ possible biases
		attended, Response rate = 70%. 247 selected for longitudinal study. Follow-up 2–3 years later.			
Bromberger et al. (1996)	N = 460	Population sample – ages 42–50 years from drivers license list. N = 541 (60% participation rate). 98% follow-up 2–3 years.	BDI	Multivariate analysis. Depressive symptoms not related to menopausal status.	Hierarchical linear regression. Short follow-up. No hormone levels included. Compared menstruating with those not menstruating for at least 3 months.
Woods and Mitchell (1996)	N = 347	Population multiethnic sample, Seattle. Ages 35–55 years. 820 eligible, 508 entered, 337 completed 1st year, Eligibility; menses in prior year, no HRT, not pregnant, intact uterus and at least 1 ovary Follow-up = 2 years.	CES-D, SCL 90	Menopausal status did not differentiate women with patterns of depressed mood from others.	Follow-up only 2 years. Discriminant analysis used.
Dennerstein et al. (1997)	N = 405 Follow-up = 4 years	Population sample of Australian-born women. Ages 45–55 years.	Affectometer, FSH, oestradiol, inhibin	Negative mood rose from early in the transition and was highest in the 2 years after FMP after	Pooled analysis. Only 4 years of longitudinal data available so only

Study	N	Sample	Measures	Results	Comments
		Inclusion: menstruating in first 3 months, not taking HRT or oral contraceptives, intact uterus and at least 1 ovary. $N = 438$, 56% of those eligible participated.		adjusting for effects of age and hot flushes. No relationship to hormones E2, FSH, FAI.	10% of observations were postmenopausal.
Dennerstein et al. (1999)	$N = 354$	Population sample Melbourne. Ages 45–55 years. Inclusion: menses in prior 3 months, uterus and ovary, no hormones. $N = 438$, (Response rate $= 56\%$ for participation from baseline). Retention rate for 6 years of follow-up $= 90\%$.	Affectometer 2 FSH, E2, inhibin	MT had indirect effect on depressed mood, amplifying the effect of stressors. No relationship of mood to hormone levels.	Repeated measures multivariate analysis of covariance. Early and late MT combined together for menopausal status analysis.
Dennerstein et al. (2000)	$N = 172$	Population sample Melbourne, $N = 2001$ at baseline. Ages 45–55 years. Inclusion longitudinal: menses in prior 3 months, uterus and ovary, no hormones. $N = 438$ (Response rate $= 56\%$ for participation). Retention rate at year $7 = 89\%$.	SCL, FSH, E2	No significant changes in any psychological symptoms when premenopause + early MT compared to late MT + postmenopause.	By grouping pre and early MT groups this analysis may have missed any increase in symptoms occurring from pre to early MT.

(Continued)

Table 11.2. (*Continued*)

Citation	Size	Admission criteria	Measures	Results	Comments/possible biases
Avis et al. (2001a)	$N = 309$	Population sample Massachusetts. Ages 43–53 years baseline. $N = 427$ (79% Response rate to baseline). Response rate 3 years follow-up = 59%.	CES-D, E2	CES-D not associated with menopausal status, not with log E2, after hot flushes and trouble sleeping adjusted for.	Logistic regression. Short follow-up (27 months). 3 years follow-up completed by only 181 women. Ages of sample during this study not described. Did not look at relationship to early MT.
Maartens et al. (2002)	$N = 2103$	Dutch population. Ages 47–53 years. Excluded HT users and hysterectomized.	Edinburgh Depression Scale	Transition from pre to MT to post, significantly related to higher depression scores.	Multiple logistic regression. 3–5 years follow-up. Attrition of various steps (analysed year 4 of original sample). No hormone levels.
Dennerstein et al. (2002)	$N = 226$	Population sample Melbourne. $N = 2001$ at baseline Ages 45–55 years, Inclusion: menses in prior 3 months, uterus and ovary, no hormones. (56% Response rate for participation). $N = 438$. 88% retention rate after 8 years follow-up.	Affectometer FSH, E2, T, FTI, DHEAS annually	No correlation of positive or negative mood scores with any hormone measures.	Floor effect for T and oestradiol assays.

Woods et al. (2002)	N = 201	Population multiethnic Seattle sample. Ages 35–55 years baseline. 820 eligible, 508 entered. Inclusion: menses in prior year, no HRT, not pregnant, intact uterus & at least 1 ovary. Follow-up = 6 years.	CES-D	Women with resolving depression more likely to be menopausal. Those with emerging depression (24/201) more likely to be in early MT. No relationship with hormone levels.	Cluster analysis. Follow-up short considering age at baseline.
Harlow and Wise (2003)	N = 728	Population sample, Boston. Ages 36–45 years. 4161 eligible. Enrolled: N = 332 met DSM-IV criteria Major Depression, N = 644 without DSM-IV Major Depression Inclusion menstrual regularity, no hormone use, not pregnant or breast-feeding, FSH <20 IU/L follow-up 3 years, >80% retention.	Hamilton Rating Scale for Depression, LH, FSH, Oestradiol	Women with history of depression at risk for MT earlier than those without. Lifetime history of depression associated with higher FSH, LH and lower oestradiol at enrollment and subsequently.	Did not test the research question in the standard way.

(Continued)

Table 11.2. (*Continued*)

Citation	Size	Admission criteria	Measures	Results	Comments/ possible biases
Freeman et al. (2004)	$N = 436$	Population-based stratified sample of African-American and Caucasian. Ages 35–47 years baseline. Inclusion regular menses, no hormone use, healthy; six assessments over 4 years.	CES-D. Major depressive disorder by interview. FSH, LH, DHEAS, T, oestradiol	Depression increased during MT and decreased postmenopausal. Changing hormone levels contribute to dysphoric mood during transition. Increasing oestradiol significantly associated with depression. Increasing FSH associated with decreasing risk of depression.	Short follow-up and younger age at baseline means this study is of the effects of the early part of the MT. Very few reached late MT or postmenopause.
Dennerstein et al. (2004)	$N = 314$	Melbourne population-based cohort measured in 11th follow-up year. Ages 45–55 years baseline.	CES-D, Affectometer, FSH, oestradiol, testosterone	Women still menstruating and surgical menopause had highest depression scores. Negative mood reduced for all groups from baseline but less for surgical menopause.	CES-D not used annually although Affectometer was.

BDI: Beck depression inventory; CES-D: Centre for Epidemiological Studies Depression scale; DHEAS: Dehydroepiandrosterone sulphate; DSM: Diagnostic and Statistical Manual of Mental Disorders; FAI: functional assessment inventory; FMP: final menstrual period; FSH: follicle stimulating hormone; GHQ: general health questionnaire; HRT: hormone replacement therapy; LH: luetinizing hormone; MAACL: multiple affect adjective checklist; OR: odds ratio; SCL: symptom checklist scores (rated on the CES-D) were not associated with menopausal status or with annual change in oestradiol. There was a significant negative association between log oestradiol and CES-D score, but this became non-significant after adjusting for symptoms. Vasomotor symptoms and trouble sleeping were strongly positively associated with CES-D scores.

The Melbourne Women's Midlife Health Project (MWMHP), a population-based study of Australian-born women, used the Affectometer, a validated affect balance scale that provides sub-scale measures for both positive and negative moods. The project found that over the 9-year duration of the study, positive moods increased with time while negative moods decreased (Dennerstein et al., 1999, 2000, 2002). The MWMHP found that women who were still in the MT at the eleventh year of follow-up had higher CES-D depression scores than those who had become postmenopausal (Dennerstein et al., 2004).

In contrast, an increased risk of depression associated with the MT is reported by a number of other studies (Hunter, 1992; Maartens et al., 2002). For example, the Pennsylvania study (Freeman et al., 2004) and the Seattle study (Woods et al., 2002) are among the few to evaluate women from the time of late reproductive stage as they transit into the menopause. Interestingly, the Pennsylvania study reported that as women enter the early MT, CES-D scores increase even after adjusting for other factors. The risk for new depression was maximal in the early phase of the MT. The highest CES-D scores (high scores indicate more depressed mood) appeared to coincide with the late MT. However, as most of the sample had not reached their final menstrual period at the time of analysis, it may be premature to conclude this.

Freeman et al. (2004) found that CES-D scores did not correlate in a linear way with oestradiol levels, but there was a significant association using cubic or quadratic statistical methods. This was interpreted as indicating that depressed mood is linked to changes in oestradiol rather than to actual level. The study also reported that symptoms of depressed mood resolved as the women aged, and as they became postmenopausal. A pre-existing history of depression, or premenstrual syndrome, significantly increased the risk of being diagnosed with major depressive disorder during the five years of the study. Other risk factors for the development of depression were poor sleep, lack of paid employment and African-American ethnicity. These findings corroborate earlier reports from the Melbourne Women's Midlife Health Project that depressed mood lessens as women pass through the transition and become postmenopausal and highlight the importance of premorbid depression and problematic premenstrual mood complaints as predictors of later depression (Dennerstein et al., 1999). The Melbourne study had reported that although depressed mood was not directly related to menopausal phase or hormone levels, women were more susceptible to becoming depressed in response to stressors occurring while they were in the MT (Dennerstein et al., 1999).

Avis et al. (1994) found that prior depression was the variable most predictive of subsequent depression as measured by the CES-D (OR = 9.6 for baseline CES-D score). Harlow and Wise (2003), in a case controlled study in Boston, suggest that women with a history of depression could be at risk for a decline in ovarian function. They found that women with history of depression were at risk for reaching MT earlier than those without such a history. Lifetime history of depression was associated with higher FSH, LH and lower oestradiol at enrolment and subsequently.

A number of studies support a domino or symptom hypothesis suggesting that depressed mood is caused by the relationship between hormone levels, sleep problems and vasomotor symptoms (Avis et al., 2001a; Dennerstein et al., 1999). For example, data from the Seattle Midlife Women's Health Study was used to examine patterns of depressed mood in women during the MT, which was not a time of onset of new depression. The most prevalent pattern was that of non-depressed mood across the transition. However, life stressors, perceived poor health and vasomotor symptoms were associated with depressed mood (Woods et al., 2002).

Mood changes may be mediated by sleep disruption. In a detailed study of 28 women aged 40–55 years, Baker et al. (1997) examined the sleep and mood differences between premenopausal and perimenopausal women. Perimenopausal subjects had greater sleep disruption and mood alterations compared to premenopausal women. Perimenopausal subjects scored higher on the State-Trait Anxiety Inventory and lower on the Vigor sub-scale than premenopausal subjects.

Clinical implications

Findings concur that although the majority of women do not become depressed with the MT, some women may be particularly vulnerable to depression at this life stage. Identifying which women are at risk for depression is important for clinicians, as these women may need extra support during the MT (Dennerstein et al., 1999).

The Melbourne Women's Midlife Health Project (Dennerstein et al., 1999) found that women at risk for depressed mood during the MT were those with prior history of depression or premenstrual mood complaints, current smokers, with lack of exercise, interpersonal and other stress, being single, and having to contend with health problems or other symptoms during the transition. There is a suggestion that those who have a longer MT or who undergo surgical menopause may be more at risk of depression (Dennerstein et al., 2004).

Diagnostic and treatment approaches for the perimenopausal woman presenting with mood complaints

The symptomatic perimenopausal and early postmenopausal woman may present with mild complaints of mood lability and "just not feeling like herself" or with more significant complaints consistent with dysthymia or major depression. She may also complain of symptoms associated with cognitive function and a decline in her perceived ability to process information. She may report new onset of panic attacks or generalized anxiety. It is very helpful to establish premorbid psychiatric history, whether previously diagnosed or not, so as to look at the issue of recurrence of illness and exacerbation or magnification of pre-existent illness, known or unbeknownst to the patient. The patient may or may not recognize that she has had these symptoms before, to a greater or lesser degree. The importance of explaining to the patient that the MT may have exacerbated or caused a recurrence is vital to validating the patient's personal experience and perspective that the menopause per se has brought on her complaints leading to her current presentation for care. It is useful to explain to the patient the mixed results from research on the role of menopause in mood problems and that it is very likely that her previous problems with mood are playing a role in her current problems.

The diagnosis of chronic untreated problems such as mild to moderate attention deficit disorder and generalized anxiety disorder may help explain the magnitude of complaints of cognitive, information processing and memory problems she is having in the context of hot flashes and sleep loss secondary to thermoregulatory instability. To stabilize this woman it may be necessary to treat both the hot flashes and the underlying problem. In some women it may be adequate to simply treat the hot flashes and observe for the tolerability and magnitude of the underlying problem when the hot flashes have been resolved.

For mood problems or mood lability, the range of symptoms can be from mild to significant. A previously tolerable sub-syndromal premenstrual dysphoric disorder may worsen though occur less frequently. The woman with a history of mood disorder associated with phases of hormonal change may have a recurrence of that mood disorder. The woman on antidepressants who has been largely stable may become unstable on the same dose during the MT. With these patients it is important to treat the underlying disorder while attempting to treat any symptoms related to the MT that would exacerbate the underlying disorder. These include hot flashes and sleep disturbance secondary to thermoregulation problems. In some patients who have an exacerbation of their treated illness that has not been responsive to an increase in medication and/or a mood problem refractory to medication, it may be necessary to augment the antidepressant strategy with oestrogen in the form of a patch or gel (Schneider et al., 2001; Soares et al., 2003). Percutaneous oestradiol is preferred as it provides steady oestradiol levels as well as minimal impact on free testosterone levels (Martin et al., 1979).

Women who have or have had breast cancer, a family history of breast cancer, who cannot or do not wish to take oestrogen, or women with a history of blood clotting problems, may not be candidates for oestrogen replacement as an augmenting strategy or as a strategy to reduce thermoregulatory problems. In these women it would be important to use antidepressants that have been shown to impact hot flashes as well as mood. The most robust data are for venlafaxine, with less impressive data for paroxetine and fluoxetine (Loprinzi et al., 2000, 2002; Stearns et al., 2003). Another strategy that may be helpful is paced breathing for daytime hot flash control (Freedman et al., 1992). This technique was shown to be equally effective with hot flash control as venlafaxine (Freedman et al., 1992; Loprinzi, et al., 2000). It would not be helpful for nighttime hot flashes and the consequent sleep loss. Lastly, there is some mixed and conflicting evidence that soy protein is helpful as well as black cohosh (Albertazzi, 1998; Drapier Faure et al., 2002; Han et al., 2002; Liske et al., 2002). These treatments would not have the global effect on brain functioning associated with oestrogen augmentation, but would be more specific for hot flashes or thermoregulation problems.

Conclusion

In general, though the data are conflicting as to the exact role of menopause in the development and the exacerbation of pre-existing mood problems, it is clear that those women most at risk for depression will be those with a previous history of mood problems or psychiatric illness, as well as with a very symptomatic perimenopause. For this reason, the perimenopausal patient requires a dual approach, with the clinician taking into account current research and treatment approaches to menopause and related symptoms, as well as the known research and treatment strategies for mood disorders.

REFERENCES

APA (1994). *Diagnostic and statistical manual of mental disorders*. 4th edn. Washington, DC: American Psychiatric Association.

Albertazzi, P., et al. (1998). The effect of dietary soy supplementation on hot flushes. *Obstetric Gynecology*, *91*(1), 6–11.

Avis, N., Kaufert, P., Lock, M., McKinlay, S., & Vass, K. (1993). The evolution of menopausal symptoms. In: H. Burger (Ed.), *Bailliere's clinical endocrinology and metabolism* (pp. 17–32), London: Bailliere Tindall.

Avis, N., Brambilla, D., McKinlay, S., & Vass, K. (1994). A longitudinal analysis of the association between menopause and depression. *Annals of Epidemiology, 4,* 15–21.

Avis, N., Crawford, S., Stellato, R., & Longcope, C. (2001a). Longitudinal study of hormone levels and depression among women transitioning through menopause. *Climacteric, 4,* 243–249.

Avis, N., Stellato, R., Crawford, S., Bromberger, J., Ganz, P., Cain, V., & Kagawa-Singer, M. (2001b). Is there a menopausal syndrome? Menopausal status and symptoms across racial/ethnic groups. *Social Science and Medicine, 52,* 345–356.

Baker, A., Simpson, S., & Dawson, D. (1997). Sleep disruption and mood changes associated with menopause. *Journal of Psychosomatic Research, 43,* 359–369.

Ballinger, B. (1975). Psychiatric morbidity and the menopause: Screening of general population sample. *British Medical Journal, 3,* 344–346.

Barentsen, R., van de Weijer, P., van Gend, S., & Foekema, H. (2001). Climacteric symptoms in a representative Dutch population sample as measured with the Greene Climacteric Scale. *Maturitas, 38,* 123–128.

Boulet, M., Oddens, B., Lehert, P., Vener, H., & Visser, A. (1994). Climacteric and menopause in seven south-east Asian countries. *Maturitas, 19,* 157–176.

Bromberger, J., & Matthews, K. (1996). A longitudinal study of the effects of pessimism, trait anxiety, and life stress on depressive symptoms in middle aged women. *Psychology and Ageing, 11,* 207–213.

Bromberger, J.T., Meyer, P.M., Kravitz, H.M., Sommer, B., Cordal, A., Powell, L., Ganz, P.A., & Sutton-Tyrrell, K. (2001). Psychologic distress and natural menopause: A multiethnic community study. *American Journal of Public Health, 91,* 1435–1442.

Burger, H.G., Cahir, N., Robertson, D.M., Groome, N.P., Dudley, E., Green, A., & Dennerstein, L. (1998). Serum inhibins A and B fall differentially as FSH rises in perimenopausal women [erratum appears in *Clinical Endocrinology* (Oxford), 1998, *49*(4), 550]. *Clinical Endocrinology, 48,* 809–813.

Burger, H.G., Dudley, E.C., Hopper, J.L., Groome, N., Guthrie, J.R., Green, A., & Dennerstein, L. (1999). Prospectively measured levels of serum follicle-stimulating hormone, estradiol, and the dimeric inhibins during the menopausal transition in a population-based cohort of women. *Journal of Clinical Endocrinology and Metabolism, 84,* 4025–4030.

Burger, H.G., Dudley, E.C., Cui, J., Dennerstein, L., & Hopper, J.L. (2000). A prospective longitudinal study of serum testosterone, dehydroepiandrosterone sulfate, and sex hormone-binding globulin levels through the menopause transition. *Journal of Clinical Endocrinology and Metabolism, 85,* 2832–2838.

Burrows, G., & Dennerstein, L. (1981). Depression and suicide in middle age. In: J. Howells (Ed.), *Modern perspectives in the psychiatry of middle age* (pp. 220–250), New York: Brunner/Mazel.

Cagnacci, A., Volpe, A., Arangino, S., Malmusi, S., Draetta, F.P., Matteo, M.L., Maschio, E., & Vacca, A.M.B. (1997). Depression and anxiety in climacteric women: Role of hormone replacement therapy. *Menopause: The Journal of The North American Menopause Society, 4,* 206–211.

Cawood, E., & Bancroft, J. (1996). Steroid hormones, the menopause, sexuality and well-being of women. *Journal of Psychological Medicine, 26,* 925–936.

Collins, A., & Landgren, B. (1995). Reproductive health, use of estrogen and experience of symptoms in perimenopausal women: A population-based study. *Maturitas, 20,* 101–111.

Dennerstein, L. (1999). Psychosexual effects of hormonal contraception. *Gynaecology Forum*, *4*, 13–16.

Dennerstein, L., Morse, C., & Varnavides, K. (1988). Premenstrual tension and depression is there a relationship? *Journal of Psychosomatic Obstetrics and Gynecology*, *8*, 45–52.

Dennerstein, L., Lehert, P., & Riphagen, F. (1989). Post partum depression risk factors. *Journal of Psychosomatic Obstetrics and Gynecology*, *10*, 53–67.

Dennerstein, L., Smith, A.M., Morse, C., Burger, H., Green, A., Hopper, J., & Ryan, M. (1993). Menopausal symptoms in Australian women. *Medical Journal of Australia*, *159*, 232–236.

Dennerstein, L., Gotts, G., Brown, J., Morse, C., Farley, T., & Pinol, A. (1994a). The relationship between the menstrual cycle and female sexual interest in women with PMS complaints and volunteers. *Psychoneuroendocrinology*, *19*, 293–304.

Dennerstein, L., Smith, A., & Morse, C. (1994b). Psychological well-being, mid-life and the menopause. *Maturitas*, *20*, 1–11.

Dennerstein, L., Dudley, E., & Burger, H. (1997). Well-being and the menopausal transition. *Journal of Psychosomatic Obstetrics and Gynecology*, *18*, 95–101.

Dennerstein, L., Lehert, P., Burger, H., & Dudley, E. (1999). Mood and the menopausal transition. *Journal of Nervous and Mental Disease*, *187*, 685–691.

Dennerstein, L., Dudley, E.C., Hopper, J.L., Guthrie, J.R., & Burger, H.G. (2000). A prospective population-based study of menopausal symptoms. *Obstetrics and Gynecology*, *96*, 351–358.

Dennerstein, L., Randolph, J., Taffe, J., Dudley, E., & Burger, H. (2002). Hormones, mood, sexuality, and the menopausal transition. *Fertility and Sterility*, *77*, S42–S48.

Dennerstein, L., Guthrie, J., Clark, M., Lehert, P., & Henderson, V. (2004). A population-based study of depressed mood in mid-aged Australian-born women. *Menopause*, *11*, 563–568.

Drapier Faure, E., et al. (2002). Effects of a standardized soy extract on hot flushes: A multicenter, double-blind, randomized, placebo-controlled study. *Menopause: The Journal of The North American Menopause Society*, *9*(5), 329–334.

Evans, M.L., Pritts, E., Vittinghoff, E., McClish, K., Morgan, K.S., Jaffe, R.B. Management of postmenopausal hot flushes with venlafaxine hydrochloride: a randomized controlled trial. *Obstet Gynecol* 2005; 105(1): 161–6.

Freedman, R.R., et al. (1992). Behavioral treatment of menopausal hot flushes: Evaluation by ambulatory monitoring. *American Journal of Obstetrics and Gynecology*, *167*, 436–439.

Freeman, E.W., Sammel, M.D., Liu, L., Gracia, C.R., Nelson, D.B., & Hollander, L. (2004). Hormones and menopausal status as predictors of depression in women in transition to menopause. *Archives of General Psychiatry*, *61*, 62–70.

Garamszegi, C., Dennerstein, L., Dudley, E., Guthrie, J.R., Ryan, M., & Burger, H. (1998). Menopausal status: Subjectively and objectively defined. *Journal of Psychosomatic Obstetrics and Gynecology*, *19*, 165–173.

Gath, D.O.M., Bungay, G., Iles, S., Day, A., Bond, A., & Passingham, C. (1987). Psychiatric disorder and gynaecological symptoms in middle aged women: A community survey. *British Medical Journal*, *294*, 213–218.

Greene, J., & Cooke, D. (1980). Life stress and symptoms at the climacterium. *British Journal of Psychiatry*, *136*, 486–491.

Hallstrom, T., & Samuelsson, S. (1985). Mental health in the climacteric. *Acta Obstetricia et Gynecologica Scandinavica*, (Suppl 130), 13–18.

Han, K.K., et al. (2002). Benefits of soy isoflavone therapeutic regimen on menopausal symptoms. *Obstetrics and Gynecology*, *99*(3), 389–394.

Harlow, B., Cramer, D., & Annis, K. (1995). Association of medically treated depression and age at natural menopause. *American Journal of Epidemiology*, *141*, 1170–1176.

Harlow, B., & Wise, L. (2003). Depression and its influence on reproductive endocrine and menstrual markers associated with perimenopause: The Harvard study of moods and cycles. *Archives of General psychiatry*, *56*, 418–424.

Holte, A., & Mikkelsen, A. (1982). Menstrual coping style, social background and climacteric symptoms. *Psychiatry Social Science*, *2*, 41–45.

Hunter, M. (1992). The South-East England longitudinal study of the climacteric and postmenopause. *Maturitas*, *14*, 117–126.

Hunter, M., Battersby, R., & Whitehead, M. (1986). Relationships between psychological symptoms, somatic complaints and menopausal status. *Maturitas*, *8*, 217–228.

Jaszmann, L., van Lith, N., & Zaat, J. (1969). The perimenopausal symptoms: The statistical analysis of a survey part A. *Medical Gynecology Society*, 268–277.

Joffe, H., Hall, J.E., Soares, C.N., Hennen, J., Reilly, C.J., Carlson, K., & Cohen, L.S. (2002). Vasomotor symptoms are associated with depression in perimenopausal women seeking primary care [see comment]. *Menopause*, *9*, 392–398.

Judd, H.L., Judd, G.E., Lucas, W.E., & Yen, S.S. (1974). Endocrine function of the postmenopausal ovary: Concentration of androgens and estrogens in ovarian and peripheral vein blood. *Journal of Clinical Endocrinology and Metabolism*, *39*, 1020–1024.

Kaufert, P., Gilbert, P., & Tate, R. (1992). The Manitoba Project: A re-examination of the link between menopause and depression. *Maturitas*, *14*, 143–155.

Khan, S.A., Pace, J.E., Cox, M.L., Gau, D.W., Cox, S.A., & Hodkinson, H.M. (1994). Climacteric symptoms in healthy middle-aged women. *British Journal of Clinical Practice*, *48*, 240–242.

Kuh, D., Wadsworth, M., & Hardy, R. (1997). Women's health in midlife: The influence of the menopause, social factors and health in earlier life. *British Journal of Obstetrics and Gynaecology*, *104*, 923–933.

Lehert, P., & Dennerstein, L. (2002). Statistical techniques for the analysis of change in longitudinal studies of the menopause. *Acta Obstetricia et Gynecologica Scandinavica*, *81*, 581–587.

Liske, E., et al. (2002). Physiological investigation of a unique extract of black cohosh (cimicifugae racemosae rhizome): A 6-month clinical study demonstrates no systemic estrogenic effect. *Journal of Women's Health and Gender-Based Medicine*, *11*(2), 163–174.

Loprinzi, C., et al. (2000). Venlafaxine in management of hot flashes in survivors of breast cancer: A randomized controlled trial. *The Lancet*, *356*, 2059–2063.

Loprinzi, C., et al. (2002). Phase III evaluation of Fluoxetine for treatment of hot flashes. *Journal of Clinical Oncology*, *20*(6), 1578–1583.

Maartens, L.W., Knottnerus, J.A., & Pop, V.J. (2002). Menopausal transition and increased depressive symptomatology: A community based prospective study. *Maturitas*, *42*, 195–200.

Martin, P.L., et al. (1979). Systemic absorption and sustained effects of vaginal estrogen creams. *Journal of the American Medical Association*, *242*(24), 2699–2700.

Matthews, K., Wing, R., Kuller, L., Meilahn, E., Kelsey, S., et al. (1990). Influences of natural menopause on psychological characteristics and symptoms of middle aged healthy women. *Journal of Consulting and Clinical Psychology, 58,* 345–351.

McKinlay, J., McKinlay, S., & Brambilla, D. (1987). The relative contributions of endocrine changes and social circumstances to depression in mid-aged women. *Journal of Health and Social Behavior, 28,* 345–363.

Morse, C.A., Smith, A., Dennerstein, L., Green, A., Hopper, J., & Burger, H. (1994). The treatment-seeking woman at menopause. *Maturitas, 18,* 161–173.

Neugarten, B., & Kraines, R. (1965). Menopausal symptoms in women of various ages. *Psychosomatic Medicine, 27,* 266–273.

O'Connor, V., Del Mar, C., Sheehan, M., Siskind, V., Fox-Young, S., & Cragg, C. (1995). Do psycho-social factors contribute more to symptom reporting by middle-aged women than hormonal status? *Maturitas, 20,* 63–69.

Oldenhave, A., Jaszmann, L., Haspels, A., & Everaerd, W. (1993). Impact of climacteric on wellbeing. *American Journal of Obstetrics and Gynecology, 168,* 772–780.

Pop, V.J., Maartens, L., Leusink, G., Van Son, M.J., Knottnerus, A., Ward, A., Metcalfe, R., & Weetman, A. (1998). Are autoimmune thyroid dysfunction and depression related? *Journal of Clinical Endocrinology and Metabolism, 83,* 3194–3197.

Porter, M., Penney, G., Russell, D., Russell, E., & Templeton, A. (1996). A population based survey of women's experience of the menopause. *British Journal of Obstetrics and Gynaecology, 103,* 1025–1028.

Punyahotra, S., Dennerstein, L., & Lehert, P. (1997). Menopausal experiences of Thai women. Part 1: Symptoms and their correlates. *Maturitas, 26,* 1–7.

Punyahotra, S., & Dennerstein, L. (1997a). Menopausal experiences of Thai women – Part 1: symptoms and their correlates. *Maturitas, 26,* 1–7.

Sarrel, P., & Whitehead, M. (1985). Sex and menopause: Defining the issues. *Maturitas, 7,* 217–224.

Schneider, L.S., et al. (2001). Estrogen replacement therapy and antidepressant response to sertraline in older depressed women. *American Journal of Geriatric Psychiatry, 9*(4), 393–399.

Shifren, J.L. (2002). Androgen deficiency in the oophorectomized woman. *Fertility and Sterility, 77,* S60–S62.

Soares, C.N., et al. (2003). Efficacy of citalopram as a monotheapy or as an adjunctive treatment to estrogen therapy for perimenopausal and postmenopausal women with depression and vasomotor symptoms. *Journal of Clinical Psychiatry, 64,* 473–479.

Soules, M.R., Sherman, S., Parrott, E., Rebar, R., Santoro, N., Utian, W., & Woods, N. (2001). Executive summary: Stages of reproductive ageing workshop (STRAW) [comment]. *Fertility and Sterility, 76,* 874–878.

Stadberg, E., Mattsson, L.A., & Milsom, I. (2000). Factors associated with climacteric symptoms and the use of hormone replacement therapy. *Acta Obstetricia et Gynecologica Scandinavica, 79,* 286–292.

Stearns, V., et al. (2003). Paroxetine controlled release in the treatment of menopausal hot flashes. *Journal of the American Medical Association, 289*(21), 2827–2834.

Taffe, J., & Dennerstein, L. (2000). Retrospective self-report compared with menstrual diary data prospectively kept during the menopausal transition. *Climacteric, 3,* 183–191.

Tam, L., Stucky, V., Hanson, R., & Parry, B. (1999). Prevalence of depression in menopause: A pilot study. *Archives Women's Mental Health*, *2*, 175–181.

Woods, N., & Mitchell, E. (1996). Patterns of depressed mood in midlife women: Observations from the Seattle midlife women's health study. *Research in Nursing and Health*, *19*, 111–123.

Woods, N., & Mitchell, E. (1997). Pathways to depressed mood for midlife women: Observations from the Seattle midlife women's health study. *Research in Nursing and Health*, *20*, 119–129.

Woods, N., Mariella, A., & Mitchell, E. (2002). Patterns of depressed mood across the menopausal transition: Approaches to studying patterns in longitudinal data. *Acta Obstetricia et Gynecologica Scandinavica*, *81*, 623–632.

Zhao, G., Wang, L., Yan, R., & Dennerstein, L. (2000). Menopausal symptoms: Experience of Chinese women. *Climacteric*, *3*, 135–144.

12

Anxiety and depression in women in old age

Robert C. Baldwin[1] and Jane Garner[2]

[1] Manchester Mental Health and Social Care Trust, York House,
Manchester Royal Infirmary, Manchester, UK
[2] Department of Old Age Psychiatry, Chase Farm Hospital, The Ridgeway, Enfield, UK

One is not born a woman: one becomes one.

Simone de Beauvoir,
Le Deuxieme Sexe (1949)

Gender, age, ethnicity and class are major dimensions of social inequality in human societies. Mental illness adds to this inequality and to stigmatisation. Gender and age, although with roots in biology, are both understood within a social context. Women in later life may be seen as compounded of the negative myths which surround the feminine sex and old age.

In classical mythology the three Fates were conceived of as old women at a spinning wheel determining men's lifespans and destinies. Clotho draws out the thread of life, Lachesis measures it out and Atropos cuts it off. This duality of women, the weaker sex but with a dark and powerful side is evident in religions, pseudoscience, art and literature. Old age similarly attracts fables which emerge from and influence deeply ingrained fears and attitudes. Old age rarely attracts positive epithets, usually it is denigratory or patronising – grumpy old; boring old; sweet old............ We praise old people not for ageing well but for seeming younger than their years.

This negative perception is reflected in the way older people view themselves. Ageing is a wound to one's narcissism and self-esteem. To counteract it, it is possible to enumerate many who have overcome the barriers and handicaps of age, but an idealisation of a few biographies (Garner & Ardern, 1998) does not adequately redress the balance in a culture where most would fail by comparison with the youth centred norm. Elders are defined as a "minority" group, except of course numerically where the expectation is that services will be overwhelmed, and the (younger) tax-payer will be burdened by this tide of need and dependence. Stereotypes of masculinity and femininity change with advancing years. The loss of "men are strong and women are beautiful" simplicities may be felt as a personal blow to the older person who struggles to seem younger. The inequalities between the genders may seem more unfair to older women. The Jungian Archetype "senex" seems very male. Old women do not command the adjective "wise". The mature man will be seen as having character lines, the old woman wrinkles. The lusty old man with an eye for the ladies is admired for his energy and continued libido, the elderly woman with sexual interests is seen pejoratively. The dominant cultural storyline is of asexual older women (Jones, 2002).

Old people being part of society have incorporated these concepts into their own view of themselves. Few clinicians have questioned the prevailing myths about women, old age and even psychological disorders. Freud regarded the feminine as a lack of a penis and old age as the castration of youth: old women associated with images of absence.

Psychiatrists have not been immune from myths and misconceptions regarding clinical disorders in old age. It is thought that depression in later life is symptomatically different, more common, more chronic, more difficult to treat and more often caused by psychological factors. The evidence does not bear this out (Blazer, 2003). These ideas, untruths, among lay and professional people generate a pessimism which does a disservice to older people suffering from depression and anxiety disorders. The majority of women in late life are not depressed but still the doctor may say or think "you are old, widowed, arthritic, living on only a pension – what do you expect?" As for any "minority" group it is easy to categorise them together with general descriptions, to stereotype older women rather than look at the unique individual personal history and experience each brings to their current situation. Old women are more than their age and their gender.

Old age psychiatrists see people born over four decades with inevitably different experiences and cohort effects. External socioeconomic factors leave their psychological mark in the internal world. Contemporary post-modern Western society with its self-absorbed emphasis on youth, beauty, fashion, lifestyle and individuality is a difficult place to be old, particularly old and ill (Garner, 2004). The increased sexualisation of society does no favours for older women, supposed to be asexual but who nevertheless may be struggling with unmet needs (Garner & Bacelle, 2004). In younger life thinking about old age there will have been anticipated roles and activities. However, rapid societal changes, social mobility for family members, marital problems in retirement, becoming a carer, widowhood or financial problems may change and upset plans. The prospect of some freedom in later life will also be blighted if the woman herself becomes ill. Chronic and multiple handicaps may accumulate, either increasing isolation or forcing a change of accommodation.

When does old age begin? The popular saying is that a man is as old as he feels, a woman as old as she looks. From ancient literature to contemporary times most authorities have located the beginning of old age around 60 (some much earlier) but with women consistently viewed as ageing more rapidly and sooner than men (Covey, 1992). Psychiatry services for older people tend to be organised around the age of 65 and above.

Psychological development and old age

For Freud, development was a childhood task only. Jung (1931) spoke of the "morning" of life being different from the "afternoon" of life which was governed by distinct principles, a focus on culture and spirituality and the necessity of giving serious attention to the self to achieve individuation. Erikson (1959) also saw development continuing beyond early libidinal stages throughout the life cycle with specific tasks to be negotiated in each of the eight phases he described. His framework was the person's attitude to and interaction with the world, emphasising cultural as well as intrapsychic factors; the life cycle is charted through social science and psychoanalysis. The final developmental stage is of "ego-integrity versus despair and disgust". The person with integrity sees their personal life and history to be as it had to be. Their route through life was the only possible one for them. The one without emotional integration is despairing that there is no more time to try out different paths, death is near, the fear is of "not being" rather than valuing the experience one has had. In addition to this task the mark left by the previous seven stages may be stimulated by the exigencies of old age.

The challenges of later life for women particularly involve accepting bodily changes with equanimity; reconsidering the marital relationship in retirement, the children having left; perhaps feeling one has failed as a mother, paradoxically worse for those who are childless; coming to terms with increasing dependency, perhaps also forced dependency in residential or nursing home care; retirement which may or may not live up to expectations; widowhood; financially straitened circumstances, particularly if one were dependent on the husband to make pension contributions on her behalf; the cultural expectation of an asexual old age; and the sexism and ageism which is a part of sociocultural existence.

The assumption that older women do not have libido is just that. Of a surveyed group of reasonably healthy women ranging in age from 80 to 102, 70% still fantasised about intimacy with men, 64% engaged in touching and caressing their men, 40% masturbated and 25% had a regular sexual partner (Bretschneider & McCoy, 1989). If women do experience a decline in libido this tends to start at or around the menopause rather than late in life. Subsequent to this, sexual interest is influenced less by age than health, medication and availability of a partner (Bretschneider & McCoy, 1989). Sexual needs across the lifespan may not differ dramatically, although older women voice more concerns about their partner's sexual difficulties (Nusbaum et al., 2004). Even these contemporary findings date quickly in societies where attitudes to same-sex relationships are undergoing rapid change, a subject hardly touched when considering later life partnerships. Many older women would welcome the opportunity to discuss sexual concerns at consultation but few physicians seem willing to initiate this (Nusbaum et al., 2004).

Positive factors in old age are predominantly the adaptive personality traits, strengths and coping strategies one brings into the senium. For those with sufficient internal resources ageing itself may be a creative process in developmental adaptation (Garner, 2004); coming to terms with one's own inevitable death is a task for middle age (Knight, 1986) which if successfully accomplished eases later years. The capacity to make mutual and sharing relationships with family but particularly with friends will help women deal with this time of their life. There is a need for intimate connectedness whatever the age. Indeed, Fooken (1994) suggests that sexuality promotes health in later life. For those whose pension is sufficient, the removal of the pressure for paid employment may be helpful but only if sufficient activity of some sort fills the available time. Exercising body and mind extends the span of healthy life.

Epidemiology

Depression

Nearly twice as many women as men suffer from major depressive disorder (see Chapter 7). This difference continues into extreme old age but the differential decreases. The higher prevalence of depression among women is due to a higher risk of first onset rather than differential persistence or recurrence (Kessler, 2003). The cause of the gender difference in rates is not known but speculation covers cognitive styles, psychosocial and economic stress, an increased rate of abuse in childhood and in the work place, an increase in the incidence of hypothyroidism and other biological factors related to the effects of endogenous and exogenous gonadal steroids (there is no sex difference in incidence before adolescence). However, these differences only pertain to unipolar depression. For bipolar disorder the male/female ratio is equal (Blehar et al., 1998) although women have more depressive and fewer manic episodes (see Chapter 10).

The rate of depressive disorder in residential and nursing homes where the population is predominantly female is two to three times higher than in community surveys. There may be a number of reasons why this is so. Inevitably the population will have many with physical illness and handicaps; there may also be co-morbidity with dementia.

Anxiety

There are difficulties in arriving at estimates of prevalence for anxiety in old age. First, the most widely used classificatory systems for psychiatric disorder are hierarchical and tend to subsume symptoms of anxiety under depressive disorders. Second, judging whether symptoms of anxiety are "understandable" is not easy. What may start as an appropriately cautious response to threat, for example fear of falling or fear of crime, can spiral into disabling fear and phobic avoidance. Fear of falling has even been proposed as a form of agoraphobia in the elderly (Kay, 1988).

Lindesay et al. (1989) found that the prevalence of generalised anxiety disorder was 3.7% and of phobias 10% amongst community-living elderly people. Among those with phobic disorders, specific phobias were often longstanding and agoraphobia associated with physical disability. Save for specific phobias, which were equally distributed between the sexes, the rates for women were two to three those of men. Using a symptom checklist, a recent study found that 15% of older people were anxious, rising to 43% in those who were concurrently depressed (Mehta et al., 2003). Again women predominated.

Classification and diagnosis

With the exception of increased hypochondriasis and a greater preoccupation with poor memory with age, the symptoms of major depression do not alter dramatically over the adult lifespan (Baldwin, 2002). An unanswered question though is whether the term "major depression" adequately encompasses all clinically relevant forms of mood disorder in later life. A clue comes from epidemiological studies which show that for every older woman with major depression between two and four more have "subthreshold" symptoms (Beekman et al., 1999). There is no perfect way to classify these new syndromes, but terms such as "minor" depression and "subsyndromal" depression are used. "Minor" depression is not trivial depression; it is associated with considerable morbidity (Katon et al., 2003).

A factor analysis using a depression rating scale in 14 European countries identified two factors that represented the main classes seen in older people. One was called "affective suffering", characterised by depression, tearfulness and a wish to die; this was associated with female gender. The second, a "motivation" factor, comprised loss of interest, poor concentration and anhedonia; this showed a positive correlation with age but not gender. Speculatively, this latter form may be linked to the emerging concept of vascular depression, a form of late-onset depression associated with vascular disease and more "deficit" depressive symptoms such as poor motivation (Alexopoulos et al., 1997).

These modest age-related differences in symptoms are outweighed by more general factors which may mask the presentation or detection of late-life depression. These include poor physical health, alcohol misuse, medication effects and co-morbid psychiatric disorder, notably dementia. Significant depressive symptoms are found in around a fifth of patients with dementia (Allen & Burns, 1995).

Detection can be difficult. Medical co-morbidity may obscure the interpretation of physical depressive symptoms such as appetite change or reduced energy. It is unusual for a neurotic illnesses to present de novo in later life. Where marked symptoms of anxiety, obsessive–compulsive symptoms or phobia newly present the underlying cause is usually depressive disorder. Hysteria, the latter-day classical condition of women, is rare in old age. Most hysterical symptoms arise from organic disorder or depression.

Burden of depression

Depression is predicted to be the second leading illness associated with negative impact and disease burden by 2020 (Lopez & Murray, 1998). As a cause of morbidity depression ranks alongside most major disabling medical conditions (Wells et al., 1989).

After a decline lasting several decades, the suicide rate for people age 65 years and over rose 9% between 1980 and 1992 (CDC, 1996). The increase was most dramatic for men and women aged 80–84 years, the fastest growing segment of the population, for whom the rate rose over 35%. Among young adults, those who commit suicide have a heterogenous mixture of psychotic, mood and substance use disorders. In middle age, affective and addictive disorders predominate. Elderly victims constitute a more homogeneous population in which non-affective psychoses are rare, addictive disorders are less common, and late-onset major depression is the rule (Conwell et al., 1996). Substance misuse, whilst less common than among younger adults who kill themselves, is not rare. In the survey of Conwell et al. (1996) of older adults, almost half of those who killed themselves had both depressive disorder and substance (mainly alcohol) misuse.

Depressive disorder adds to disability from physical disorder when present and is associated with greater physical decline (Penninx et al., 2000). Depressed older women are at increased risk of hip fracture (Whooley et al., 1999). They are less compliant with medical treatments (Dimatteo et al., 2000). Conversely, poorer health is associated with a worse prognosis for depression (Lyness et al., 2002), emphasising the two-way nature of the interaction. This is a complex subject, involving putative mechanisms such as immune function, hypothalamic hormones, turnover of substances such as homocysteine, cytokines and vascular processes and is beyond the scope of this chapter. To give a flavour though, a group of older adults (mean age 71 years) were rated for depressive symptoms before being given an influenza vaccination. Those with even a modest number of depressive symptoms had a significantly greater and longer inflammatory response (assessed by interleukin 6 levels) compared to those who were not depressed (Glaser et al., 2003).

Depressive symptoms in older women are associated with both poor cognitive function and subsequent cognitive decline (Yaffe et al., 1999) and female gender is a risk factor for both depression and Alzheimer's disease. In a study of 2000 patients with Alzheimer's disease (the MIRAGE study; Green et al., 2003) depression contributed significantly to the risk for up to 25 years, even after controlling for other factors.

Mortality is increased in older patients with depressive disorders (Murphy et al., 1988). Although much of this is due to co-morbid physical disorders, depression is an independent risk factor (Blazer, 2003). This may be more true of men than women (Arfken et al., 1999). In one study women with subthreshold depression, as opposed to depressive disorder or no depression, had significantly reduced mortality (Hybels et al., 2002). This counter-intuitive finding may accord with suggestions that some forms of depression may be adaptive (Nesse, 2000). Speculatively this may reflect in women a biological drive to retreat from external threats in order to focus on more immediate protective functions (Hybels et al., 2002).

The economic health burden of depression in late life is high. In a large study of older people living at home, the total outpatient costs were 47–51% higher in depressed compared with non-depressed elderly patients after adjustment for chronic medical illness. This increase was seen in every component of health care costs, with only a small proportion due to mental health treatment. No differences in costs were seen between those with subthreshold depressive syndromes compared to those with major depression (Katon et al., 2003).

Risk and protective factors

Predisposing factors

Age on its own does not appear to be a risk factor for women in the development of depression or anxiety, nor is a family history (Baldwin, 2002). A history of depression, suicide attempts or other psychiatric disorders increases the likelihood of a further depressive episode. Co-morbid medical illness is a major risk factor in late-onset depression. Up to 50% of elderly general hospital patients may also be depressed, and there is an association with a variety of systemic medical and neurological disorders as well as medication (Szewczyk & Chennault, 1997) (Table 12.1). Depression may mimic dementia, herald it or increase the risk of developing it (Green et al., 2003).

In refining the impact of physical illness as a risk factor for depression, Prince et al. (1998) identified handicap, the social disadvantage that accompanies disability, as an important determinant. Two older women may share a similar degree of disability

Table 12.1. Medical conditions and central-acting drugs that may cause organic depression

Medical conditions	Central-acting drugs
Endocrine/metabolic	*Anti-hypertensive drugs*
Hypo/hyperthyroidism	Beta-blockers
Cushing's disease	Methyldopa
Hypercalcaemia	Reserpine
Pernicious anaemia	Clonidine
	Nifedipine
Organic brain disease	Digoxin
Stroke	
CNS tumours	*Steroids*
Parkinson's disease	*Analgesic drugs*
Alzheimer's disease and vascular dementia	Opioids
Multiple sclerosis	Indomethacin
Systemic lupus erythematosus	
	Anti-Parkinson
Occult carcinoma	L-dopa preparations
Pancreas	Amantadine
Lung	Tetrabenazine
Chronic infections	*Psychiatric drugs*
Neurosyphilis	Neuroleptics
Brucellosis	Benzodiazepines
AIDS	
	Miscellaneous
	Sulphonamides

from arthritis. If one has inadequate local transport then she is the more handicapped. The concept of handicap lends itself to practical remedies.

Widowhood, divorce, stressful life events and poor social support are also risk factors (Kivela et al., 1998; LePine & Bouchez, 1998). Social isolation and a lack of a close confiding relationship predispose to late-life depression. The latter appears to be a personality trait rather than simply a lack of opportunity (Murphy, 1982). Early loss, maternal loss among men and an early loss of the father among women are risk factors for depression (Kivela et al., 1998). Poverty and lower social class are linked to depression but probably via poorer health, itself a major risk factor (Murphy, 1982).

Whether age-related brain changes increase the susceptibility to depression in later life is of great interest. Some, but by no means all, brain biochemical changes associated with ageing are similar to those seen in depression. For example, both are associated with decreased brain concentrations of serotonin, dopamine, noradrenaline and their metabolites, and increased mono amine oxidase isoform-B (MAO-B) activity (Veith & Raskind, 1988). A variety of neuroendocrine changes are associated with ageing (Veith & Raskind, 1988). Ageing is associated with increasing cortisol levels and cortisol non-suppression (Alexopoulos et al., 1984). It seems likely that normal ageing is associated with enhanced limbic–HPA axis activity, perhaps related to neuronal degeneration in the hippocampus, and that this may be exacerbated by raised glucocorticoid secretion, caused either by depression or repeated stressful life events or both (the "feed forward cascade" – Sapolsky et al., 1986).

However, the much touted term "age-related" is probably inaccurate. Many, perhaps most, geriatric syndromes are due to pathology rather than age. Recent research into the relationship between late-onset depression and vascular pathology supports this assertion (Baldwin & O'Brien, 2002).

Risk factors for suicide in later life include depression, chronic illness, social isolation and alcohol misuse. These have been discussed. Older women with depression and longstanding anxiety may also be at risk (Waern et al., 2002).

Precipitating factors

Loss life events often precipitate depression in susceptible individuals. In later life, especially for women, the major example is the loss of a life partner. However, other painful losses include health deterioration, loss of function, death of a pet, role changes at retirement, children or friends moving away and the loss of one's home. Some losses may re-awaken earlier grief. Among the long-term widowed, rates of depression decline, suggesting that a majority of elderly widows do eventually adjust. However, this may take a number of years (Turvey et al., 1999).

Going into a residential or nursing home may seem to others the right and logical decision but to the older person it often signifies a loss of independence, choice, privacy and the familiarities of one's own home, street and neighbourhood. Moving home is immensely stressful (Holmes & Rahe, 1967) and particularly if it is seen as the last move one will make. If clinical assessments prior to the move are not comprehensive, failure to function at home may not be recognised as depression. Achterberg et al. (2003) found that low social engagement was very common in newly admitted nursing home residents in the Netherlands and that depression was an important independent risk factor.

The role of less obviously catastrophic life events ("daily hassles") are greater than is generally realised, especially if occurring close to other significant losses (Murdock et al., 1998).

As both a risk factor and a precipitant, caregiving deserves a special mention. By virtue of traditional roles and because of their longevity, women are the main caregivers. A high proportion of those caring for someone with dementia will become depressed; the majority are women (Ballard et al., 1996), yet female carers attract less formal and informal support than male ones.

Protective factors

True to the stereotype of old age as uniformly bleak, little has been written about factors that are likely to be protective against depression such as the arrival of grandchildren, improved financial security or "fresh start" experiences including new friendships.

Whether or not a woman's marital state is a risk or protective factor is a matter of much debate. It would seem that marital dissatisfaction is uniquely related to major depression and post-traumatic stress disorder for women (Whisman, 1999). However, being happily married protects more than the single life. Other protective factors include the ability to make confiding relationships and friendships, and being able to maintain them over time. This includes having the ability to accept appropriate help when increasing difficulties occur and to make relationships with formal and informal carers. Having a religious conviction has been shown to be protective from depression in later life (Blazer, 2003). Older women may take on particular roles in different religions.

The higher rate of depression in women is found across cultures. The prevalence of depression in African-American and Hispanic women is twice that in men. Major depression seems to be diagnosed less frequently in African-American women and more frequently in Hispanic than in Caucasian women. Different groups may express depression and anxiety in different ways. Harralson et al. (2002) explored similarities and differences in depression among black and white nursing home residents in Philadelphia, USA. White residents were more likely to report psychological symptoms and black people to report somatic symptoms. Functional disability was an important predictor of depression in both groups.

Compared to depression, less is known about risk factors for anxiety disorders in old age, but women are more at risk than men (Kay, 1988). As with depression, white race is associated with greater risk than black (Mehta et al., 2003). Several physical disorders may cause anxiety. The more common include thyroid disorder, chronic obstructive pulmonary disease, pulmonary embolism, Meniere's disease, hypoglycaemia and paroxysmal tachyarrhythmias (Kay, 1988). In women urinary incontinence is a neglected cause (Mehta et al., 2003). Hypochondriasis is closely linked to depression but in Europe is also classified separately as one of the somatoform disorders. In psychotic depression hypochondriacal delusions are common (Baldwin, 2002). Interestingly, in older women hypochondriasis does not correlate with the extent of physical illness (Kramer-Ginsberg et al., 1989).

Management

Depression

Assessment

Until recently, rating scales to measure depression were not ideally suited to older adults. The most widely used, the Hamilton Rating Scale for Depression (Hamilton, 1960), contains a number of somatic symptoms which may be hard to interpret in the older adult. The Montgomery Asberg Depression Rating Scale is perhaps more appropriate (Mottram et al., 2000). The Geriatric Depression Scale (GDS) is specifically designed for older people (Yesavage et al., 1983). This self- or assisted-rated tool is available in versions from 4 to 30 items and has been translated into a number of languages, most of which can be found on a free website (http://stanford.edu/~yesavage/GDS.html). The GDS works reasonably well in cases of mild to moderate dementia but loses sensitivity in patients with severe dementia (Baldwin, 2002). The GDS is reproduced in Table 12.2. The Cornell Depression Rating scale (Alexopoulos et al., 1988) has been developed to detect depression in those with dementia. It utilises information from a caregiver as well as the patient.

Bearing in mind the earlier discussion of sexuality in later life, of the three scales mentioned only the Hamilton rates libido, under the unsatisfactory item "genital symptoms" which includes "menstrual disturbance".

Screening for depression is useful but is not a substitute for clinical skills. The history should include medical illness, medication (including over-the-counter drugs such as analgesics), alcohol intake and information about recent life events. Modifications to the interview (shorter sessions, slower pace) may be required if there is sensory impairment, poor physical health, or pain. A cognitive assessment should be included: the Mini-Mental State Examination (MMSE; Folstein et al., 1975) is appropriate.

A physical examination should be conducted. As mentioned, ill-health is often the trigger for severe depression (Table 12.1) and is linked closely to prognosis. Laboratory investigation should include haemoglobin, full blood count, bio-chemical profile, B_{12} and folate levels. Severe depression can rapidly lead to under-nutrition. Elderly people have less physiological reserve than younger adults. In a frail 80-year-old woman it may lead to serious metabolic derangement in a short time.

Specialist referral should be considered:
- for patients where dementia is suspected;
- when depression is severe, as evidenced by psychotic depression or suicidality;
- where risk is present through failure to eat or drink; or
- when patients have not responded to first line treatment.

Table 12.2. Geriatric depression scale

Instructions: Choose the best answer for how you have felt over the past *week*.

1. Are you basically satisfied with your life? No

2. Have you dropped many of your activities and interests? Yes

 3. *Do you feel your life is empty?* Yes

 4. *Do you often get bored?* Yes

 5. Are you hopeful about the future? No

 6. Are you bothered by thoughts you can't get out of your head? Yes

 7. *Are you in good spirits most of the time?* No

8. Are you afraid something bad is going to happen to you? Yes

9. Do you feel happy most of the time? No

10. Do you often feel helpless? Yes

11. Do you often get restless and fidgety? Yes

12. *Do you prefer to stay at home, rather than going out and doing new things?* Yes

13. Do you frequently worry about the future? Yes

14. *Do you feel you have more problems with your memory than most?* Yes

15. *Do you think it is wonderful to be alive now?* No

16. Do you often feel downhearted and blue (sad)? Yes

17. *Do you feel pretty worthless the way you are?* Yes

18. Do you worry a lot about the past? Yes

19. *Do you find life very exciting?* No

20. Is it hard for you to start on new projects (plans)? Yes

21. *Do you feel full of energy?* No

22. *Do you feel that your situation is hopeless?* Yes

23. *Do you think most people are better off (in their lives) than you are?* Yes

24. Do you frequently get upset over little things? Yes

25. Do you frequently feel like crying? Yes

26. Do you have trouble concentrating? Yes

27. Do you enjoy getting up in the morning? No

28. Do you prefer to avoid social gatherings (get togethers)? Yes

29. Is it easy for you to make decisions? No

30. Is your mind as clear as it used to be? No

Notes: (1) Answers refer to responses which score "1"; (2) bracketed phrases refer to alternative ways of expressing the questions; (3) questions in italics comprise the 15-item version. Cut-off scores for *possible* depression: 10/11 (GDS30); 5/6 (GDS15); 1/2 (GDS4). * = 4-item GDS questions

Treatment principles

The treatment of late-life depression should be multimodal and multidisciplinary. General principles are outlined in Table 12.3. As at other times of life, full remission is the goal. In a review of treatments available to older adults with depression (Baldwin

Table 12.3. Management goals

Goal	Ways to achieve
Risk reduction – of suicide or harm from self-neglect	• A risk assessment and monitoring of risk • Prompt referral of urgent cases to a specialist
Remission of all depressive symptoms	• Providing appropriate treatment (usually an antidepressant and/or a psychological treatment) • Giving the patient and his/her supporters timely education about depression and its treatment
To help the patient achieve optimal function	• Enable practical support • Ensure access to appropriate agencies which can help
To treat the whole person, including somatic problems	• Treat co-existing physical health problems • Reduce wherever possible the effects of handicap caused by factors such as chronic disease, sensory impairment and poor mobility • Review medication and withdraw unnecessary ones
To prevent relapse and recurrence	• Educate the patient about staying on medication once recovered • Continuation treatment (12 months after recovery, see text) • Maintenance treatment (preventive treatment, see text)

et al., 2003), there is evidence of efficacy for antidepressants, psychological treatments (notably Cognitive Behaviour Therapy (CBT) and Inter-Personal Therapy) and psychosocial interventions.

Antidepressants

There is no difference between men and women in terms of antidepressant response (Quitkin et al., 2002). Selective Serotonin Reuptake Inhibitors (SSRIs) are nowadays usually the first line choice. They are probably as effective as tricyclics antidepressants and somewhat better tolerated. However, there has been some concern about an increased risk of upper gastrointestinal bleeding in older patients prescribed SSRIs who are taking aspirin or non-steroidal anti-inflammatory drugs (NSAIDs) (De Abajo et al., 1999). Altered pharmacodyamics and kinetics coupled with frailty mean that initial antidepressant dosages may be half those recommended for younger adults but with the newer antidepressants the target dose is often the same. Antidepressants are effective in patients with depression complicating dementia and stroke and are tolerated satisfactorily by patients in nursing homes, although no adequate trials of efficacy have been conducted. Average starting and therapeutic dosages along with side-effect profiles are shown in Table 12.4.

Table 12.4. Suggested starting and therapeutic dosages of antidepressants

Drug	Mode of action or class	Antimuscarinic	Antihistaminic	α_1 adrenergic blocking	Starting dosage (mg)	Average therapeutic dose (mg)
Amitriptyline	Tricyclic	4	3	4	25–50	75–100
Imipramine	Tricyclic	3	2	3	25	75–100
Nortripyline	Tricyclic	3	2	2	10–30	75–100
Dothiepin (dosulepin)	Tricyclic	3	2	2	50–75	75–150
Lofepramine	Tricyclic	1	1	1	70–140	70–210
Trazodone	Tricyclic-related	0	3	1	100	300
Fluvoxamine	SSRI	0/1	0/1	0	25–100	100–200
Sertraline	SSRI	0/1	0	0	25–50	50–100
Fluoxetine	SSRI	0/1	0	0	10	20
Paroxetine	SSRI	0/1	0	0	10–20	20–30
Citalopram	SSRI	0	0	0	10–20	20–30
Escitalopram	SSRI	0	0	0	5–10	10
Phenelzine	Monoamine oxidase inhibition (non-reversible)	0/1	0	2	15	30–45 (divided dosages)
Moclobemide	Reversible Inhibitor of Monoamine oxidase A (RIMA)	0/1	0	0	300	300–400
Venlafaxine	NA/5HT reuptake inhibitor	0/1	0	0/1	37.5–75	75–150
Mirtazepine	Presynaptic α_2 antagonist	0	2	0	7.5–15	15–30

Note: Numbers 0–4 indicate magnitude of effect from none (0) to marked (4). Adapted from Baldwin, R.C., Chiu, E., Katona, C., & Graham, N. (2002). Guidelines on depression in older people: Practising the evidence. Martin Dunitz, London, with permission. 5HT: Serotonin; NA: Noradrenaline; SSRI: Selective Serotonin Reuptake Inhibitor

Psychological and psychotherapeutic interventions

Psychological treatments are as effective as antidepressants for mild and moderate depressive disorder (Baldwin et al., 2003) and may be preferred by older patients over medication (Unützer et al., 2002). However, they are seldom readily available, and a belief that medicine alone will eradicate depression may increase feelings of helplessness and dependence with poor long-term effects (Heifner, 1996). Combining medication with a psychological intervention gives the best results (Reynolds et al., 1999).

There are few studies examining the psychotherapies with older people and the results are rarely distinguished by gender. The most common theme is loss. Losses accumulate with age although each one is particular and specific (Knight & Satre, 1999). Pollack (1982) writes of the psychodynamic work in mourning leading to liberation and the possibilities of future freedoms. However, from some losses, for example the loss of an adult child, it may be impossible to recover.

Other analysts too have eschewed Freud's (1905) dictum that people over 50 are no longer educable and have drawn on the work of Erikson (1959) and King (1974, 1980). In the UK, Hildebrand (1982) pioneered workshops aimed at helping younger therapists see patients who were struggling with the developmental tasks and difficulties of later life. Good supervision helps the therapist deal with powerful countertransferential feelings evoked by working with older patients (Garner, 2004). The biological and social realities of the patients' lives need to be acknowledged. Physical pain and disability will not be alleviated by psychotherapy but the effects on the patient's life and relationships may be understood and changed. There are a number of accounts of group psychotherapy with older patients (Evans, 2004).

The lack of social interaction in nursing and residential homes described earlier (Terry, 1997) is a potential focus for psychosocial interventions. Although the task may feel overwhelming, something can be done about the level of social engagement. Jones (2003) writes of the success of a nurse-led group, using a modified reminiscence technique, on the level of depression in elderly women in long-term care. Reminiscence therapy, as well as being a treatment in its own right, also increases the engagement and contact between staff and residents. Perhaps more attention needs to be given to admitting friends or couples together (Dayson et al., 1998), and to increasing the emotional engagement and understanding of the staff (Garner, 1998).

In a large scale meta-analysis of psychosocial and psychotherapeutic interventions with older adults, Pinquart and Sorensen (2001) found CBT to improve depression and subjective well-being, an effect which was greater if the therapist had had specialised training in work with older adults. A number of adaptations to CBT have seemed helpful when treating this patient group (Koder et al., 1996) particularly with emphasis on rationale of the treatment at the beginning with thoughts such as "I am too old to change" challenged early on.

Life review is involved in many psychotherapeutic models and particularly in modifications which may be made for older adults. Creatively reminiscing, the patient may constructively re-evaluate failures, achievements and relationships. In a comparison of a life-review group and a cognitive therapy group both treatments were as effective, as evidenced by improved scores on the Beck Depression Inventory and Life Satisfaction in the Elderly Scale; the results were also true for an old–old group (Weiss, 1994).

Miller et al. (1994) used Interpersonal Psychotherapy (IPT) for spousal bereavement related depression in late life with some success, and IPT may hold promise in the treatment of dysthymia in the elderly.

Resistant depression

Resistant depression should be approached in the same way as with younger patients. In older adults white matter abnormalities in the brain may be an additional factor in poor treatment response (Baldwin & O'Brien, 2002). Lithium augmentation has a reasonable (albeit incomplete) evidence-base (Baldwin, 2002) but is often not well tolerated in older people. Age should not be a barrier to Electroconvulsive Therapy (ECT) in the right cases (generally to save life or prevent serious deterioration). It is generally well tolerated (Tew et al., 1999) but relapse rates are high.

Other promising but not fully evaluated avenues for treatment in elderly women are folate supplementation (Coppen & Bayley, 2000), transcranial magnetic stimulation and oestrogen. As yet, despite intense media interest there is no definitive evidence that Horomone Replacement Therapy either protects against depression in older women or can be successfully used to treat it (Cutter et al., 2003; Whooley et al., 2000).

Anxiety

As at other ages, for panic disorder, generalised anxiety disorder, obsessive–compulsive disorder (rare de novo in older people) and agoraphobia first line treatment is CBT with SSRIs the second-line choice.

Anxiolytic drugs

Used in the lowest possible dose for the shortest period of time, benzodiazepines are highly effective in the short-term treatment of moderate-to-severe symptoms of anxiety. Treatment beyond 2–4 weeks risks dependency. As with antidepressants, starting dosages and therapeutic dosages are roughly half that of the younger adult (Table 12.5). Falls, sedation and ataxia may occur in older adults and some may even develop a reversible dementia. Benzodiazepines are relatively contraindicated in patients with respiratory depression, sleep apnoea and severe hepatic impairment.

Buspirone acts on $5HT_{1A}$ receptors and has a low risk of dependence but may take a number of days to weeks before it is effective. It does not counteract benzodiazepine withdrawal. Beta-blockers reduce somatic symptoms of anxiety but can be problematic in older patients because there is a risk of aggravating underlying physical problems such as bronchospasm, hypotension, heart failure and diabetes. Water-soluble beta-blockers such as atenolol are less likely to cross the blood–brain barrier and may be associated with fewer central nervous system side effects such as sleep disturbance and nightmares. The use of low dose phenothiazines in the treatment of anxiety in older women is not recommended because of the risk of

Table 12.5. Drugs used in anxiety

Drug	Mode of action or class	Important interactions or precautions	Starting dosage (mg)	Average therapeutic dosage (mg)
Diazepam	Long-acting benzodiazepine	• Sedation (enhanced with antidepressants and antipsychotics) • Ulcer healing drugs (may inhibit benzodiazepines) • May impair epilepsy control	2 bd	6–15
Alprazolam	Medium half life benzodiazepine	Ditto	0.25 bd	0.25 bd or tds
Oxazepam	Short-acting benzodiazepine	Ditto plus greater risk of withdrawal	10	20
Lorazepam	Short-acting benzodiazepine	Ditto plus greater risk of withdrawal	0.5 bd	1–2
Buspirone	Specific $5HT_{1A}$ agonist	• Diltiazem, verapamil (may enhance effect of buspirone) • Does not prevent benzodiazepine withdrawal	5 bd	15–30
Propranolol	Non-selective beta-blocker	• Co-prescription with chlorpromazine enhances concentration of both drugs • Hypotension with tricyclics and some antipsychotics	40	80–120
Atenolol	Water soluble beta-blocker	Generally fewer central nervous system side effects	25–50	50–100

tardive dyskinesia. The role of the newer atypical antipsychotics in this clinical scenario remains to be evaluated.

Non-pharmacological interventions

In a large US survey of prescriptions, 7.5% of older people were prescribed anti-anxiety drugs (Aparasu et al., 2003) while in Europe 15% were taking benzodiazepines even though they had no diagnosed mental disorder (Kirby et al., 1999). Higher prescription rates have been reported among widows and those who are socially isolated (Hartikainen et al., 2003), and older women are significantly more likely to be prescribed anti-anxiety drugs than are men (Aparasu et al., 2003). Older women taking such medication are one and a half times more likely to have falls than non-users, with no evidence that shorter-acting anxiolytics are safer in this regard (Ensrud et al., 2002).

There is therefore growing interest in non-pharmacological approaches to the treatment of anxiety disorders in older women. Evidence is sparse but best for CBT. Barrowclough et al. (2001) demonstrated sustained benefit for CBT over counselling for anxiety in older adults living at home. Single session CBT was effective in reducing symptoms of anxiety and depression in older patients with chronic obstructive pulmonary disease (Kunik et al., 2001). Using CBT, patients with panic disorder achieve a decrease in symptoms and in physiological arousal (Swales et al., 1996) as do those with generalised anxiety disorder (Stanley et al., 1996). Lastly, a psychoeducational programme was effective in reducing both anxiety and depressive symptoms in older women (Schimmel-Spreeuw et al., 2000). The course included relaxation training.

Prognosis

In the hands of psychiatrists about 60% of older women with major depression recover completely, or recover but have treatable relapses. The remainder either stay unwell or only partially recover. Ill-health is a major adverse predictor (Cole & Bellavance, 1997). The prognosis in community settings and in medical wards is poorer than this (Cole & Bellavance, 1997), with low rates of treatment an important factor.

Barriers to care

Depression and anxiety are under-treated in old age to the extent that it presents a serious public health problem but depressed or anxious older women are unlikely to create a political or public relations furore about it. The under-treatment occurs for a number of reasons. Depression impairs the ability to seek help by inducing a lack of energy and motivation and feelings of worthlessness. Old people are less likely to report feelings of worthlessness and dysphoria, and attribute them to the ageing process – as do the doctors. Evans (1998) writes of elderly patients mirroring others' attitude to them – they are quite aware of society's prejudice and stereotyping which they share and project onto other older people.

The rapid throughput in primary care may mitigate against a thorough assessment, as those who are old and those who are depressed need time to express themselves. Clinicians may regard the signs and symptoms of depression as "normal ageing" or attribute them to the "inevitable decline of dementia" or they may have the diagnosis veiled by the psychosocial situation, multiple losses, deteriorating physical health or sensory impairment. Depression may amplify physical problems and so increase attention given to them. The clinician may correctly diagnose depression in an elderly woman but is prevented from doing anything about it either by ignorance or attitude.

As well as societal stereotypes of ageing there are also societal values. Children would always command sympathetic and active care and treatment whereas the old woman "has had her innings". In England, money has been put into the National Service Framework for Mental Health but this stops at 65 years of age.

Organisational and financial barriers are erected to continuing care in a society where independence is prized and dependence treated with contempt (Bell, 1996). Policy makers are undoubtedly influenced by personal and societal attitudes and no doubt the wish for a quiet life. Depressed old women are likely to create less bother than young men with forensic problems. It is up to clinicians to endeavour to redress the balance.

Prevention: Primary and secondary

Little is known about primary prevention except that keeping active and stimulated is beneficial for mind and body. The co-morbidity of depression and physical illness suggests that keeping physically as fit as possible through "healthy living" – diet, exercise, limiting alcohol intake, etc. – is likely also to decrease the likelihood of depression. Some find that education and life long learning in old age keeps them interested in life in all its facets and reduces feelings of depression. There is some concern now in the UK that the pressure on older people not to retire but continue to support themselves by working will increase the pressures on, and decrease the pleasures for, those in later life. "Make them work" could be the new ageism.

Continuation therapy after major depression should be for a minimum of 12 months in older patients. Both tricyclics and SSRIs have been proven effective in the prevention of relapse and recurrence (Baldwin et al., 2003). Longer term treatment should be considered, after discussion with the patient, for those experiencing their third or more recurrence (Baldwin et al., 2003). Importantly, of older people who kill themselves a majority will have consulted their primary care physician recent to the act (Harwood et al., 2001). The correct identification of depression in primary care therefore offers a prospect of influencing suicide rates among older people.

Cuijpers and van Lammeren (2001) studied secondary prevention of depressive symptoms in elderly inhabitants of residential homes. Staff were trained in detecting depression and in supporting depressed residents. Information was given to residents and their relatives and group interventions offered. Their results suggest that general approaches within a residential home are capable of influencing depressive symptoms in the residents. Early intervention seems to be successful and avoids the need for more extensive treatment.

Looking to the future and to unanswered questions

Societies need to consider how to react positively to major demographic change and to be more accepting and embracing of diversity which increases with age. From the point of view of research there is a need to consider why so little is known about anxiety in old age. Charting physiological changes in emotion in ageing may illuminate mood disorders and anxiety in older people. Prevention research is needed throughout the life cycle. Gender differences in depression in late life are poorly understood. Something may be learned from the biological, psychological and social situation of women in considering the higher suicide rate in men and the greater incidence of vascular depression in older males. The narrowing of the gender gap in the incidence of depression in old age needs to be understood, as well as the intriguing suggestion (Hybels et al., 2002) that older women with subthreshold depression are more likely to live longer than those who are not depressed.

One would be hard-pressed to produce evidence that the new antidepressants developed over the past 20 years have led to any improvement in the outcome of depression in older women. Rather, attention is turning to new ways of delivering existing treatments, as well as to improve their uptake. Combining treatments offers considerable advantages over single modalities. In primary care, collaborative management offers significant advantages for outcome over usual care. The key components are a care manager based in primary care and timely access to specialist advice. The emerging trial data are encourageing (Unützer et al., 2002).

Consideration is needed as to why despite professionals' avowed adherence to evidence-based medicine, myths about old age, women and mental disorders nevertheless persist. An attitude needs to be promoted which makes the world and its health services a reasonable place for today's young women to grow old.

REFERENCES

De Abajo, F.J., Garcia Rodríguez, L.A., & Montero, D. (1999). Association between selective serotonin reuptake inhibitors and upper gastrointestinal bleeding: Population based case–control study. *British Medical Journal, 319*, 1106–1109.

Achterberg, W., Pot, A.M., Kerkstra, A., Ooms, M., Muller, M., & Ribbe, M. (2003). The effects of depression on social engagement in newly admitted Dutch nursing home residents. *Gerontologist, 43*, 213–218.

Alexopoulos, G.S., Young, R.C., & Kocsis, J.H. (1984). Dexamethasone suppression test in geriatric depression. *Biological Psychiatry, 19*, 1567–1571.

Alexopoulos, G.S., Abrams, R.C., & Young, R.C. (1988). Cornell scale for depression in dementia. *Biological Psychiatry, 23*, 271–284.

Alexopoulos, G.S., Meyers, B.S., Young, R.C., Campbell, S., Silbersweig, D., & Charlson, M. (1997). "Vascular depression" hypothesis. *Archives of General Psychiatry, 54*, 915–922.

Aparasu, R.R., Mort, J.R., & Brandt, H. (2003). Psychotropic prescription use by community-dwelling elderly in the United States. *Journal of the American Geriatrics Society, 51*, 671–677.

Allen, N.H.P., & Burns, A. (1995). The non-cognitive features of dementia. *Reviews in Clinical Gerontology, 5*, 57–75.

Arfken, C.L., Lichtenberg, P.A., & Tancer, M.E. (1999). Cognitive impairment and depression predict mortality in medically ill older adults. *Journals of Gerontology Series A – Biological Sciences and Medical Sciences, 54*(3), M152–M156.

Baldwin, R.C. (2002). Depressive illness. In: R. Jacoby, & C. Oppenheimer (Eds.), *Psychiatry in the elderly*. 3rd edn. Oxford, England: Oxford University Press.

Baldwin, R.C., & O'Brien, J. (2002). Vascular basis of late-onset depressive disorder. *British Journal of Psychiatry, 180*, 157–160.

Baldwin, R., Anderson, D., Black, S., Evans, S., Jones, S., Wilson, K., & Iliffe, S. (2003). Guideline for the management of late-life depression in primary care. *International Journal of Geriatric Psychiatry, 18*, 829–838.

Ballard, C.G., Eastwood, C., & Gahir, M. (1996). A follow-up study of depression in carers of dementia sufferers. *British Medical Journal, 312*, 947.

Barrowclough, C., King, P., Colville, J., Russell, E., Burns, A., & Tarrier, N. (2001). A randomized trial of the effectiveness of cognitive-behavioral therapy and supportive counseling for anxiety symptoms in older adults. *Journal of Consulting & Clinical Psychology, 69*, 756–762.

Beekman, A.T., Copeland, J.R., & Prince, M.J. (1999). Review of community prevalence of depression in later life. *British Journal of Psychiatry, 174*, 307–311.

Bell, D. (1996). Primitive mind of state. *Psychoanalytic Psychotherapy, 10*, 45–57.

Blazer, D. (2003). Depression in the elderly: Review and commentary. *Journal of Gerontology Series A – Biological Sciences and Medical Sciences, 58*, M249–M265.

Blehar, M., De Paulo, R., Gershon, E., Reich, T., Simpson, S., & Nurnberger, J. (1998). Women with bipolar disorder: Findings from the NIMH genetics initiative sample. *Psychopharmacology Bulletin, 34*(3), 239–243.

Bretschneider, J., & McCoy, N. (1989). *Sexual interest and behavior in healthy 80- to 102-year-olds. Our Sexuality Update*, Benjamin/Cummings Publishing, Spring 1989, pages 5–6.

CDC (1996). Suicide among older persons-United States, 1980–1992. MMWR Morbidity Mortal Weekly Report, 45, 3–6.

Cole, M.G., & Bellavance, F. (1997). The prognosis of depression in old age. *American Journal of Geriatric Psychiatry, 5*, 4–14.

Conwell, Y., Duberstein, P.R., Cox, C., Herrmann, J.H., Forbes, N.T., & Caine, E.D. (1996). Relationships of age and Axis I diagnoses in victims of completed suicide: A psychological autopsy study. *American Journal of Psychiatry, 153*, 1001–1008.

Coppen, A., & Bailey, J. (2000). Enhancement of the antidepressant action of fluoxetine by folic acid: A randomised, placebo controlled trial. *Journal of Affective Disorders, 60*, 121–130.

Covey, H.S. (1992). The definitions of the beginnings of old age in history. *International Journal of Ageing and Human Development, 34*(4), 325–337.

Cuijpers, P., & van Lammeren, P. (2001). Secondary prevention of depressive symptoms in elderly inhabitants of residential homes. *International Journal of Geriatric Psychiatry, 16*, 702–708.

Cutter, W.J., Norbury, R., & Murphy, D.G.M. (2003). Oestrogen, brain function, and neuropsychiatric disorders. *Journal of Neurology Neurosurgery and Psychiatry, 74*, 837–840.

Dayson, D., Lee-Jones, R., Chahal, K.K., & Leff, J. (1998). The TAPS project 32: Social networks of two group homes … 5 years on. *Social Psychiatry and Psychiatric Epidemiology*, *33*, 438–444.

Dimatteo, M.R., Lepper, H.S., & Croghan, T.W. (2000). Depression is a risk factor for non-compliance with medical treatment: Meta-analysis of the effects of anxiety and depression on patient adherence. *Archives of Internal Medicine*, *160*, 2101–2107.

Ensrud, K.E., Blacwell, T.E., Mangione, C.M., Bowman, P.J., Whooley, M.A., & Bauer, D.C. (2002). Central nervous system-active medications and risk of falls in older women. *Journal of the American Geriatrics Society*, *50*, 1629–1637.

Erikson, E.H. (1959). *Identity and the life cycle. Psychological issues monograph No. 1*. New York: International Universities Press.

Evans, S. (1998). Beyond the mirror: A group analytic exploration of late life and depression. *Ageing and Mental Health*, *2*, 94–99.

Evans, S. (2004). Group Psychotherapy: Foulkes, Yalom, Bion and others. Chapter 7. In: S. Evans, & J. Garner (Eds.), *Talking over the years: A handbook of psychodynamic psychotherapy with older adults*. London: Brunner-Routledge, 87–100.

Folstein, M.F., Folstein, S.E., & McHugh, P.R. (1975). "Mini-Mental State": A practical method for grading the cognitive state of patients for the clinician. *Journal of Psychiatric Research*, *12*, 189–198.

Fooken, I. (1994). Sexuality in the later years – the impact of health and body image in a sample of older women. *Patient Education and Counselling*, *23*, 227–233.

Freud, S. (1905). *On Psychotherapy*. Standard Edition 7.

Garner, J. (1998). Open letter to Director General of Fair Trading. APP Newsletter. *Psychoanalytic Psychotherapy*, *22*, 4–5.

Garner, J. (2004). Growing into old age: Erikson and others. Chapter 6. In: S. Evans, & J. Garner (Eds.), *Talking over the years: A handbook of psychodynamic psychotherapy with older adults*. London: Brunner-Routledge, 71–85.

Garner, J., & Ardern, M. (1998). Reflections on old age. *Ageing and Mental Health*, *2*, 92–93.

Garner, J., & Bacelle, L. (2004). "Sexuality". Chapter 17. In: S. Evans, & J. Garner (Eds.), *Talking over the years: A handbook of psychodynamic psychotherapy with older adults*. London: Brunner-Routledge, 247–263.

Glaser, R., Robles, T.F., Sheridan, J., Malarkey, W.B., & Kiecolt-Glaser, J.K. (2003). Mild depressive symptoms are associated with amplified and prolonged inflammatory responses after influenza virus vaccination in older adults. *Archives of General Psychiatry*, *60*, 1009–1014.

Green, R.C., Cupples, A., Kurz, A., Auerbach, S., Go, R., Sadovnick, D., Duara, R., Kukull, W.A., Chui, H., Edeki, T., Griffith, P.A., Friedland, R.P., Bachman, D., & Farrer, L. (2003). Depression as a risk factor for Alzheimer disease: The MIRAGE study. *Archives of Neurology*, *60*, 753–759.

Hamilton, M. (1960). A rating scale for depression. *Journal of Neurology, Neurosurgery and Psychiatry*, *23*, 56–62.

Harralson, T., White, T., Regenberg, A., Kallan, M., Have, T.T., Parmelee, P., & Johnson, J. (2002). Similarities and differences in depression among black and white nursing home residents. *American Journal of Geriatric Psychiatry*, *10*, 175–184.

Hartikainen, S., Rahkonen, T., Kautiainen, H., Sulkava, R., & Kuopio. (2003). 75+ study: Does advanced age predict more common use of psychotropics among the elderly? *International Clinical Psychopharmacology*, *18*(3), 163–167.

Harwood, D., Hawton, K., Hope, T., & Jacoby, R. (2001). Psychiatric disorder and personality factors associated with suicide in older people: A descriptive and case–control study. *International Journal of Geriatric Psychiatry*, *16*, 155–165.

Heifner, C.A. (1996). Women, depression and biological psychiatry: Implications for psychiatric nursing. *Perspectives in Psychiatric Care*, *32*, 4–9.

Hildebrand, H.P. (1982). Psychotherapy with older patients. *British Journal of Medical Psychology*, *55*, 19–28.

Holmes, T.H., & Rahe, R.H. (1967). The social readjustment rating scale. *Journal of Psychosomatic Research*, *11*, 213–218.

Hybels, C.F., Pieper, C.F., & Blazer, D.G. (2002). Sex differences in the relationship between sub-threshold depression and mortality in a community sample of older adults. *American Journal of Geriatric Psychiatry*, *10*, 283–291.

Jones, E.D. (2003). Reminiscence therapy for older women with depression. Effects of nursing inter-vention classification in assisted-living long term care. *Journal of Gerontological Nursing*, *29*, 26–33.

Jones, R. (2002). That's very rude, I shouldn't be telling you that: Older women talking about sex. *Narrative Inquiry*, *12*, 121–142.

Jung, C.G. (1931). *The stages of life. Collected works*, Vol. 8, 387–403.

Katon, W.J., Lin, E., Russo, J., & Unützer, J. (2003). Increased medical costs of a population-based sample of depressed elderly patients. *Archives of General Psychiatry*, *60*, 897–903.

Kay, D.W.K. (1988). Anxiety in the elderly. In: R. Noyes, M. Roth, & G.D. Burrows (Eds.), *Handbook of Anxiety, Vol. 2. Classification, etiological factors and associated disturbances.* Elsevier Science Publications BV.

Kessler, R.C. (2003). Epidemiology of women and depression. *Journal of Affective Disorders*, *74*, 5–13.

King, P.H.M. (1974). Notes on the psychoanalysis of older patients. *Journal of Analytical Psychology*, *19*, 22–37.

King, P.H.M. (1980). The life-cycle as indicated by the transference in the psychoanalysis of the middle aged and elderly. *International Journal of Psychoanalysis*, *61*, 153–160.

Kirby, M., Denihan, A., Bruce, I., Radic, A., Coakley, D., & Lawlor, B.A. (1999). Benzodiazepine use among the elderly in the community. *International Journal of Geriatric Psychiatry*, *14*, 280–284.

Kivela, S.L., Luukinen, H., Koski, K., Viramo, P., & Pahkala, K. (1998). Early loss of mother or father predicts depression in old age. *International Journal of Geriatric Psychiatry*, *13*(8), 527–530.

Knight, B.G. (1986). *Psychotherapy with older adults.* London: Sage.

Knight, B.G., & Satre, D.D. (1999). Cognitive behavioural psychotherapy with older adults. *Clinical Psychology: Science and Practice*, *6*, 188–203.

Koder, D.A., Brodaty, H., & Anstey, K.J. (1996). Cognitive therapy for depression in the elderly. *International Journal of Geriatric Psychiatry*, *11*, 97–107.

Kramer-Ginsberg, E., Greenwald, B.S., Aisen, P.S., & Brod-Miller, C. (1989). Hypochondriasis in the elderly depressed. *Journal of the American Geriatric Society*, *37*, 507–510.

Kunik, M.E., Braun, U., Stanley, M.A., Wristers, K., Molinari, V., Stoebner, D., & Orengo, C.A. (2001). One session cognitive behavioural therapy for elderly patients with chronic obstructive pulmonary disease. *Psychological Medicine*, *31*, 717–723.

LePine, J.P., & Bouchez, S. (1998). Epidemiology of depression in the elderly. *International Clinical Psychopharmacology*, *13*(Suppl 5), S7–S12.

Lindesay, J., Briggs, K., & Murphy, E. (1989). The guy's/age concern survey. Prevalence rates of cognitive impairment, depression and anxiety in an urban elderly community. *British Journal of Psychiatry*, *155*, 317–329.

Lopez, A.D., & Murray, C.C. (1998). The global burden of disease, 1990–2020. *Nature Medicine*, *4*, 1241–1243.

Lyness, J.M., Caine, E.D., King, D.A., Conwell, Y., Duberstein, P.R., & Cox, C. (2002). Depressive disorders and symptoms in older primary care patients: One-year outcomes. *American Journal of Geriatric Psychiatry*, *10*(3), 257–282.

Mehta, K.M., Simonssick, E.M., Penninx, B.W.J.H., Schultz, S., Rubin, S.M., Satterfield, S., & Yaffe, K. (2003). Prevalence and correlates of anxiety symptoms in well-functioning older adults: Findings from the health ageing and body composition study. *J American Geriatrics Society*, *51*, 499–504.

Miller, M., Frank, E., & Cornes, C. (1994). Applying interpersonal psychotherapy to bereavement – related depression following loss of a spouse in late life. *Journal of Psychotherapeutic Practise Research*, *3*, 149–162.

Mottram, P., Wilson, K., & Copeland, J. (2000). Validation of the Hamilton depression scale and montgomery and Asberg rating scales in terms of AGECAT depression cases *International Journal of Geriatric Psychiatry*, *15*, 1113–1119.

Murdock, M.E., Guarnaccia, C.A., Hayslip Jr, B., & McKibbin, C.L. (1998) The contribution of small life events to the psychological distress of married and widowed older women. *Journal of Women & Ageing*, *10*, 3–22.

Murphy, E. (1982). Social origins of depression in old age. *British Journal of Psychiatry*, *141*, 135–142.

Murphy, E., Smith, R., Lindesay, J., & Slattery, J. (1988). Increased mortality rates in late-life depression. *British Journal of Psychiatry*, *152*, 347–353.

Nesse, R.M. (2000). Is depression an adaptation? *Archives of General Psychiatry*, *57*, 14–20.

Nusbaum, M.R.H., Singh, A.R., & Pyles, A.A. (2004). Sexual healthcare needs of women aged 65 and older. *Journal of American Geriatric Society*, *52*, 117–122.

Penninx, B.W., Deeg, D.J., van Eijk, J.T., Beekman, A.T., & Gurainik, J.M. (2000). Changes in depression and physical decline in older adults: A longitudinal perspective. *Journal of Affective Disorders*, *61*, 1–12.

Pinquart, M., & Sorensen, S. (2001). How effective are psychotherapeutic and other psychosocial interventions with older adults? A meta-analysis. *Journal of Mental Health and Ageing*, *7*, 207–243.

Pollack, G. (1982). On ageing and psychoanalysis. *International Journal of Psychoanalysis*, *63*, 275–281.

Prince, M.J., Harwood, R.H., Thomas, A., & Mann, A.H. (1998). A prospective population-based cohort study of the effects of disablement and social milieu on the onset and maintenance of late-life depression. The Gospel Oak Project VII. *Psychological Medicine*, *28*, 337–350.

Quitkin, F.M., Stewart, J.W., McGrath, P.J., Taylor, B.P., Tisminetzky, M.S., Petkova, E., Chen, Y., Ma, G., & Klein, D.F. (2002). Are there differences between women's and men's antidepressant responses? *American Journal of Psychiatry*, *159*, 1848–1854.

Reynolds III, C.F., Frank, E., Perel, J.M., Imber, S.D., Cornes, C., Miller, M.D., Mazumdar, S., Houck, P.R., Dew, M.A., Stack, J.A., Pollock, B.G., & Kupfer, D.J. (1999). Nortriptyline and interpersonal psychotherapy as maintenance therapies for recurrent major depression: A randomized controlled trial in patients older then 59 years. *Journal of the American Medical Association*, *281*, 39–45.

Sapolsky, R., Krey, L., & McEwen, B. (1986). The neuroendocrinology of stress and ageing: The glucocorticoid cascade hypothesis. *Endocrine Reviews, 7,* 284–301.

Schimmel-Spreeuw, A., Linssen, A.C., & Heeren, T.J. (2000). Coping with depression and anxiety: Preliminary results of a standardized course for elderly depressed women. *International Psychogeriatrics, 12,* 77–86.

Stanley, M., Beck, G., & Glassco, J.D. (1996). Treatment of generalised anxiety in older adults: A preliminary comparison of cognitive-behavioural and supportive approaches. *Behaviour Therapy, 27,* 565–581.

Swales, P., Solfvin, J., & Sheikh, J. (1996). Cognitive-behavioural therapy in older panic disorder patients. *American Journal of Geriatric Psychiatry, 4,* 46–60.

Szewczyk, M., & Chennault, S. (1997). Depression and related disorders. *Primary Care (Women's Health), 24,* 83–101.

Terry, P. (1997). *Counselling the elderly and their carers.* London: Macmillan Press.

Tew, J.D., Mulsant, B.H., Haskett, R.F., Prudic, J., Thase, M.E., Crowe, R.R., Dolata, D., Begley, A.E., Reynolds III, C.F., & Sackeim, H.A. (1999). Acute efficacy of ECT in the treatment of major depression in the old–old. *American Journal of Psychiatry, 156,* 1865–1870.

Turvey, C.L., Carney, C., Arndt, S., Wallace, R.B., & Herzog, R. (1999). Conjugal loss and syndromal depression in a sample of elders aged 70 years or older. *American Journal of Psychiatry, 156,* 1596–1601.

Unützer, J., Katon, W., Callahan, C., Williams, J.W., Hunkeler, E., Harpole, L., Hoffing, M., Della Penna, R.D., Noel, P.H., Lin, E.H.B., Arean, P., Hegel, M., Tang, L., Belin, T.R., Oishi, S., & Langston, C. (2002). Collaborative care management of late-life depression in the primary care setting. *Journal of American Medical Association, 288,* 2836–2845.

Veith, R.C., & Raskind, M.A. (1988). The neurobiology of ageing: Does it predispose to depression? *Neurobiology of ageing, 9,* 101–117.

Weiss, J.C. (1994). Group therapy for older adults in long term care settings, research and clinical cautions and recommendations. *Journal for Specialists in Group Work, 19,* 22–29.

Waern, M., Runeson, B.S., Allebeck, P., Beskow, J., Rubenowitz, E., Skoog, I., & Wilhelmsson, K. (2002). Mental disorder in elderly suicides: A case–control study. *American Journal of Psychiatry, 159,* 450–455.

Wells, K.B., Stewart, A., & Hays, R.D. (1989). The functioning and well being of depressed patients: Results from the medical outcomes study. *Journal of American Medical Association, 262,* 914–919.

Whisman, M.A. (1999). Marital dissatisfaction and psychiatric disorders: Results from the National Comorbidity Survey. *Journal of Abnormal Psychology, 108,* 701–706.

Whooley, M.A., Kip, K.E., Cauley, J.A., Ensrud, K.E., Nevitt, M.C., & Browner, W.S. (1999). Depression, falls and risk of hip fracture in older women. *Archives of Internal Medicine, 159,* 484–490.

Whooley, M.A., Grady, D., & Cauley, J.A. (2000). Postmenopausal estrogen therapy an depressive symptoms in older women. *Journal of General Internal Medicine, 15,* 535–541.

Yaffe, K., Blackwell, T., Gore, R., Sands, L., Reus, V., & Browner, W.S. (1999). Depressive symptoms and cognitive decline in nondemented elderly women: A prospective study. *Archives of General Psychiatry, 56,* 425–430.

Yesavage, J.A, Brink, T.L., Rose, T.L., & Lum, O. (1983). Development and validation of a geriatric depression screening scale: A preliminary report. *Journal of Psychiatric Research, 17,* 37–49.

Index